Key to Localized Pr

Cradle Cap and Dandruff (50)
Head Injuries (10)
Headache (63)
Hair Loss (35)

Eye Burning (78)
Foreign Body (79)
Eye Pain (79)
Styes (80)
Decreased Vision (81)

Earaches (20)
Ear Discharges (21)
Sudden Hearing Loss (22)

Acne (43)

Colds and Flu (18)
Runny Nose (23)
Nosebleeds (29)

Swollen Glands (28)

Shoulder Injuries (9)

Croup (25)
Wheezing (26)
Hoarseness (27)

Sore Throat (19)
Mouth Lesions (31)
Toothaches (32)
Bad Breath (30)
Swallowed Foreign Objects (73)

Elbow Injuries (9)

Cough (24)
Chest Pain (75)
Shortness of Breath (76)
Palpitations (77)

Acute Abdominal Pain (84)
Recurrent Abdominal Pain (85)
Colic (86)
Nausea and Vomiting (82)

Low-back Pain (60)

Constipation (66)
Rectal Pain (87)
Diarrhea (83)

Wrist Injuries (9)

Smashed Fingers (15)

Painful Urination (88)
Bloody Urine (88)
Vaginal Discharge (89)
Vaginal Bleeding (91)
Menstrual Problems (91)
Problems with the Penis (90)
Jock Itch (45)

Knee Injuries (8)
Pain in the Muscles or Joints (59)
Scrapes and Abrasions (4)
Bowlegs and Knock-Knees (61)

Is a Bone Broken? (6)

Ankle Injuries (7)

Athlete's Foot (44)
Pigeon Toes and Flat Feet (62)
Puncture Wounds (2)

Important Telephone Numbers

Emergency Room _____

Poison Control Center _____

Ambulance _____

Family Doctor _____

Pediatrician _____

Specialist _____

Dentist _____

Dental Emergency Number _____

Hospital _____

Other _____

_____

_____

_____

Taking Care of Your Child

A Parents' Guide to Medical Care

Robert H. Pantell, M.D.

James F. Fries, M.D.

Donald M. Vickery, M.D.

ADDISON-WESLEY PUBLISHING COMPANY

Reading, Massachusetts • Menlo Park, California
London • Amsterdam • Don Mills, Ontario • Sydney

Library of Congress Cataloging in Publication Data

Pantell, Robert H   1945-
   Taking care of your child.

   Includes index.
   1. Children--Care and hygiene. 2. Children--Dis-
eases. I. Fries, Robert H., 1938-   joint author.
II. Vickery, Donald M., joint author. III. Title.
[DNLM: 1. Pregnancy--Popular works. 2. Labor--
Popular works. 3. Infant care--Popular works.
4. Child care--Popular works. WS113 P195t]
RJ61.P215   618.9'2'0024   77-81635

ISBN 0-201-08122-9
ABCDEFGHIJ-DO-7987

Dedication

To our parents, who first taught us about health;
To our mentors, Floyd Denny, M.D., and Clarence McIntyre, M.D.,
who first taught us how to care for children, and
To our children, patients, and their parents, who continue to teach us.

How to Use Decision Charts

Your child has a medical problem . . . and you're worried. For the great majority of problems, this book can help; ninety-one of the most common problems are described in detail in Part II, beginning on page 137. Here is what you do:

- FIND the problem number on the inside cover, in the table of contents, or in the index at the back of the book.

- READ about the problem on the page facing the chart. The information there will help you understand the reasons for the instructions on the chart, will tell you exactly what you can do at home, and will describe what to expect at the doctor's office.

- LOOK at the decision chart to determine if immediate action is needed, if an appointment with the doctor should be scheduled, or if home treatment is advised.

This is a decision chart. Start with the first box and answer the question inside. Depending on the answer, follow the arrow to the next box and then to the next until you get to an instruction. If the instruction reads "Apply home treatment," then read the detailed instructions for home treatment on the facing page. If the instruction refers you to the doctor, then read the description on the facing page of "what to expect at the doctor's office."

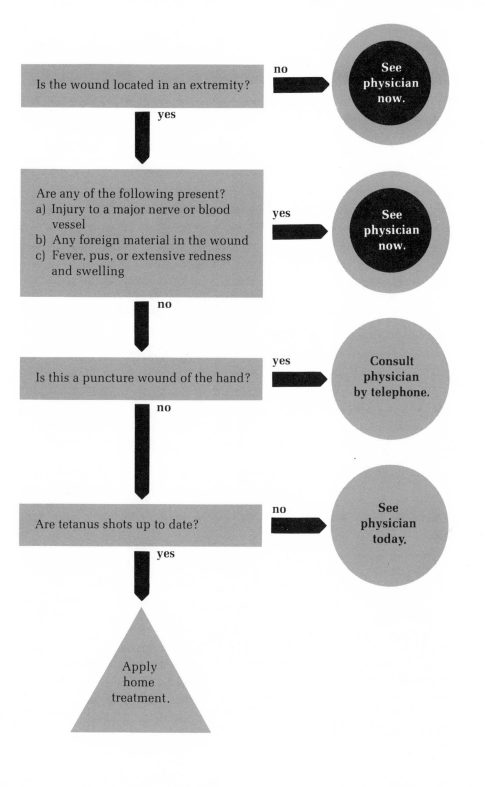

Contents

Part I
Parent Skills

1

1
A Child Is Coming

3

I'm pregnant, we're pregnant 3
Becoming pregnant 6
Taking care of yourself during pregnancy 6
Breast feeding or bottle feeding? 12
Childbirth preparation classes 15
Home delivery, hospital delivery, or something else? 17

2
The Big Event

19

Rupture of the membranes 22
Medications used during labor 22
Anesthesia 22
Pitocin and "induced births" 23
Fetal heart monitoring 24
Preparation procedures 24

Delivery room procedures 24
Premature births 25
Newborn procedures 26
Circumcision 28
Taking your child home 29

3

Your First Concerns 33

The first child 33
The second time around 36
Activity 39
Breathing 40
The skin and birthmarks 40
The head 41
The eyes 41
The nose 42
The mouth 42
The face 43
The hands 43
The chest 43
The abdomen 43
The genitalia 43
The feet 44
Feeding 44

4

Growth and Development 51

Your child's weight 52
Your child's height 53
Growth at puberty 53
Your child's development 55
Toilet training 57
What is normal development? 60

5

Personality Development 63

Infancy: birth to one year 63
Toddlers 65
The preschool years 70
The early school years (6–11) 71
Adolescents 72
Sexuality 75

6

School Days 79

Day-care centers 79
School readiness 80
Failing in school 81
Intelligence testing (I.Q.) 84
School avoidance 85
Childhood athletics 86

7

The Medical Encounter 91

Finding someone to care 91
Well-baby examinations 93
The first pelvic examination 95
Routine laboratory tests for children 97
Screening for the cause of frequent illness 99
Surgery 99

8

Staying Healthy 103

Accidents 103
Immunizations 109
Dental care 118
Preventing adult diseases 121

9

The Home Pharmacy 127

Allergy 128
Cold preparations 129
Constipation 130
Diarrhea 131
Eye irritations 131
Pain and fever 131
Poisoning 132
Sterilizing agents and antiseptics (hydrogen peroxide and iodine) 133
Vaporizers 133
Vitamins 133
Giving medicine 133
Tincture of time 135

Part II
The Child and the Common Complaint

137

A
Interpretation of Childhood Complaints

139

How to use this part 139
The sick child 141

B
Emergencies

143

C
Common Injuries

147

1 Cuts (lacerations) 148
2 Puncture wounds 150
3 Animal bites 152
4 Scrapes and abrasions 154
5 Tetanus shots 156
6 Is a bone broken? 158
7 Ankle injuries 160
8 Knee injuries 162
9 Wrist, elbow, and shoulder injuries 164
10 Head injuries 166
11 Burns 168
12 Infected wounds and blood poisoning 170
13 Insect bites or stings 172
14 Fishhooks 174
15 Smashed fingers 176

D
Poisons

179

16 Oral poisoning 180

E
Fever

183

17 Fever 184

F

Allergies   191

    Food allergy 192
    Asthma 193
    Allergic rhinitis (hay fever) 195
    Atopic dermatitis (eczema) 196
    Allergy testing and hyposensitization 197

G

The Ears, Nose, and Throat   199

    Is it a virus, bacteria, or an allergy? 200
18 Colds and flu 202
19 Sore throat 204
20 Earaches 206
21 Ear discharges 208
22 Hearing loss 210
23 Runny nose 212
24 Cough 214
25 Croup 216
26 Wheezing 218
27 Hoarseness 220
28 Swollen glands 222
29 Nosebleeds 224
30 Bad breath 226
31 Mouth lesions 228
32 Toothaches 230

H

Common Skin Problems   233

    Skin symptom table 236
33 Baby rashes 238
34 Diaper rash 240
35 Hair loss 242
36 Impetigo 244
37 Ringworm 246
38 Hives 248
39 Poison ivy and poison oak 250
40 Skin lumps, bumps, and warts 252
41 Eczema (atopic dermatitis) 254
42 Boils 256
43 Acne 258
44 Athlete's foot 260
45 Jock itch 262
46 Sunburn 264
47 Lice and bedbugs 266

48 Ticks and chiggers (redbugs) 268
49 Scabies 270
50 Dandruff and cradle cap 272
51 Patchy loss of skin color 274

I

Childhood Diseases   277

52 Mumps 278
53 Chicken pox 280
54 Measles (red measles, seven- or ten-day measles) 282
55 German measles (rubella, three-day measles) 284
56 Roseola 286
57 Scarlet fever 288
58 Fifth disease 290

J

Bones, Muscles, and Joints   293

59 Pain in the muscles or joints 294
60 Low-back pain 296
61 Bowlegs and knock-knees 298
62 Pigeon toes and flat feet 300

K

Common Concerns   303

63 Headache 304
64 Hyperactivity 306
65 Bedwetting 308
66 Constipation and soiling 310
67 Overweight 312
68 Underweight 314
69 Stress, anxiety, and depression 316
70 Weakness and tiredness 318
71 Dizziness and fainting 320
72 Seizures (convulsions, fits, falling-out spells) 322
73 Swallowed foreign objects 324
74 Frequent illnesses 326

L

Chest Pains, Shortness of Breath,   329
and Palpitations

75 Chest pain 330
76 Shortness of breath 332
77 Palpitations 334

M

Eye Problems 337

78 Eye burning, itching, and discharge 338
79 Foreign body in eye/eye pain 340
80 Styes and blocked tear ducts 342
81 Decreased vision and crossed eyes 344

N

The Digestive Tract 347

82 Nausea/vomiting 348
83 Diarrhea 351
84 Acute abdominal pain 354
85 Recurrent abdominal pain 356
86 Colic 358
87 Rectal pain, itching, or bleeding 360

O

The Urinary Tract 363

88 Painful, frequent, or bloody urination 364

P

The Genitals 367

89 Vaginal discharge 368
90 Problems with the penis 370
91 Vaginal bleeding and menstrual problems 372

Q

Contraception 375

Part III
Family Records 379

Index 390

Introduction

You can do more for your child's health than your doctor can. Your care and judgment are the most important ingredients for fostering a lifetime of health for your child. A sound diet, a clean environment, and sensible living habits are the best way to reach this goal. However, illnesses and accidents are a part of growing up. While some of these problems will require professional assistance, many can be handled at home. The purpose of this book is to help you manage the common problems of childhood, and to enable you to make better decisions about when to see a medical professional.

Medical science encompasses a body of knowledge so vast and a technology so intricate that no one person can maintain command of it. It is easy to become intimidated by the complexity of modern medicine and to feel uncomfortable making common-sense medical decisions for your family. The most commonly encountered medical problems, however, are usually uncomplicated and inevitably get better by themselves. Each day you make sound decisions requiring good judgment in caring for your child. But there will always be a time when you are confronted with a new problem or an illness that is not typical. This book should help you in these times of uncertainty and improve your ability in judging how best to use your physician.

There is an expression used by many medical educators: "When you hear hoofbeats, don't think of zebras." This has been our guiding principle. We have tried to focus in *Taking Care of Your Child* not on rare events that might happen, but on what probably will occur. Our own children have encountered the majority of the problems outlined in this book. Most of these problems can be successfully managed at home.

This book is divided into three sections: Part I provides information helpful in understanding the several subject areas that we have found to be of greatest concern to parents. You will find discussions of pregnancy, birth, physical development, personality development, and school problems, as well as advice for staying healthy and for stocking the medicine cabinet. We have tried to give you both sides of such controversies as breast versus bottle feeding, home versus hospital birth, circumcision, and immunizations. Part I provides background information for your role as parent and will assist you in developing a long-range strategy aimed at ensuring a healthy life for your child.

Part II is the heart of this book; it provides specific guidance for 91 of the medical problems most likely to be encountered by infants, children, and adolescents. The charts in this section present step-by-step guidelines to help you decide on a program of home treatment or whether to make a telephone call or visit to your physician. These charts are useful as an aid to your common sense and not as a substitute; you know your child best.

Part III provides a place to record growth, development, and medical information for each child.

As parents, we preside over the maturation of our children from complete dependence at birth to complete independence less than two decades later. In gaining independence, a young adult needs to learn how to make personal and medical decisions with confidence. Teaching children to make independent decisions about their own health is one of the most important things a parent can do. The decision guidelines in this book can help you and your child with these important skills.

The tasks of a parent are many. Besides the obvious feeding, clothing, and teaching, there are the countless hours of caring activities which are so natural that we hardly ever realize their importance. But the time spent in touching, holding, looking, and smiling at children is a crucial part of their development. In attempting to capture the complex feelings that develop between parent and child, we have relied on parents' statements of their experiences throughout the book.

The typical child sees a physician four times a year and has many more problems managed at home. Your family's experience with these scores of inevitable illnesses and accidents provides an opportunity for your children to learn, directly or by example, skills that will last a lifetime. The information presented in this book is intended to help you increase your confidence in the common-sense decisions you must make. In this process you may save time and money, to be sure, but the real goal is to assist you in helping your child become a healthy adult.

Stanford, California   R. H. P.
Herndon, Virginia   J. F. F.
August 1977   D. M. V.

Acknowledgments

The following parents contributed to the development of this book and their help was invaluable: Anne and Dave Bergman, Val Blanchette, Jani Butler, Susan Charles, Libby and Milton Clapp, Linda Collins, Audrie Engbretson, Lee Hall, Mary Ann and Arthur Hanlon, Lenore and Larry Horowitz, Lois Kazmer, Michalline Krey, Shirley Lewis, Irmhild and Matthew Liang, Pit Lucking, Margaret Olebe, Kay Neumann, Suzanne Pennycook, Rosa Delgadillo Reilly, Marni Smith, Melissa Thornhill, Heather Van Nostrand, and Anne Wilkins.

We would also like to thank the following individuals for conceptual assistance and review: G. Robin Beck, M.D.; John Beck, M.D.; Irene Cannon, M.D.; Mark Constantz; Doris Denney, R.Ph.; June Fisher, M.D.; Victor Fuchs, Ph.D.; Judy Geisinger, M.S.W.; Dewleen Hayes; Halsted R. Holman, M.D.; Larry Horowitz, M.D.; Charles Irwin, M.D.; Al Jacobs, M.D.; Matthew Liang, M.D., M.P.H.; Jane Morton, M.D.; Bev Kusler; Tom McMeekin, M.D.; Pat Moylan, R.N.; Bonnie Obrig; Margaret Olebe; Shirley Rudd, R.N.; Alan Shapiro, M.D.; John Slane, R.Ph.; Elihu Sussman, M.D.; John Wasson, M.D.; and Anne Wilkins. We include special thanks to David Bergman, M.D.

The clerical assistance of Carolyn Hinkle, Ruth Lynn, Sharon Joseph, Bonnie Obrig, and Catherine Williams made this book possible.

Finally, for continuing advice, review, and encouragement we should like to acknowledge our wives Marcia, Sarah, and Shelley, and our children Andrew, Elizabeth, Gregory, and Meredith. Their daily input and effort make this as much their book as ours.

To Our Readers

This book can be of great help to you and your family. The medical advice is as sound as we can make it. Many doctors have reviewed each section, and we have tried to capture for you the essence of the standard medical recommendations for each problem. But the advice will not always work. Like medical recommendations of all kinds, it will not always prove successful. There is also a dilemma: If we don't give you direct advice for taking care of your children, we may not be helpful. If we do, we will sometimes be wrong. So here are some qualifications: If your child is under the care of a physician and if you receive advice contrary to that given in this book, follow the physician's advice; the individual characteristics of your child's problem can then be taken into account. You know your child best; do not hesitate to follow your own judgment as to when to seek professional assistance. If your child has an allergy or a suspected allergy to a medication, check with your doctor, at least by phone. With any medication, read the label instructions carefully; instructions vary from time to time and you should follow the latest. And if your child's problem persists beyond a reasonable period, you should usually make an appointment with a doctor.

Part

I

Parent Skills

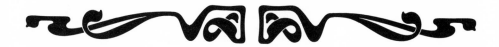

Chapter

1

A Child Is Coming

Pregnancy is as complex as any natural event in our lives. It is exciting, exhausting, fulfilling, fatiguing, happy, sad, simple, creative, and many more contradictions for both mother and father. In a few pages we cannot do justice to a subject about which poets, parents, philosophers, and physicians have written extensively. Taking care of your child, however, begins with pregnancy. In this chapter, we will cover some of the most relevant topics that may concern you at this important time.

I'M PREGNANT, WE'RE PREGNANT

There is no such thing as an unnatural feeling during pregnancy. Most parents find that they experience a variety of emotions, from uncertainty and anxiety to satisfaction and exhilaration. We have tried to capture some of these feelings by collecting written accounts and recording conversations with parents. These statements, and those in the following chapters, are only a sampling. You will certainly experience feelings not found on these pages. Indeed, many will be concerned if they initially have no feelings about such an important occurrence. This, too, is a common experience, especially before the first movements of the developing infant are felt. It is difficult to appreciate the transition in feelings that occurs by reading isolated statements. Many of the parents, however, who expressed tremendous anxiety about child raising during pregnancy have found that the actual task is natural and rewarding. The advice of one mother is important to remember: "In having children and raising children, nobody is likely to experience something that hasn't happened to someone else. All of the emotions, from terrible fear to joy, have been shared by millions of others many times before.''

Before our first child was born, I hadn't given very much thought to what our lives would be like after the birth itself, which occupied most of my attention. If I thought at all about it, I guess I had a subconscious picture of myself in a Woman's Day ad, one of those slightly out of focus pictures of a beautiful young mother in a pastel dressing gown nursing her baby in a pose of peaceful fulfillment. I must have imagined that she took care of her baby in her spare time. Was I surprised!

Mother of two

Libby kept asking me, "Aren't you excited about it?" She, of course, already was, and I had to admit to her disappointment that it was just hard to realize that we now had a baby on the way and I really had no solid feelings or comprehensions about the child. She did come home wearing one of those tacky T-shirts with "baby" bold across the front. My shy Libby did this. At first I wasn't too interested in being seen at the A & P with her and her new brazen shirt. But she was and still is proud of her tummy. I begrudgingly gave her my hand which she pressed firmly on her tummy. I told her not to press too hard. I could hurt the baby. I still have a feeling of slight uneasiness when pressing on her tummy.

Expectant father

He said, "I'm so glad you are going to have your baby at last," and I said, "But it isn't me having mine, it's us having ours," and he said, "But the baby is so much more the mother's thing." And something went cold, and I often wish I had walked away then, found someone who wanted to share it with me.

Mother of six

We seem to blunder into most of the major decisions in our lives with no facts and no experience. We're going into childraising with a lot of ignorance and a lot of trepidation. My cousins asked us to babysit for their four kids recently and we realized for the first time we had very discordant philosophies about raising children. I always thought that I would naturally know how to raise kids—it never occurred to us we might have very different philosophies.

Expectant father

We had been trying for several months before Lenore got pregnant. When each month came and went with no pregnancy, we were filled with both relief and anxiety and I think it is the mixture of the two emotions that is important. When Lenore did become pregnant my first reaction was one of great exhilaration and excitement. But there must have been subconscious underpinnings of uneasiness or uncertainty because within a very few days these feelings surfaced. The exhilaration of starting a family was tempered by the uncertainty of not knowing what kind of change in our lives was to be forthcoming. Would we lose freedom? Would our new life-styles be as comfortable as our present ones? Would the rewards justify the work? What was parenting all about anyway? We tended to try to cram many things into the nine-month pregnancy period. We had the feeling that each trip we took, each vacation, each special activity, each late-night dinner might be the last for a very long time. This ambivalance continued throughout the pregnancy, but as Lenore changed physically, I felt more sure that this was a very positive thing. The anxieties over the unknown were still present, but somehow less important. Maybe they were replaced by the anxieties surrounding pregnancy and delivery. Would the baby be healthy? Would the delivery be easy? Would Lenore be well?

Father of two

I was totally unprepared for being almost solely responsible for her care . . . Why did I waste 9 months thinking about a birth that lasted only 20 hours instead of how to live with a dependent human being for another 20 years? I did not even see or hold a newborn in the time I was pregnant. I never saw breast milk or bottle milk stuff. And none of the people who were professional helpers seemed to think it was important.

Mother of two

Being brought up as a woman you see child care as your responsibility and being brought up as a man, John doesn't even conceive of some of the things that could fall apart or could possibly go wrong.

Mother of one

The one big thing that was taught in the Catholic Church was that in the event of a problem at birth, you were supposed to save the child. The doctors aren't allowed to make the decision and they come out and ask the husband and he's supposed to say "save the child." And I woke up upset and told David if that happened, I would really like a chance to try again.

Mother of two

We've hired a person to do full-time child care. The first month we hope to share tasks of childraising. I hope to get a feeling of what it will be like to leave the child with her before I actually do it. It really will be an experimental time. I hope it won't be a competition. Other working mothers who have had this arrangement have reassured me that the children know who mommy is.

Expectant mother

I feel much more protected and cared for. Bob shares work a lot more than he did.

Expectant mother

BECOMING PREGNANT

Planning your family size has only recently become a matter of choice. Changing attitudes and contraceptive technology have permitted couples to decide on if they want children, and if so, how many to have and when. Discussion of the subject recently has centered almost entirely on how *not* to become pregnant. However, here is some important "how to" information for those who want to have children.

Although women may become pregnant after first intercourse, this is the exception and not the rule. The average delay in becoming pregnant during unprotected intercourse is between six and nine months. For women younger than 18 or older than 27, an even longer time is required. The conception rate for men also decreases with age. Highest rates occur with men younger than 25. The more frequent the intercourse, the more likely the chances for conception.

The most likely time for conception is during ovulation, at the time when the egg leaves the ovary. This time is approximately midway between menstrual periods, but it may vary from as much as a few days after to a few days before the menstrual period. The time of ovulation varies from woman to woman and from month to month, but the average time is the fourteenth day before the start of the next menstrual period. Often you can become pregnant by timing intercourse with ovulation, but this technique is not uniformly successful. The most practical way to estimate the time of ovulation is to take your temperature. Body temperature usually drops slightly just before ovulation and will then rise about one degree Fahrenheit. This is the time when you are most likely to become pregnant. You can detect this temperature change by taking your temperature at about the same time every morning, and making a chart of it. An oral thermometer is fine. Remember, some months there may be no ovulation. Also, your temperature change may occur at any time between two days before and two days after ovulation; hence this provides only an approximation of ovulation time.

The use of vaginal lubricants can interfere with fertility. Washing or urinating after intercourse will empty the vagina of a significant number of sperm and decrease the likelihood of conception. Failure to achieve female orgasm has absolutely no influence on fertility. There is some evidence that exposure to significant heat can hamper sperm, so prolonged, hot baths (male before intercourse, female after) may impair fertility somewhat.

Besides a missed menstrual period, fatigue, nausea, breast tenderness, and frequent urination are all signs of pregnancy. Pregnancy can be confirmed by a urine test, which checks for chorionic gonadotropin, a hormone present early in pregnancy.

TAKING CARE OF YOURSELF DURING PREGNANCY

Taking care of yourself during pregnancy is just like living sensibly at other times, with one obvious exception: You are now providing for two individuals. Your bad habits—smoking, drinking, taking drugs or medications—now affect a second life. Most things that you have done before becoming pregnant can con-

tinue without interruption. We will spend some time now discussing exceptions
to this rule and some current misconceptions.

Diet

A well-balanced diet is always advisable and your nutritional status at the
beginning of pregnancy is probably as important as what you eat during
pregnancy. The exact amount that you need to eat during this time will vary
according to your individual requirements, but common sense tells us that
extremes are harmful. Weight gain should be between 20 and 25 pounds. As
our understanding of maternal nutrition has improved, the practice of restricting
weight gain to less than 20 pounds has ended. However, gaining more than 25
pounds makes it harder to get back in shape after delivery. During pregnancy,
you will need about 15 percent more calories, on the average, each day. This is
only the equivalent of a pint of milk, so you can see how easy it is to overshoot.

Most women do not need elaborate dietary changes and caloric bookkeep-
ing during pregnancy; common sense and a normal diet will usually suffice. The
increased nutritional requirements you will need throughout your pregnancy will
continue during breast feeding.

The majority of the extra calories you eat should come from increased
protein (milk, meat, fish, poultry, etc.), the basic building blocks of fetal development. *Carbohydrates,* such as bread, potatoes, and cereals, provide
energy for the developing fetus. Restricting carbohydrates forces your body to
rely on other sources of energy such as fat; too heavy a reliance on fat produces
chemical by-products known as ketones, which alter your mood and are potentially harmful to both mother and fetus. *Fats,* however, are also required for fetal
development; they aid in the absorption of important vitamins. *Vitamins and
minerals* are largely provided by fruits and vegetables. The requirements for
Vitamins A and C increase considerably in pregnancy, but are usually met by an
ordinary diet. Folic acid, found in milk and green vegetables, is an important
requirement for the creation of blood, and the need for folic acid doubles during
pregnancy. It is sometimes difficult to meet this increased need during pregnancy; therefore, this is the most frequently prescribed nutritional supplement. In
general, a proper diet will supply all nutritional requirements but many physicians rely on vitamin supplements if they are uncertain of your diet. The body
requirement for calcium, important for maintaining sound bones and preventing
muscle spasms, also increases considerably. Calcium is best supplemented by an
intake of milk, cheese, or eggs. Broccoli and oranges are also rich in calcium.
More iron, needed for blood building , is also required. Foods rich in iron include
meats, cereals, and many vegetables, such as peas, spinach, lima beans, and
lentils.

The human fetus is remarkable in its ability to obtain nutrition from the
mother. If there is a shortage of the necessary nutrient, the fetus will receive
preferential treatment in getting what is available. Improper nutrition is thus
detrimental first to the mother, and then to the fetus.

Many mothers report cravings for fruits and vegetables during pregnancy;
these are undoubtedly the body's way of telling you what you need. Feel free to

follow your cravings. Eat sensibly and review your diet with a nutritionist or physician should any questions arise.

During the first three months of pregnancy, nausea and vomiting may interfere with your normal pattern of eating. Morning sickness occurs in many mothers, while others are most nauseated at suppertime. Having frequent small feedings is often the best way to obtain nutritional requirements in these circumstances. Many drugs used to treat nausea are potentially dangerous during pregnancy and should be avoided unless absolutely necessary and after full discussion with your physician.

Foods to avoid

The only food to be avoided is beef liver. Beef liver may contain levels of diethylstilbestrol, an artificial hormone that increases weight in cattle and is not considered safe in pregnancy. Diethylstilbestrol was used years ago to prevent miscarriages, and mothers taking the drug produced daughters with a higher risk of developing vaginal cancer than daughters of mothers not exposed to the drug. Despite the 1972 recommendations by the Food and Drug Administration, 1976 legislation passed by the Senate, and testimony by the Director of the National Cancer Institute that the levels found in beef liver may potentially be hazardous to humans, beef liver is still being consumed by the American public.

On 3 December 1960, the Food and Drug Administration published an order prohibiting the use of sassafras in foods because it was found to cause cancer of the liver in animals. Sassafras is still widely available in many parts of the country as a tea. It should be avoided during pregnancy. In 1977, the FDA raised concern about artificial sweeteners; they should also be avoided during pregnancy.

Exercise

Feel free to continue any physical exercise that you enjoyed before becoming pregnant. Because of the ability of the fetus to preferentially obtain an adequate blood supply, some of your physical reserves for strenuous exercise may be lost during pregnancy. Consequently, you may tire more quickly and feel faint, particularly at high altitudes. Basically, your body will tell you when to stop. You should also use your own judgment about certain types of physical exercise that involve the possibility of abdominal injury—for instance, skiing and hockey.

Traveling

With one exception, there are no traveling restrictions except those dictated by common sense. As you approach the expected day of the birth, you should avoid trips that will place you out of striking distance of the site you have chosen for delivery. If you are planning on flying in your ninth month, commercial airlines request a letter in triplicate from your physician, stating that he or she feels it is safe for you to fly.

Sex

Occasionally, conventional wisdom is not very wise. Such is the case with the frequent statements about avoiding intercourse for six weeks before and after delivery. There is no evidence that intercourse poses any risk to mother or fetus.

There is better evidence that abstinence for prolonged periods is stressful for both partners. Except for instances of vaginal bleeding, possible premature labor, or premature rupture of the amniotic fluid sac, intercourse is possible whenever both partners are willing and able. After delivery, an episiotomy incision that is healing may cause discomfort with intercourse for several weeks.

Amniocentesis

Amniocentesis is a procedure in which amniotic fluid is removed from the uterus by means of a needle inserted through the abdominal wall. The purpose of obtaining the amniotic fluid is to evaluate the risk of a child having an inherited disease. It is usually done between the twelfth and fourteenth week of pregnancy. The procedure is complex, is expensive, requires a skilled physician, and has complications. It is not for everyone.

Amniotic fluid can be evaluated for the presence of a metabolic disease like Tay-Sachs disease or a chromosomal disease like mongolism. In families with known metabolic diseases, the risk of a child having the disease is usually one in four if both parents carry the gene for the disease. Many metabolic diseases can be diagnosed by amniotic-fluid analysis. In the process of examining for abnormal or extra chromosomes, the sex of the child can also be determined by looking for the presence of an XX chromosome pattern (female) or an XY chromosome pattern (male).

Downs syndrome (Mongolism) is one of the most common chromosomal disorders caused by an extra chromosome. As women become older, the chance of having a child with Downs syndrome increases. Only one in 2500 women at age 25, but one in 40 women at age 45, will have an affected child. Advancing age is therefore one reason for contemplating amniocentesis. Younger women with an affected child already may be concerned about having a second child with this condition. Although there are seldom recurrences, many of these parents may be interested in considering amniocentesis.

Some problems, such as hemophilia, occur only in males. Women carry the gene for hemophilia but cannot have the disease. Amniocentesis can identify a developing male, but only 50 percent of males with carrier mothers will actually have hemophilia.

Amniocentesis is relatively safe, but there are risks. Spontaneous abortions and infant blood system problems (Rh sensitization) have occurred, but in competent hands, the risk of a serious complication should be less than one percent. Occasionally no amniotic fluid is obtained and the procedure must be repeated. Sometimes the laboratory is unsuccessful in its attempt to analyze the fluid and a repeat amniocentesis may be necessary. There can also be test errors in the results.

There are also many ethical considerations. Which "disorders" should be aborted, if you accept the practice of abortion? A given inherited disease can affect one child seriously and the next child minimally. What should be done with a fetus having a 50-percent chance of a devastating disease? What do you do if you are looking for one problem and accidentally discover another minor problem? Will amniocentesis allow elimination of dread diseases or encourage abortion for even the most minor handicaps?

If you are considering amniocentesis, you should discuss it extensively at home and then with your doctor. In the end you should make a decision consistent with your own moral framework. Physicians cannot tell you whether or not you should accept or reject a child with a given disorder. Complete information is often difficult to obtain about amniocentesis, but persist until you are satisfied that you have enough information to make a decision.

Medicine

All drugs are potentially harmful and the risk of taking drugs increases during pregnancy because of potential harm to the fetus as well as the mother. Despite this, American women consume on the average 4.5 different drugs during pregnancy, and 80 percent of these drugs are not prescribed by physicians. Heavy drug use is not surprising when one considers the number of drug messages we see and hear every day. On television alone, pharmaceutical preparations are the number-one type of product advertised. Resist them!

As a general rule, any drug that a mother takes will reach the fetus, and all drugs are potentially harmful to the fetus. The majority of drugs now on the market have never had their safety tested with respect to the fetus; effects on human infants are often discovered only later. Thalidomide, for example, was tested on rodents and did not produce the limb deformities it later did in human offspring.

Below is a list of drugs to be especially avoided, along with explanations of the problems they cause. Not all of these associations are well documented. However, when considering infant safety we feel that drugs should be regarded as guilty until proven innocent. Many medications change in composition when stored on the shelf and become harmful only with increasing age. This is a good time to throw out *all* medications on your shelf. Before taking any medication, even aspirin, while pregnant or nursing, consult your physician.

Medication	Potential Problem in Infants
Aspirin (during last three months of pregnancy)	Yellow jaundice Bleeding Premature labor
Aspirin-phenacetin combination	Oxygen-carrying ability of blood decreases
Acetaminophen (Tylenol, Tempra, Validol)	Kidney problems
Alcohol—chronic abuse or high doses	Seizures Growth retardation Birth defects

Antidepressants (tricyclic)
    Impromine (Tofranil)
    Amitryptyline (Elavil, Etafron)
	Birth defects

Antihistamines Diphenhidramine (Benadryl)	Seizures
Antinausea drugs Meclizine (Bonine)	Birth defects

Medication	Potential Problem in Infants
Cyclizine (Marezine)	Birth defects
Chlorocyclizine	
Antibiotics	
Sulfa drugs	Yellow jaundice
Tetracycline	Malformed teeth
	Suppressed bone growth
	Cataracts
Kanamycin	Hearing loss
Streptomycin	Hearing loss
Bronchial medications	
Potassium iodide	Goiter
Hormones	
Estrogens (diethylstilbestrol)	Vaginal cancer
Androgens	Masculinization of daughter
Progestins	Birth defects
	Growth retardation
LSD	Limb defects
Tranquilizers	
Diazepam (Valium)	Decreased body temperature
Chlordiazepopide (Librium)	Seizures
Barbiturates	Seizures
Chlorpromazine (Thorazine)	Temperature regulation
Promethazine (Phenergan)	Bleeding
Vitamin excess	
C	Skin and intestinal problems
Pyridoxine	Birth defects
Vaginal preparations	
Flagyl	Cancer (in rats)
	Mutations (in bacteria)

Immunizations and Allergy Shots

All immunizations should be avoided during pregnancy; this is especially true for rubella (German measles) immunizations. Women receiving rubella immunizations should avoid becoming pregnant for three months afterwards. Although no birth defects have been reported in the few children born to women accidentally immunized with rubella vaccine during pregnancy, the potential for problems remains. There does not seem to be any necessity for avoiding contact with children who have recently been immunized. Also, allergy desensitization should be discontinued during pregnancy.

Pets

Cats are often feared during pregnancy; some of them carry and transmit a disease called toxoplasmosis. Toxoplasmosis, like German measles, produces few symptoms in the mother (occasionally there may be fever or lymph gland swelling), but is potentially harmful to the developing fetus. Toxoplasmosis can be transmitted in the excrement of cats. It is also found in meat, but is only transmitted in meat that has been undercooked. Toxoplasmosis is very common (30 to 40 percent of the population has had it). Congenital toxoplasmosis, a relatively rare form of this illness, appears in newborn children of women who become infected for the first time during early pregnancy. If you have cats and are concerned, your physician can do a blood test that will inform you of whether you have already had toxoplasmosis; if so, you need not concern yourself about this problem during your pregnancy. The common-sense approach is for the pregnant woman to avoid the kitty litter box and not to buy a new cat. A cat that has been in the family for a while is less hazardous, so you can keep and love your old cat during pregnancy with relatively little risk.

BREAST FEEDING OR BOTTLE FEEDING?

Decide how you are going to feed your baby before the birth; the stress of the hospital makes rational decisions difficult. Breast feeding is best for some mothers, while others will prefer bottle feeding. Either choice is fully acceptable and will be guided by *individual* circumstances.

It is unfortunate that fashion is often responsible for making a mother feel she should choose one particular method. Bottle feeding became popular fifty years ago. The society at the time wanted to do everything "scientifically," women wanted to be free to leave the home, and the female breast was shifting from being a nursing object to being a sexual object. Fortunately, social attitudes are constantly in movement and currently there is widespread acceptance of mothers nursing in public. Breastfeeding is now gaining in popularity and is currently considered to have many "scientific advantages."

Although we personally recommend breastfeeding when possible, it is important for mothers to realize that both methods supply sound nutrition and intimacy to the child. Neither choice should provoke feelings of guilt in the mother or father. Your baby is happy when you are happy. Choose the method *you* feel most comfortable with. Both breast feeding and bottle feeding require you to learn new skills. The choice is yours.

Making an informed decision requires, among other things, the availability of factual information, which we attempt to provide here. Given the proper encouragement and assistance, nearly every mother can breast-feed her child. A few rare medical conditions, such as severe breast infections or infants with a cleft palate, may make breast feeding more difficult. Many pediatricians now recommend breast feeding for most women and we do too. Here are some of our reasons.

The Advantages of Breast Feeding for the Child

- Nutrition is provided in the proper proportion, if the mother is eating a balanced diet. Proteins, carbohydrates, fats, minerals, vitamins, and iron are all provided in amounts suitable for adequate growth. Although at one time iron drops were thought necessary to supplement human milk, this is no longer felt to be true. Only vitamin D, to the best of our knowledge at this time, does not seem to be present in adequate amounts in breast milk. Although exposure to sunshine will provide some vitamin D, supplemental vitamin D is necessary.

- Breast feeding is hygienic. There is less chance of contamination of the milk than there is with bottle feeding.

- A mother can spend time being very close to her baby.

- There may be fewer respiratory and intestinal infections in breast-fed infants. In addition, maternal immunity to a number of common viral illnesses may be transferred to the infant through breast feeding.

- There may be fewer allergic disorders of the skin, respiratory tract, and intestine in breast-fed infants.

- In poverty areas in underdeveloped countries, the death rate is lower among breast-fed infants. In the United States, there does not seem to be a difference; infant death is unusual fortunately with either feeding method.

- Breast-fed babies tend not to become fat as frequently. The composition, and therefore the taste, of breast milk changes during the course of a feeding; thus infants will reject a breast after several minutes and move on to the next breast, even though the first breast still contains milk. This is one of nature's ways of preventing obesity in the newborn child.

- The stools of breast-fed babies are lighter in color and looser than those of babies who are fed a formula. This looseness should not be interpreted as diarrhea. In fact, breast-fed babies have diarrhea less often. Because the stools are soft, breast-fed babies may have fewer irritations of the rectum, and they hardly ever become constipated. A strange bonus—breast-fed babies' bowel movements smell better!

The Advantages of Breast Feeding for the Mother

- Hormone release during breast feeding causes rapid contraction of the uterus and encourages the return to normal of the uterus after delivery.

- It is a period of relaxation for the mother. In a society in which time is money, this is nature's way of forcing you to slow down and relax.

- The cost is less. Bottles, nipples, and baby formula are more expensive than the extra nutrition required by a nursing mother.

- Breast feeding is convenient. There is no need to fuss with the paraphernalia of bottle feeding. You don't have to run to the store in the middle of the night to buy milk.

- It is one means, but not a good method, of birth control. (Don't count on it!)

- Some reports suggest that breast feeding may reduce the frequency of blood clots in the legs, and some indicate that there may be a lower frequency of breast cancer in mothers who breast-feed. These findings need more study.

Myths about Breast Feeding

- Breast feeding does *not* depend on your breast size. Large breasts contain predominantly *excess* fatty tissue and in no way increase the ability to breast-feed.

- Inverted nipples are *not* an insurmountable problem.

- Breast feeding does *not* interfere with poliovirus immunization. The trivalent vaccine used in the United States is equally effective in breast-fed and artificially fed infants.

- Breast feeding does *not* cause more frequent jaundice in infants. In some instances a baby may be taken off breast milk for several days to speed the resolution of the normal jaundice that occurs at birth.

- Breast feeding does *not* cause sagging breasts. However, it is important that you wear a comfortable brassiere that gives adequate support during your period of breast feeding.

Problems with Breast Feeding

- The schedule of breast feeding may interfere with the mother's ability to spend time away from home. This problem can sometimes be solved by taking along a breast pump and emptying the breast when it becomes uncomfortable.

- The more frequent stools will require more frequent changing of the infant.

- The father may feel left out. If the father desires to feed the baby, breast milk can be emptied by pump or manually and then given from a bottle by the father. Or a supplemental bottle of formula may be given by the father.

Cautions about Breast Feeding

- Most drugs taken by the mother will be passed to the infant through breast milk. Valium, sulfa drugs, and tetracycline are particularly common and should be avoided, since they are hazardous to the infant. In general, never take any drug without consulting your physician first.

- Chemical contamination of food or water supplies has resulted in the contaminant being found in breast milk [e.g., PCB (polychlorinated biphenyls), PBB (polybrominated biphenyls), and DDT]. Such rare instances are not an argument for bottle feeding but an argument for tighter regulations against chemical poisons in our environment.

Techniques of breast feeding are discussed on pp. 44–47. A good source on breast feeding is *Nursing Your Baby* by Karen Pryor (New York: Pocket Books, 1975).

Bottle Feeding

There are many advantages to bottle feeding. The father can help and become involved in feeding very early. In addition there is somewhat more freedom of movement for the mother. Also, the intimacy and relaxation in nursing a baby can be enjoyed when bottle feeding as well. Parents who choose bottle feeding may be assured that the commercial milk available today is of high quality. Great efforts have been made to produce a product that is as close in composition to breast milk as is feasible. Millions of Americans who were bottle-fed are a testimony to its overall safety.

Sterilization is a thing of the past in all areas where tap water is safe to drink. If it is safe for you it is safe for the baby. Parents wishing to prepare several days worth of feedings in advance should consider sterilizing, however, since bacteria can grow in the formula after it has been mixed.

Bottles and nipples are all the equipment you will need. Infants obtain milk naturally by a process of squeezing with their lower jaws and gums. They use their tongues to push up on the nipple and keep it securely on the roof of their mouth. The usual bottle nipples permit milk flow more easily than the breast does, causing the infant to exercise the jaws less and forcing him or her to stick the tongue outward instead of upward to retard the rush of milk. Nuk nipples are commercial nipples that allow the infant to closely duplicate the sucking performed on the breast. Types of formula and techniques of breast feeding are discussed on pp. 44–47.

Babies will grow beautifully on breast or bottle milk. Mothers should choose the method with which they feel most comfortable. Many mothers are reluctant to try breast feeding because they feel anxious. This is a natural feeling as it is something new that appears to be complicated. In fact, breast feeding is an elegant function of the human body with which many other mothers can assist you. Nursing-mothers councils and the La Leche League are always willing to help. The best place to get help is from a friend who has successfully breast fed her baby.

CHILDBIRTH PREPARATION CLASSES

Pregnancy places different physical and psychological demands on both parents. The key elements of a successful pregnancy are adequate physical and psychological preparation. Coping with some of the physical demands for mothers can be straightforward, such as eating to meet the increased requirements. So too is exercising to strengthen back and abdominal muscles by doing sit-ups, swimming, and kicking. Standing in place for a long period of time should be avoided during pregnancy. However, there are very few exercises done every day that prepare a woman for the demands on her perineal muscles. Similarly, the breathing best suited for labor is not something women often have a chance to practice. Prepared childbirth classes teach about the special physical demands of pregnancy and the most suitable exercises.

The purpose of childbirth classes is to help the mother and father take an active part in the process of labor and birth. These classes attempt to focus the energies during birth into productive psychologic and physical activity, hence eliminating the portrait of the mother as a passive person depending on the doctor to relieve her pain and to deliver her baby.

Classes will generally discuss in detail what occurs biologically during labor and delivery. They will train you to use your body most efficiently in order to deliver your child. This will include physical and breathing exercises and demonstrations. In addition, they will teach your partner how to help. Classes generally consist of 6 to 10 two-hour sessions in the last three months of pregnancy. Many also include a tour and explanation of local delivery facilities.

The Lamaze method, probably the most discussed of the current methods, attempts to go beyond mere physical conditioning and elimination of fears. The method is based on reconditioning or changing the responses that the mother already has. The method here is to "enlighten the woman by instructing her about the phenomenon involved in childbirth, the purpose being to convert delivery from the idea of pain to a series of understood processes in which uterine contraction is the leading phenomenon." The other purpose of Lamaze teaching is to develop a new set of conditioned reflexes in an effort to block out the old set. By coupling a new breathing method with uterine contractions, it is hoped that the uterine contractions may stimulate breathing rather than pain.

It is unfortunate that Dr. Lamaze has entitled his book *Painless Childbirth*. The purpose of prepared childbirth is to help the mother, father, and infant experience a safe, nontraumatic birth, but there is often pain. It is important that family members can feel good and have the energy to enjoy the moment and begin to develop positive feelings about their infant. Pain can be terrifying if misunderstood; it is not necessarily an evil force to be eliminated at all costs by drug or psychologic anesthesia. The pain you may experience during swimming, running, or childbirth should not be hunted down and eliminated. In fact, very few natural childbirth classes have as their goal the creation of a "painless childbirth," but rather a childbirth in which the family is best prepared to deal with the event. Parents should also realize that problems such as prolonged labor will occur despite the best preparation. There are many problems that have a physiological basis and are *not* the fault of the mother.

Many of our patients have recently been concerned that childbirth preparation classes focus almost entirely on the physical aspects of delivery. There has been increasing demand from patients for further discussion of some of the emotional aspects of pregnancy and delivery. For instance, the Bradley method has done much to actively bring fathers into the birth process. Several groups are now developing childbirth preparation classes which focus on the feelings that parents experience during pregnancy as well as on the reorganization of everyday life that is brought about by the birth of a new child.

We feel that childbirth classes are helpful for many; testimonials are the best evidence for their effectiveness. A recent study compared a group of women undergoing prepared childbirth with a group that had not taken the classes. There was no difference in the medical complications for mothers or for infants in either group, but prepared mothers requested considerably fewer analgesics and anesthetics. These drugs often make mothers and infants drowsy in the first few hours and diminish the quality of the interaction between them.

To find childbirth classes in your neighborhood, ask your friends, physician, local hospital, or local nursing association. Many hospitals offer excellent classes about prepared childbirth, while other classes concentrate on how to best understand hospital routines. Be sure you know the curriculum before you enroll.

If you are having difficulty locating childbirth classes, you may write to one of the organizations below.

1. American Academy of Husband-Coached Childbirth, P. O. Box 5224, Sherman Oaks, CA 91413.
2. American Society for Psycho-prophylaxis and Obstetrics, Suite 410, 1523 L Street, N.W., Washington, DC 20005.
3. International Childbirth Education Association, P. O. Box 5852, Milwaukee, Wisconsin 53220.
4. Maternity Center Association, 48 E. 92nd St., New York, NY 10028.

ADDITIONAL READING

Robert A. Bradley, *Husband-Coached Childbirth*. New York: Harper and Row, 1974.
Fernand Lamaze, *Painless Childbirth: The Lamaze Method*. New York: Pocket Books, 1972.

HOME DELIVERY, HOSPITAL DELIVERY, OR SOMETHING ELSE?

You have a choice of where your child is born. It has always been a paradox that people will spend hours doing comparative shopping for televisions and automobiles, yet automatically accept the local hospital for something as important as the birth of their child. The hospital can be an excellent place for your child to be born, or it can create problems.

How good is your local hospital? University affiliation does not necessarily ensure safety and quality. Each hospital must be judged on its own performance. How many deliveries are done in the hospital? Who attends these deliveries? Is there a pediatrician available for emergencies? How often are Caesarean sections performed? What indications does your hospital use for a Caesarean section? What about fetal heart monitoring? Severe fetal distress is an indication for an immediate Caesarean section, but some people are now questioning whether the increased number of Caesarean sections that have resulted from better monitoring is actually improving the outcome for the infants delivered. It certainly isn't for the mother. There are no perfect guides to choosing the right hospital or for answering these difficult questions.

The hospital you choose should be willing to treat the entire family with respect. They should be supportive of your wishes for *your* childbirth. Most hospitals allow fathers in the delivery room, but some do not. If you are planning on this, be sure to inquire beforehand. Also be sure to find out what the "routine" procedures of medication and anesthesia are. Individualized care consistent with your wishes, and not "routine" care, should be provided. If you feel uncomfortable with certain hospital procedures, negotiate before delivery or look elsewhere.

More and more people are choosing home delivery for their children. In many countries, delivery of children at home is the rule and not the exception.

The experience with home deliveries in these countries is excellent. Women are followed carefully throughout their entire pregnancy and those who do not have complications are delivered at home by people with training and experience. In some countries even first deliveries are performed at home, while other countries have a policy of doing home deliveries only with the second and later pregnancies. However, the fact that home deliveries are safe in such countries as England and Holland does not mean that they are safe in your community. If you are talking to someone who is offering to assist with your child's birth at home, ask about his or her qualifications. Are they a lay or nurse midwife? Are they physicians well trained in obstetrics? How many deliveries have they done? How are they prepared to deal with an emergency in the home? What backup facilities are available?

You should also make an effort to investigate alternate facilities. As home deliveries are becoming more popular, hospitals are feeling the stimulus to innovate that competition always brings. One San Francisco hospital has set up comfortable, ''homey'' rooms for childbirth. In the event of an emergency, the mother is wheeled down the hall to the conventionally equipped delivery room. A physician in Idaho has rebuilt part of his house as a delivery area. There is a comfortable living room and two ''delivery rooms.'' All the equipment of the hospital is available in the setting of a home.

Most communities have several options for delivery of your child and you should know about them. We feel that rather than beginning with a categorical decision of ''I want a home birth'' or ''I want a hospital birth,'' you should begin with the question ''What is the best method of delivery for me and my child in my community?''

ADDITIONAL READING

Jean Marzollo (ed., written by parents), *Nine Months, One Day, One Year.* New York: Harper and Row, 1976.

Chapter

2

The Big Event

Just as in pregnancy, the big event, birth, is full of complex emotions for both mother and father. Here are some of the feelings that parents have shared with us:

. . . Great joy sweeps over you, but not on schedule. They placed my newborn son on the bed beside me . . . it was all so private having the baby born at home . . . even though it was a difficult birth . . . and I looked at the child and I did not recognize him. It's odd when you have felt his every move from the moment he started to move . . . when he has been a physical part of you for so long . . . even though you don't even know the sex of the child, you still expect to recognize him . . . and you look at this total stranger . . . you find out what his face looks like . . . a new and totally unknown face, a whole new and different person you have to get to know . . . and with the knowing comes the loving.

. . . The huge sweeping joy of giving birth . . . of the act itself . . . came with the second. The "for this was I born" feeling . . . a level of satisfaction unfelt before. It came again with the fourth and fifth . . . but not with the sixth. But then the sixth was another difficult delivery and I was too tired to feel much of anything except overwhelming relief that after all that had gone wrong in the pregnancy, the child was perfect . . . I couldn't believe it . . . that was Christmas Eve . . . what a present.

Mother of six

Although I had excellent prenatal care and access to the most enlightened and modern practices, the emotion I felt strongest after Mary's birth was anger and resentment toward myself and members of the medical and helping professions. Why specifically—too much time was spent on reading, exercising, and talking about giving birth. I got sucked in by the movie star syndrome of the big event. How I would have natural childbirth, breathing, learning about my body, the muscles and how they worked, learning about pain, about control, learning my script, being undrugged and awake so I could experience birth, so I could see another baby coming out of my body. Hey, for nine months I read about it, talked about, drove everyone nuts (and I loved every minute of it). After laboring 19 hours at home with a sunny side up presentation, I finally was driven screaming and contorted with pain to the hospital, where I expected to die. After being quickly gassed, but not soon enough to feel a midforceps delivery, I passed out and missed Mary's birth. I expected a dark haired, different baby somehow bloody and face red and contorted with squalling. Mary was so unlike the monkeyish newborn I expected. Her face with tiny eyes, tiny mouth, and huge cheeks. Like a mongoloid! Yes! For a few days, I had the uneasy feeling that she was retarded. But I loved her intensely the moment I saw her, she was really special. I could spot her the minute I walked into the nursery, she was so fair and bald and her head so lumpy. I was so proud of her and myself.

Mother of two

It is almost impossible to have any kind of relationship with the unborn baby. When I saw Peter for the very first time, he was lying in a plastic bassinet and had stopped crying very soon with his eyes wide open, seemingly looking around. I thought he was so beautiful! The fact that he was a boy which we had hoped for and was so beautiful made it so easy to accept him right away. I had been looking foward to having a child very much but this seemed so special like something you wish for but don't dare to hope for. After this initial feeling of joy, it was a matter of getting used to this little warm, cuddly and sleepy living thing. I didn't sense any immediate attachment, it was an adjustment to something very new. The feeling of wanting to protect this new presence, nurse it and take care of it was very strong—I guess this is what they meant by "motherly instinct."

Mother of three

I remember very well the earlier parts of labor and then Irmhild disappearing into the delivery room where I was intentionally excluded. The next thing I remember was that Irmhild was on a stretcher being carted back to the ward and she held up this little brown thing and said, "Guess what?" I said, "A girl" wishing it were a boy—and it was.

Father of three

My husband couldn't care less if it was a girl or a boy—he was so frightened something would happen to me—he only wanted to know "Are you all right?"

Mother of four

I had a lot of depression because it didn't go according to the book. Being a middle class person I read all the books and did all the exercises and learned how to blow but nobody prepared me for any of the things that might happen. And I felt that because I was healthy and was not 4' 10" people looked at me funny when I told them I had a C-section. They seemed to be saying what's wrong with you, you seem to be big enough to have a baby. You need to know that it's not your fault. I felt guilty for 6 months because I thought if I had only breathed right, I would not have had 60 hours of labor.

Mother of two

After Aaron was delivered I held him immediately. He nursed a bit and I just held him. The nurses (one older one) grudgingly wrapped him up. My husband Terry held him and walked around with him. All in all we had him over half an hour. When the nurse would keep trying to clean him up, he'd scream and kick. When I was alone with Aaron in my hospital room nursing him, I was thinking of my son, Gabriel, and Terry. I had never spent a night away from Gabriel. I was jealous of Terry. I wanted to be there to share in telling Gabriel about Aaron. Gabriel had been so excited about the birth of his baby.

Mother of two

The labor and delivery process ended with a feeling of great exhilaration, an indescribable feeling, unmatched by anything else I have ever known. Somehow everything was right with the world and nothing could be wrong.

Father of two

Most women begin labor in the 40th week of pregnancy, but ten to fifteen percent have premature labor. Many premature labors, however, do not proceed to delivery but end after a short period of time. For many days before delivery, the mother may experience contractions known as Braxton-Hicks contractions. The contractions are thought to prepare the uterus for delivery and thin and widen the mouth of the uterus (womb); this process is known as effacement and dilation.

The first stage of labor begins when contractions in the uterus become more regular and intense. It is often difficult to tell precisely when this stage of labor begins, and there are frequent false starts. Often a small amount of bloody mucus may show several days before labor. Contractions may be coming regularly, strongly, and at short intervals, and then suddenly they will cease. Labor has generally begun when contractions are ten minutes apart. These contractions may be felt in the lower abdomen or the lower back. Generally, the first stage of labor becomes shorter with each pregnancy. This stage often lasts from 6 to 18 hours in the first pregnancy, but from only 2 to 5 hours for the average second pregnancy. During the first stage, the mouth (cervix) of the uterus proceeds to open (dilate) more and more. The end of the first stage of labor is known as transition, and is often the most tiring stage. In transition the cervix dilates from 8 cm to 10 cm (3 in. to 4 in.), the size required for the infant's head to pass through the birth canal. It is for this stage that childbirth class preparation is often the most helpful, since relaxation is important.

The second stage of labor is usually much shorter than the first. It usually lasts about an hour for the first child and 15 minutes for subsequent births. The second stage starts when the cervix is fully dilated and ends when the child is delivered. During the early phases of the second stage, pain medications or anesthesia are usually administered.

The third stage is usually the shortest and lasts from several minutes to half an hour. During the third stage of labor the placenta or afterbirth is delivered. The physician or midwife will examine the placenta carefully to ensure that no parts still remain in the uterus. Parts of the placenta remaining in the uterus must be removed because they can become a serious cause of bleeding later on.

RUPTURE OF THE MEMBRANES

Throughout pregnancy, the developing infant rests in a pool of fluid enveloped by the amniotic sac. During the first stage of labor, this fluid cushions the child's head as the head is being pushed against the outlet of the uterus. The amniotic sac generally bursts by itself at the end of the first stage of labor. Frequently the amniotic sac will begin to leak fluid or rupture even before labor has begun; this will usually bring about the beginning of labor. The absence of fluid does not directly interfere with labor, but an amniotic sac that has been ruptured for more than 24 hours increases the chances of infection. If labor has not begun and a large rush of fluid indicates that the amniotic sac has ruptured, contact your physician.

The amniotic sac is often ruptured artificially at the end of the first stage of labor to facilitate the delivery. This is a painless procedure.

MEDICATIONS USED DURING LABOR

All medications that are given to the mother reach the child; no medications should be used automatically. For certain conditions, however, medication can be used with relative safety.

Sleep medications are sometimes used for women who are having false labor or who have been in and out of labor for several days and may have had little or no sleep. The fatigue of the mother may carry a greater risk to both mother and child than a mild sleeping medication would. Barbiturates such as Seconal, Nembutal, or Luminal are frequently used as sedatives.

Analgesics (pain medication) reduce the pain of labor, but do not completely eliminate it. Strong narcotic pain relievers and tranquilizers such as Demerol and Sparine are often used. These medications enter the infant's bloodstream and have temporary depressing effects on the infant. However, extreme pain can interfere with the progress of labor and can also affect the infant. Sleep medications and pain relievers should be used only when necessary and after careful deliberation by the physician.

ANESTHESIA

Anesthesia involves the complete elimination of pain by blocking the nerve impulses at either the local, spinal, or brain level. There are several kinds of anesthesia used in childbirth. Discuss them with your physician before labor begins.

General anesthesia is used rarely in this country today, but is sometimes used after the first stage of labor is complete. With general anesthesia, the mother has no awareness of either pain or the birth of her child. We do not believe that general anesthesia has any place in routine deliveries; it may be used in complicated deliveries where extreme relaxation of the mother's uterus and birth canal is necessary to perform a complicated obstetrical maneuver such as rotation of the infant. General anesthesia is also used when a Caesarean section must be performed.

Spinal anesthesia is administered at the end of the first stage of labor and results in complete absence of pain from the mother's waist down. This procedure had great popularity several years ago, but is being used less and less today. Complications are possible in both mother and child, and postpartum headaches often trouble the mother. Again, this is a very acceptable procedure for complicated deliveries or when the mother is experiencing moderate pain.

Caudal anesthesia is administered in the last half of the first stage of labor. It is generally given in a lower part of the spine than spinal anesthesia is, and can be given continuously by a small tube inserted into the lower portion of the back. Caudal anesthesia has many of the same problems of spinal anesthesia including the possibility of lowering the mother's blood pressure and causing portpartum headaches.

Paracervical anesthesia is administered by injecting a local anesthetic (such as Xylocaine) into the area surrounding the cervix by means of a long needle. The Xylocaine deadens the nerves going directly to the cervix. Although the Xylocaine produces a temporary decrease in infant heart rate, there are no known long-term effects.

Pudendal block anesthesia eliminates pain in the woman's external genitalia. This provides partial anesthesia during the second stage of labor and during repair of spontaneous or surgical cuts of the birth canal (episiotomy). Some episiotomy repairs require an additional local injection of Xylocaine.

PITOCIN AND "INDUCED BIRTHS"

Oxytocin is a natural hormone that produces contraction of the uterus. It is produced by the body during labor to intensify the contractions of the uterus; it is also produced after labor in order to cause contraction of the uterus and to decrease uterine bleeding. Infant sucking on the mother's breast will stimulate the production of oxytocin and hence uterine contractions.

Pitocin is synthetic oxytocin. It should not be used routinely to augment natural contractions or to produce a child at a more convenient time. It may be of great assistance during prolonged labor or in aiding uterine contraction after labor. It can be administered either intravenously or by intramuscular injection. With certain types of anesthesia, it must be used because the anesthesia diminishes the strength of the uterine contractions. Too much pitocin can cause such painful or excessively strong uterine contractions that depressant drugs must be used to counteract the force.

FETAL HEART MONITORING

Fetal heart monitoring has long been accomplished by listening to an infant's heartbeat through a stethoscope. A strong, regular heartbeat is a sign that an infant is doing well during labor. A significant, prolonged drop in rate or intensity of the heartbeat is a sign of distress of a fetus that may, on occasion, necessitate a Caesarean section in order to prevent damage to the infant.

Recently, at many hospitals, electronic monitors have replaced the stethoscope for keeping track of the infant's heartbeat. In some cases, external monitors are used to keep track of both uterine contractions and fetal heartbeat by electrodes strapped to the mother's abdomen. In other cases, internal fetal monitors are used. Electrodes are inserted during the first stage of labor and are placed directly on the infant's head. This requires rupture of the amniotic sac, if it has not already ruptured. Some of these monitors are capable of measuring the acidity (pH) of the infant's blood as well as the infant's heartbeat. The mother's uterine contractions are also measured.

The theoretical advantage of fetal monitors is the detection of early infant distress. Many women object to them on the grounds that they interfere with mobility during labor. There is, however, a more significant disadvantage to fetal monitors. With the use of fetal monitors at certain hospitals, the rate of Caesarean section has doubled. The rate of newborn complications in hospitals not using fetal monitors appears no different from the hospitals using the monitors and having a higher Caesarean section rate. The full risks and benefits of fetal monitors have yet to be clarified. It does not seem to us that they should be used routinely. We do feel, however, that they can be important in high risk or complicated pregnancies.

PREPARATION PROCEDURES

Prepping involves shaving the mother's pubic hair before delivery; whether this reduces the risk of infection to the infant is debatable. The regrowth of pubic hair can be uncomfortable and itchy and may add to the discomfort that sometimes accompanies the healing in the postpartum period. Discussion with your physician or midwife as to what will be done can avoid confusion and misunderstanding at the last moment. Preparation should certainly include a thorough washing of all parts of the body surrounding the vagina.

Enemas have also been the subject of recent debates. Some have argued that infants come in contact with a great number of bacteria in passing through the birth canal and that an enema will decrease this exposure. The true risk of an infant becoming contaminated with a mother's stool is not well understood. Many women have diarrhea for several days preceding delivery, and most women will not have a bowel movement at the time of delivery. Again, this is a subject for discussion with your physician or midwife that should not be left until the last moment.

DELIVERY ROOM PROCEDURES

Forceps are curved metal instruments designed to fit around a baby's head. They have been used for hundreds of years to make birth easier. As with all potentially dangerous interventions into the birth process, we do not believe that their use should be routine. They often must be used if anesthesia has interrupted the progress of labor, and they should be used if a prolonged or abnormal labor is causing fetal distress or if hemorrhaging is jeopardizing either mother or child. Sometimes they are used to rotate an infant's head so as to make the birth easier.

An *episiotomy* is an incision made in the skin between the lower end of the vagina and the anus to enlarge the vaginal opening and ease the birth of the child's head. Many obstetricians feel that an episiotomy minimizes damage to infant and mother. They argue that these straight incisions heal better and hurt less than the irregular tearing that might otherwise occur. Others argue that this skin is extremely elastic and usually tears only when improper techniques are used. They maintain that properly controlled deliveries will not lead to tearing. Like so many other areas of medical care, the answer is not to be found by siding with either group. There are indications for episiotomies, but not all women will need them. The need for an episiotomy diminishes with subsequent births. Discuss episiotomy with your physician or midwife beforehand so you will know what to expect.

Breech deliveries are not really "feet first"; they are actually "hips first." Although about three percent of births are breech, most of those occur in premature or multiple (twins or triplets) births. Although it is difficult to assess precisely, breech births are more complicated and carry greater risks to the fetus. Caesarean sections are often performed to deliver babies from the breech position.

A *Caesarean section* (C-section) is a surgical procedure performed under general anesthesia to remove the infant from the uterus through the abdominal wall. C-sections are performed in from 5 to 15 percent of births. Because they are performed so commonly, parents should have an understanding of the procedure in the event that it must be done. Discuss this possibility fully with your obstetrician.

There are many reasons for doing C-sections. Pelvic bones may be too small to permit the infant's head to pass through. Or labor may suddenly stop; this often occurs spontaneously, and sometimes because of drugs. Prolonged labor usually is a physiological problem and is *not* the fault of the mother doing something improperly. Less common reasons include a placenta implanted in front of the cervical opening and complications of diabetes or other illnesses. Signs of significant fetal distress or other serious problems of the developing infant are also indications for a C-section.

C-sections are relatively safe, although they carry a higher complication rate than vaginal deliveries. Because of more sensitive methods for detecting signs of fetal distress, minimum distress is being discovered more often and leading to a higher number of C-sections. The benefit of this new approach has not yet been evaluated.

PREMATURE BIRTHS

Between five and ten percent of all infants are born more than two weeks before the due date. A number of factors account for these premature births. Some are merely due to error in calculation of dates and some are due to premature inducement of labor or Caesarean section. Infections, longstanding illness, poor nutrition, and complications of pregnancy also can lead to premature labor. However, the majority of premature births are unexplained. Often, a mother who has had a good diet, exercised regularly, avoided drugs, and received proper medical help will spontaneously begin labor early. The reasons simply are not known.

Fortunately, the chances of a premature infant surviving and developing normally are excellent. Many premature infants are faced with temporary respiratory problems because of immature lungs (hyaline membrane disease or respiratory distress syndrome). Other premature infants have problems with infection. Competent medical care can do much to help the infant with these problems. Recent work suggests that corticosteroid hormones given to the mother early enough in labor can prevent some of the respiratory problems. There are methods for halting premature labor; contact your physician or midwife immediately if labor begins early.

Premature infants often surprise parents by their appearance. They are certainly not as big and cuddly as expected. They appear quite frail and are often connected to a variety of complicated devices in the nursery. Often it is difficult to locate the child among the machines. Nevertheless, you are just as important to your premature child as to your full-term child. Holding and cuddling the child is important and is encouraged in many nurseries. Premature infants who have greater human contact become stronger faster.

NEWBORN PROCEDURES

We feel that delivery room procedures should encourage the unity of the family while ensuring the safety of the infant. More and more infants are given to their mothers immediately after birth and often breast feeding starts in the delivery room. There are many reasons why we approve of this process. Stimulation of the nipples encourages uterine contraction and thus decreases bleeding. Holding the child and looking at it provides an opportunity to experience the child early and to explore your feelings about this new baby. For many mothers these are significant moments. We also encourage the father to hold the infant along with the mother. (A tremendous amount of emphasis has recently been placed on the importance of the first few moments of life. These first moments are important, but so are the first days, weeks, months, and years. If the delivery doesn't go as planned and you miss the first few minutes, don't worry needlessly. There are many more to come.) Although we agree with recent advocates that the bathing of infants in warm baths immediately after birth is soothing, we feel this is optional and that the opportunity for parents to hold their new child is more important and gratifying for all.

Hospitals vary in their newborn routines and you may want to spend some time becoming familiar with the procedures of your local hospital before delivery. Here is a list of the most common routines; all of them are designed to improve the safety of your infant's stay while in the hospital.

- Deliveries should be attended by an individual whose responsibility it is to care for the infant as soon as the infant is delivered. This need not be a pediatrician. Most delivery room nurses are skillful in managing the common problems of the first few moments of life. However, complicated pregnancies or complicated deliveries, such as breech births, should be attended by a pediatrician or other physician who will care for the baby immediately after birth.

- We have never seen an infant held up by the feet at birth and smacked in order to begin crying. That is for the movies. Most infants breathe and cry spontaneously at birth. The fact that the infant's chest is forced through a narrow birth canal removes most of the fluid from the infant's lungs. Most infants will have their mouths and upper respiratory passages suctioned in order to remove the considerable amount of fluid that has recently been in the infant's lungs, hence to facilitate breathing.

- The delivery room should be equipped with infant warmers or the infant should be wrapped snuggly in a blanket. It takes a while for a baby's temperature regulation to begin performing smoothly. One of the worst things that can happen to infants is a rapid drop in their body temperature, and this can happen if a wet infant is left exposed in a delivery room at normal room temperature.

- Babies should be examined promptly after birth for any signs of distress. The initial assessment includes evaluation of color, tone, activity, respiratory rate, and heart rate. Often this initial evaluation is expressed as a number from 1–10 known as an Apgar score. This score is *not* a predictor of your child's intelligence or health. A more thorough examination is usually performed within the first few hours of life.

- All infants should have prophylactic eye medication administered; in most states this is a legal requirement. The purpose of the eye medication is to stop infections from the gonococcus bacteria (gonorrhea). Gonococcal conjunctivitis is a major threat to the infant and is a common cause of blindness. Although most mothers are certain that they do not and have never had gonorrhea, this disease can remain hidden for many years. The most common types of eye medication are silver nitrate and neosporin; these medications may cause several days of tearing in the newborn.

- New babies should have a vitamin-K injection. Before the administration of vitamin K became routine, hemorrhaging was common in the newborn. The newborn's immature liver is often unable to produce the important vitamin K, which is necessary for the production of one of the components of the blood that prevents hemorrhaging.

- Infants should be examined daily by a physician and daily conferences should be held with the parents in order to discuss any questions or concerns.

- Upon discharge from the hospital all children should receive a blood test for phenylketonuria, a rare disease that causes mental retardation. Again, this is a legal requirement in most states. If detected at birth and treated with the appropriate diet, these children can have normal intelligence. Because many mothers are now discharged within the first 24 to 36 hours after delivery, you may need to bring your child to a physician later in the first week to have this test performed; the test is not accurate within the first 24 to 36 hours of life.

- "Rooming in" is a procedure used in many nurseries. Very simply, it means that the child is kept in your room. The advantages of rooming in are that your child is in your room at all times and you can provide most of the care for your child. In addition, rooming in can prevent the spread of infection from child to child during infectious epidemics in newborn nurseries. The disadvantage of rooming in is that you are providing the majority of care for your infant—an advantage for some, a disadvantage for others. Most hospitals offer daytime rooming in. The child is with the mother all day but returns to the nursery at night. If you are interested in rooming in, you should discuss this possibility with your physician. It is not available in all hospitals.

CIRCUMCISION

The decision to have your child circumcised should be considered carefully by both parents before the birth. Circumcising a male infant involves the surgical removal of the foreskin of the penis. The child is sometimes sent home with a small plastic ring still in place around the penis; we mention this only because physicians occasionally forget to tell the parents and the plastic ring can cause considerable anxiety.

Circumcision has its historical roots in both ritual and health. The only real reason for circumcision is to prevent *phimosis*, an infection beneath the foreskin that causes swelling of the foreskin and even obstruction of the urinary stream. Phimosis happens only if the foreskin is not retracted and cleansed regularly; it does not occur where proper hygiene is used. It is difficult and unnecessary to retract the foreskin in a newborn infant; retraction usually becomes easy after several months. Phimosis is frequently seen in children who are beginning to take responsibility for their own bathing but who do not retract the foreskin and wash the glans of the penis carefully.

Complications from circumcision can occur, although they are rare; these complications can include damage to the penis itself. In some children, the end of the penis has not completely developed and the child is unable to produce a forceful stream of urine. This problem, termed *hypospadias*, is not a dangerous medical problem, but can create difficulties if boys find that they are unable to use the urinal like everyone else. It can also be a cause of infertility. One of the surgical procedures to correct this problem requires the foreskin. Unfortunately, some foreskins are removed by circumcision without first checking for this condition. No foreskin should be removed in a circumcision without first checking to make sure the child does not have hypospadias.

Other arguments for and against circumcision have been made, but they are not well substantiated. Cancer of the penis has been said to be more common in uncircumcised males and cancer of the cervix more common in the sexual partners of uncircumsized males. Sexual pleasure for the male has been said by some to be enhanced by the presence of a foreskin and by others to be diminished; neither argument has been substantiated.

Finally, there are those who worry, "Will he be like *everyone else*"? or "Will he be like his *father*"? Circumcision is an optional procedure and there will be plenty of circumcised and uncircumcised boys around. We feel medical procedures should be for medical reasons and not to make boys look like somebody else.

TAKING YOUR CHILD HOME

The joy of taking your child home can be limited by many petty details. Here are some of the things you should prepare for in coming home from the hospital.

- *Discharge details.* Hospital paperwork must be completed. Generally, the husband can attend to this, although many hospitals now have someone from the financial office drop by the hospital room so the mother can make the arrangements herself.

- *Hospital routine.* While most hospitals permit unlimited visiting by fathers, young children usually are not allowed on maternity wards. A young child can be anxiously looking forward to mother's return only to be restrained from embracing the mother by hospital rules. The mother usually will be provided with a wheelchair while leaving the maternity ward (like it or not) and generally will not be allowed contact with her older children while leaving the maternity ward. While there are many compelling humane arguments against these procedures, the rules are there and should be anticipated.

- *Junk they will send home with you.* Many hospitals provide a package of goodies for the parents to take home for their new child. These goodies are supplied by the companies making the products and not by the hospital or your physician. They are advertising samples. While some of these products may be useful, many are unnecessary. Although they are free, they can cost you money in the long run, and can get some bad habits started. We have spent many hours personally discarding many of the items from these packages.

  A typical package will include the following:
  □ *Infant formula.* This is fine if you are going to bottle-feed your child. Very often the formula included is the prepared liquid or a liquid concentrate. These are handy to have and have a long shelf life. If you do choose to use infant formulas, however, remember that use of the powdered formulas is the more economic route. Check in your local supermarket to see which formula has the lowest local price. (It is probably *not* the one you get a free sample of.) There is no difference between any of the major commercial products now available on the market.
  □ *Lotions, creams, and oils.* Keep these and use them on yourself if you like lotions, creams, and oils. Most infants do not need these prepa-

rations. We do not recommend routine use of any skin preparation for children. While some preparations can protect skin in the diaper area from urine and consequently diaper rash, these same preparations usually should not be used after a diaper rash has developed since they keep air away from the skin and prolong the rash.

☐ *Powders.* Baby powders have been used for centuries in order to keep babies dry. But the best way to dry the baby's bottom is to dry the baby's bottom. As soon as the child urinates, the effect of the powder is gone. Powders do help dry the perspiration that occurs underneath a warm diaper. If you choose to powder your child, place the powder in your hand and *then* place it on the child's bottom. Shaking powder from a distance of a foot or so will spread a cloud of powder around your child; this is dangerous because the infant can inhale the powder particles. Powders with talc in them have been incriminated as a cause of serious lung disease. Use these powders cautiously or avoid them.

☐ *Q-tips.* We have never really understood what Q-tips should be used for! For one thing, Q-tips should *never* be used to clean the inside of children's ears. Wax is produced within the ear canal for a purpose, and usually becomes a problem only when it is impacted in the ear canal by the use of Q-tips. We tell parents never to put anything smaller than their elbow in a child's ear.

☐ *Vitamins.* All infant formulas are supplemented with all vitamins necessary for your child's proper growth and development and several more. For mothers choosing to breast-feed their infants, only a vitamin-D supplementation is necessary.

■ *Driving home.* The number-one killer of children in this country is accidents. The leading accidental killer is the automobile. The risk to your child from the automobile is greater than the risk from childhood infectious diseases and childhood cancer together. You may want to hold your baby in your arms on your way home from the hospital, but this is not in anyone's best interest. The driver will probably be excited about the baby coming home for the first time, and will be less attentive to road conditions than usual. We know of several tragic accidents in this setting. Have an infant seat ready to use on the way home. Discussion on infants' seats can be found on p. 106.

■ *Arriving home.* Upon arriving home you need time and attention for yourself, your new infant, and your other children who are anxious to see that you still love them. These are the most important items on your agenda. Contact with friends and relatives is secondary. If a friend or a relative will be staying with you, we advise that they help with the household chores and free you for time with your children. Well-meaning relatives too often come between older children and their mother. Older children need reassurance from their mother, as well as their grandmother, that mother still loves them. Mothers who have no relative or no husband to help at home can seek help from neighbors, friends, social agencies, and employment agencies.

ADDITIONAL READING

Jean Marzollo (ed., written by parents), *Nine Months, One Day, One Year.* New York: Harper and Row, 1976.

Boston Women's Health Book Collective Touchstone, *Our Bodies, Ourselves.* New York: Simon and Schuster, 1976.

Chapter

3

Your First Concerns

Is there life after birth? Becoming a new family is a major physical and emotional adjustment for everyone. Here are some thoughts on this new experience from parents we know.

THE FIRST CHILD

The first several weeks made it very clear that our lives had changed fundamentally and unalterably, partially for the better, partially not. We were tied to the breast feeding schedule. Our freedom of movement was over. Our nights were continually interrupted. There were times I resented the change, resented the baby for bringing them about and felt guilty because it seemed unconscionable to hold such feelings towards such a small, adorable, helpless infant. On the whole, however, the changes were positive. The process of interaction with the baby was fantastic. It exceeded my expectations. Walking her to sleep became a cherished event. Feeding her her first cereal. Listening to her sounds develop. There were many things I couldn't do, but many new things I was doing for the first time. There is also a sense of fulfillment of purpose and of family in a sense that I had never understood before. We were both able to work and enjoy the baby and get out and felt strongly that our lives, although radically different, were on the whole better.

Father of two

No one told me what I was going to feel like afterwards.

Mother of one

I found myself being very dependent during birth for support, also after we took Suzie home. I had no one else to talk to and was worried about whether I was overreacting to things like too much or too little crying, how much clothing, small things but so constant they made my day seem like a mass of indecisions and insecurity. Artie was really my only friend. I also was physically dependent. I was unable to cook or clean for at least a week and depended on Artie for meals, laundry and going out. This topic was the subject of almost all of our fights which increased sharply in number after Suzie's birth. I was spending literally 24 hours a day with the baby, while Artie was in school for most of the time. He didn't understand why I had to get away from her sometimes.

Mother of two

As Peter grew, I tried to remind myself over and over again that husbands and new fathers are supposed to be jealous of the baby and I tried to take this into consideration by letting Matt be involved and giving me advice in the care of our son. The latter was the hardest and still is today. I was quite unsure about the care of our first child and relied heavily on my mother's advice, but I also asked a lot of other people. I was confident that I would someday learn.

Mother of three

During the early months I don't remember feeling as close physically or emotionally to the baby as I do now. Was it because Irmhild had everything so under control and was breast feeding? Or, was it because I was still working? I don't know. The first time I held the baby, even though I had held others before, was a fairly nervous time. He seemed very small and fragile and I was afraid of letting his neck fall down for fear of causing some whiplash injury.

Father of three

After four years of peaceful dinners enjoyed after hectic days, my husband and I resented the interruption. I felt an obligation toward the baby but also sympathy for my husband. We felt guilty that we were being selfish. After discussions with friends, we decided that our feelings were shared by many couples adjusting to a new member in their family.

Mother of one

With the first there is "the buck stops here" . . . the responsibility lasts for 24 hours each day, and the decisions are all yours . . . there is no escape . . . you can't put the problem aside or pass it on . . . I believe this is the essence of the trapped feeling so common in new parents, much more than the fact that they can't go to the party because there is no sitter available tonight.

Mother of six

This is the first time in my life that any individual had the right—not the privilege—to call on me 24 hours a day any place—and I had the obligation to go. Nobody had ever done that to me before. I was a schoolteacher and my husband used to say "Ha! This one doesn't go home at 4:30" and it was true—he was sympathizing. Another big shock was that mothers of little children don't get sick—you can have a 104° temperature and vomiting and you still have to be there. And my husband feels the same way. Whenever the children are sick at night he's also up with them.

Mother of two

The first baby is the hardest. Now that I have four I find I have time to get things done. With my first baby we were living abroad and even had two maids but I still had no time to make even Jello for dessert and I asked myself what was I doing? It seemed that I had no time for a bath. Now that I have four, everything is organized and there's plenty of time.

Mother of four

Coming from a large family—the oldest—I knew the mechanics of caring for babies but somehow I didn't remember babies as so small and weak. I had a feeling of nervous anxiety, not depression. Sue's breathing was so irregular I found myself checking her constantly, really expecting to find her dead from crib death or suffocation from not being able to lift her head up high enough. After two weeks she snapped out of her depression and developed colic. Jim and I would sit silently through supper and listen to her scream until nine, when suddenly and what seemed miraculously she stopped. Being angry at her because we really tried all the remedies— burping stomach down, warm bath, extra burping, tipping up and down, longer feedings. Picking her up made her cry harder. I felt my husband thought I was neglecting her or being mean to her or taking the whole thing too lightly at first. Do something, don't just sit there and listen. We didn't realize it was colic, until it ended two weeks later.

Mother of two

You worry about unnecessary things with the first baby, you don't with the second. You take a diaper off the top of the pile and your husband says "That one is dusty." With the first baby you waste a lot of unnecessary time on things like that.

Mother of four

Nursing too, followed the same pattern. A lot of propaganda from the La Leche league. "People who don't nurse are downright degenerate and those who nurse less than a year or 2 or 3 or 4 are shirkers and crummy mothers." I nursed Tally for 6 months and once again felt anger at those women who had full breasts at the right time instead of the 3 months of engorgement, leaking, pain, PAIN? Maybe I was the only one, maybe I wasn't relaxed enough, not in tune with my body, something must be wrong with me. Only after talking with other mothers, some successful, some not, did I discover that the "letdown reflex" is often painful. OK. So I was willing to accept it. But why not say that nursing is really hard sometimes?

Mother of two

I used to drive in the car and plan for hours what would happen if we drove into a river—how I would get everyone out. I don't think I ever realized how fragile life was until I had Danny.

Mother of one

THE SECOND TIME AROUND

This is what the days were like:

6 A.M.	*Feed/change Jeremy*
8 A.M.	*Dress Mirah/breakfast/clean up*
10 A.M.	*Feed/bathe Jeremy; change Mirah*
12 P.M.	*Change Mirah; lunch/clean up*
2 P.M.	*Feed/change Jeremy; change Mirah for nap*
3 P.M.	*End of Mirah's nap*
4 P.M.	*Change Mirah*
6 P.M.	*Feed/change Jeremy; dinner for Mirah*
6:30 P.M.	*Larry burps Jeremy/I fix dinner*
7 P.M.	*Dinner/clean up*
8 P.M.	*Bath for Mirah/dress for bed*
8:30 P.M.	*Ice cream for Mirah*
9 P.M.	*Bed for Mirah*
10:30 P.M.	*Feed/change Jeremy/pray he sleeps through the night*
11:30 P.M.	*Fall exhausted into bed*

If I thought of childbearing primarily in terms of its rewards before my children were born, I seem now to describe it largely in terms of its work. Both are lopsided views. At the same time that my days seem to turn into an endless series of jobs—like a string of paperclips—they also become filled with sudden pleasures—Mirah's smiles and kisses, her delight in running, climbing high on the slide, her excitement in reading books and going to the Bookmobile for book time.

Mother of two

I guess the second time around it is all more real . . . you know about the new person arriving . . . and the joy is easier. And then you discover they never both sleep at the same time.

Mother of six

*The first night home I put Rick down and went to bed. I woke up a short
while later because I realized I had not checked on Alan and tucked him in
again—something I always did. I forgot Alan was in the house. That made
me feel strange and also sad.*

*About three nights after Rick was born, I was playing with Alan and feeling
very close to him. We were enjoying ourselves when Rick started crying. I
had to leave Alan to feed Rick and I felt myself resenting Rick because he
had broken in on a special time.*

*When we first brought Rick home, Alan started taking out a lot of frustration
on my husband—hitting, yelling, refusing to do anything. I hadn't thought
he would react to Rick like that. But it only lasted two days. I guess it was
better that he acted it out rather than keep it all in. I felt myself feeling less
tense and pleased at how easily Rick became a family member. But one
night my husband said "You're enjoying him more than you thought you
would." I guess I felt relieved at that.*

*I feel badly that Rick, Alan, housework, etc., have taken so much time—
time that I would like to share with my husband. He never complains and
just pitches in to take care of the children and to help out.*

Mother of two

*After the first baby, I never cried once and I thought there was no such thing
as the postpartum blues. When Emily was born—I brought her home and I
woke up one morning and burst into tears and I rolled over and David was
still in bed and he put his arms around me and said what's wrong and I said
"I'm very unhappy about that baby" and he said "I know" and we both
decided wrongly that since we had had another little girl we were very
disappointed. I felt terribly guilty. It was a big thing in the Navy—everybody
was very macho—and wanted little boys. I told myself as long as it was
healthy I'd be happy and I really am happy and she really is healthy so why
in the name of heaven am I crying and I felt so mad at myself for being so
unhappy over the fact that I had 2 daughters. It wasn't until a year later
when I thought maybe it was postpartum blues. Since I hadn't experienced
postpartum blues the first time I didn't expect it the second time. Even
though David said "her plumbing's on the inside and not on the outside" I
couldn't understand why I was so sad when I really was so happy.*

Mother of two

*By the second time you learn to cope with your own reactions. I would
breast feed the baby and hand him to his father who would rock him and
put him back to sleep. I did 20 minutes, he did 20 minutes and the baby
was back to sleep.*

Mother of four

*I felt and was completely trapped, unable to change their diapers fast
enough. I felt guilty because Sarah was so jealous of her sister and I was
hard pressed to devote an "hour," as my pediatrician had recommended,*

to her exclusively. I also felt badly that I was not so involved in the new baby's personality as I was in Sarah's. The little things like rolling over that Sarah did that thrilled Will and me seemed less exciting the second time around.

Mother of two

Caring for kids in the first year is not too great and we've tried to share it between the two of us, but obviously my wife gets the brunt. Doing every other diaper when I'm home we thank God for a well formed stool. In traveling I am much more sympathetic to parents with children, but am still uptight when our kids cry in public.

Father of three

I look back on the past three months as both swift and interminable— punctuated for so long by four-hour wakings, changings, and feedings. I have almost unconsciously learned to use my left hand while the baby is cuddled and nursing on the right. It's amazing how I can now manage to eat my dinner, not quickly it is true, during two-year-old tantrums and three-months-old cranky crying, talking to one and holding the other. I sometime think that hardening on the eardrums must be estrogen related.

Mother of two

Other couples talked about it, but we never had the experience of feeling restricted by our new addition. In fact, it was pretty nice to have an excuse to stay home.

Father of two

The second baby was a very different experience. The peaks of exhilaration were lower although present, the valleys of anxiety were not nearly as deep although they too were present. A different kind of uncertainty confronted us. To what degree would our lives be more restricted? What additional increment of work would be involved? Was a second child a quantum leap in work and change of life-style from the first child? Or, would only a minor modification have to be made? Several times, I wondered if it was a mistake at all to enlarge our family. Delivery and birth were much easier with Jeremy, and he proved to be an easier baby to take care of even than Mirah, but my God what an added increment of work. Two sets of diapers. Two car seats. Two feeding schedules. Two sleeping schedules. But not that much more restriction. We were able to accommodate to it. We resumed our other lives more easily.

Father of two

Sam really wasn't as much work as Mandy. We were less attentive to his every move. We didn't listen as closely to his grunts in bed. We didn't carefully measure every step we took. We were more relaxed. We were more natural. And I think the reason Sam has been easier is that we were easier on him than we were on Mandy. At no point did the addition of Sam provoke the kind of reaction that the first several weeks with Mandy did. Never did I feel, "My God, what have we done?" Yet, there are times when I still resent being tied down, get angered because there is very little quiet time and together time for Lori and me, but I wouldn't change it—not for anything.

Father of two

We found that we were spending most of our time with people who had children—they understood the constant interruption and irrational and seemingly destructive behavior of our children.

Mother of two

We take on a 24-hour-a-day job with a pathetic lack of skills with which to cope . . . and for the mother and father who have been accustomed to being effective and successful at their own work, the feeling of gross incompetence leads to a great resentment of the role inflicted upon them . . .

Mother of six

It is more important for the child to feel loved than for the house to look good. The three-year-old will remember you sitting down and drawing silly faces for him with a warm glow. He won't feel the same about you mopping the floor and his not being allowed in until it is dry . . . eventually one has to, but not too often. It's now he needs you, mop the floors later if you must . . . anyway, drawing silly faces is much more fun than mopping floors. I remember the Montreal taxi driver who said it always worried him if he came home to a tidy house . . . it made him wonder if his kids had had any fun at all that day.

Mother of five

In the first few days at home, new parents often spend a great deal of time checking their new baby. Perfectly normal infants often appear strange in some way, causing concern to new parents. The purpose of this section is to describe the sometimes surprising features found in normal newborns.

ACTIVITY

Infants spend much of their time sleeping. The newborn may spend 18 or even 22 hours in sleep, the six-month-old will spend from 16 to 18 hours sleeping, and the one-year-old child from 14 to 15 hours. You may observe several types of sleep states. In one state, the child will be very, very motionless and have regular breathing. In another sleep state, the breathing will be irregular, the eyes will be seen to be fluttering, and there will be motion of the hands.

There are also different stages of being awake, the least satisfying of which is crying. This is the infant's most obvious way of communicating needs, frustrations, and discomforts, but there are other subtle ways of communicating that parents can learn to recognize. Infants spend much of their quiet time looking and watching. In this stage the infant is exploring the world with his or her eyes and will stare intently into the parents' faces and follow them across the room. Babies have certain likes and dislikes in shapes, patterns, and even colors, and these preferences have been demonstrated even in the first few hours after birth. In the "active alert" state, the infant is looking around actively, as well as moving arms and legs. Newborn babies are often disappointing to parents who expect laughing, gurgling infants. The image most of us have is actually when they are four to eight months old. Newborns are exciting but you must remember that it will be many months before they laugh and gurgle.

BREATHING

Infant breathing patterns are often irregular. There may be periods of five to ten seconds when infants will stop breathing; this is known as an *apneic spell*. Normal infants outgrow this pattern within the first few months of life. This breathing pattern is characteristic of a certain state of sleep; it is a normal phenomenon in the newborn, and should not be of concern to parents unless it persists for a number of months.

THE SKIN AND BIRTHMARKS

At birth, most infants are covered by a protective, white, thick material known as the vernix caseosa. This covering is generally washed off within the first day. Often some of the material is missed, especially behind the ears and in the ear folds. You should not be disturbed to find white, sticky material behind your child's ears. In addition, the baby's skin will frequently peel in the first week or two of life; this is another normal phenomenon of the newborn period. There are a number of other rashes that are extremely common in the newborn and not serious. (See Problem 33, Baby Rashes.)

About 50 percent of babies will be born with a birthmark. The most common type of birthmark is called a "salmon patch." This patch, when located in the center of the forehead, is known as an "angel's kiss"; if located on the back of the neck it is a "stork bite." Virtually all salmon patches disappear in the first few months, although occasionally a stork bite will remain.

Many babies have a dark discoloration around their buttocks; this will be found in about 95% of black babies, 80% of Oriental babies, 70% of Mexican-American babies, and 10% of white babies. It also disappears.

Strawberry marks are often barely visible at birth. If they can be seen, they are red and white. They gradually enlarge, achieving their biggest size at about six months of age. Occasionally they are quite large. They always get smaller and should never be treated with surgery or X-rays. An *extremely* rare occurrence is when these strawberry marks trap some of the blood cells (platelets) that assist in preventing bleeding problems. In such circumstances medicine (steroids) will be administered by physicians. Virtually all strawberry marks will disappear if left alone; large persistent ones can be surgically removed after the child is much older (over six years old).

Portwine stains are large purple marks that occur in about 3 of every 1000 babies. They are cosmetically disturbing if they are on the face. There are currently no good methods for removing the color, which will persist. X-rays are harmful and must be avoided. Adults find that cosmetics often cover these spots quite well. If a portwine stain covers an entire eyelid, there may occasionally be an associated problem of seizures, which will require medical help.

Finally, there are brown and black hairy and nonhairy moles. More than 2% of white babies and 20% of black babies have these moles, which do not disappear. Because there is a risk of large moles developing into cancer, many physicians recommend their removal soon after birth. You should discuss a problem of large moles with your physician.

THE HEAD

The head is the largest part of the infant's body at birth. As such, the head will frequently show signs of damage from its passage through the birth canal. Infants often have a circular swelling on the back of their heads where a beanie or a yarmulke might rest; this swelling is known as a *caput succedaneum*. It is a result of pressure while the child's head is pushing against the mother's pelvis during labor. It generally disappears within two to three days. Another type of swelling that may appear in the same area is known as a *cephalohematoma*; this is due to a small amount of superficial bleeding from the scalp. It can be distinguished from the caput succedaneum in that it generally does not cross the midline of the scalp so that it is found only on one side or the other. Cephalohematomas generally take longer to disappear than do caputs, but are of no concern unless they are of such large size that there may have been significant blood loss.

In addition, the head may have marks from the pressure of forceps, if forceps were used in the delivery. Again, these marks are very, very common and should resolve within a few days. The size of the fontanels, the two soft spots on the infant's head, may vary greatly. Normal fontanels may range in size from one to three inches. When the infant is asleep they will ordinarily be flat. When the infant is crying, the fontanel will bulge upward. It also rises and falls regularly with the infant's heart rate. The front fontanel, on top of the head, closes at about twelve months of age, the smaller back one before six months.

THE EYES

Infants can see quite well from birth, although they do have some difficulty focusing for the first few months of life. One of the most frequently asked questions is what color the child's eyes will be. Most newborns have the same eye color—bluish-gray. Eye color generally cannot be determined accurately until some time after the third month. Yellowness of the "whites" of the eyes, also known as jaundice, is usual in newborns. The newborn liver is not as capable as the adult liver of handling the normal waste products of human red blood cells, and this causes a certain amount of jaundice for the first few days of life. An extremely high level of jaundice can be a problem. If you are concerned about jaundice after you go home, call your physician promptly. Sunlight has been discovered to be beneficial in reducing the amount of jaundice in newborns, but use caution since infant skin is extremely sensitive to the sun. A special type of lighting is used in most hospitals to reduce the jaundice level.

Occasionally the eyelids may be swollen because of pressure placed on them in the birth canal. This swelling usually resolves by three days of age.

Excess tearing in newborns is usual. Tears are absorbed by tear ducts located in the inner aspect of the eyes; excess tearing on one side may signal a blocked tear duct on that side. Frequently, excess tearing on both sides in the first few days of life is the result of the silver nitrate drops placed in the newborn's eyes to protect against infection. Doctors usually examine the newborn's eyes carefully at birth, including a test for vision. Frequently, however, physicians arrive on the scene when the infant is sleeping or crying. The test for vision is not adequate under these conditions and it is mothers who usually confirm that their infants have good vision. Infants will follow your face and your eyes as you move from side to side. Physicians examine the lens of the eye and make sure that there are no cataracts present. In addition, they use an ophthalmoscope to examine the back of the eye, known as the retina, for signs of infection. They also examine the retina for any blackening, which will alert the physician to the presence of a retinoblastoma, an extremely rare but treatable tumor of the eye in newborns.

Crossed eyes are common in newborn babies and are discussed further in Problem 81.

THE NOSE

Most textbooks tell us that infants must breathe through their noses, and much attention has been paid to clearing the nostrils of excess mucus and debris in order to make breathing easier. Seldom does mucus completely block the nostrils, and even then we have found that infants adapt quickly to mouth breathing, so parents need not worry excessively about clearing the nose. Babies also have protective reflexes that enable them to turn away from potentially suffocating situations. Newborns also spend a great deal of their time sneezing; the sneeze is an indication of neither a respiratory infection nor an allergy. Sneezing is a normal reflex of newborns.

THE MOUTH

Frequently parents will notice little white spots on the roof of the infant's mouth directly in the midline, known as *Ebstein's pearls*. These pearls are normal findings in almost all newborns. Many parents, especially years ago, used to worry about their infant being tongue-tied, meaning that the frenulum, the piece of tissue on the bottom of the tongue that attaches to the floor of the mouth, is short. A short frenulum will *not* interfere with the child's speech. However, it will interfere with a child's ability to stick his or her tongue out as far as friends can, will interfere with the ability to catch M & M's thrown in the air, and occasionally may interfere with the ability to lick an ice cream cone down to nothing as fact as friends can. Inability to do these acts can be troublesome, and a frenulum can be cut in order to enable the child to participate in these childhood activities. This is a simple procedure, but should not be carried out until the child is much older and actually experiences some handicap.

THE FACE

The face is subjected to a considerable amount of pressure coming through the birth canal. This pressure may cause a dotted, purple rash over the face known as *petechiae*. Petechiae are caused by ruptures in very tiny blood vessels that occur because of the high pressure. These purple dots will generally resolve within two weeks.

In addition, infants often have white dots with red bases all over their faces. This is known frequently as newborn acne. If there is a widespread rash, your physician may tell you that your child has *erythema toxicum neonatorum*. Again, this is a harmless rash of the newborn period, discussed in Problem 33 (Baby Rashes).

THE HANDS

Infants ordinarily keep their fists clenched. You may notice that your baby has long fingernails. An infant's fingernails are generally soft, but nonetheless can scratch the infant's skin. If the fingernails appear long or scratch marks seem to be appearing on the infant (or on you when the infant is held close to you), the nails may be cut. Almost any nail-clipping instrument or even teeth will do so long as you are careful.

THE CHEST

Many parents are surprised to find that their infants have swollen breasts, boys as well as girls. This is a response to the mother's hormones, which have crossed the placenta and are found in the fetal blood. The swelling of the breasts usually disappears within the first month of life, but may last for two to three months. Occasionally a breast discharge may occur.

THE ABDOMEN

The umbilical cord is of frequent concern to parents; this cord consists of a white gelatinous material through which run two arteries and one vein. The cord will dry up in a period of about one week, but the decaying process usually smells. The smell comes from ordinary bacteria on the cord. Put a little alcohol on the cord; this will destroy the bacteria and also hasten the drying process. The cord will eventually become smaller, develop a brownish color, and fall off in one to three weeks. Often there is a slight amount of bleeding after the cord falls off. If an area of redness develops on the skin surrounding the cord, your doctor should be consulted. Swelling or hernias of the navel are very common in black babies, and far less common in white babies. Almost all of these disappear by themselves. The hernia is really a separation in the muscles of the abdominal wall. See the further discussion of hernias on pp. 101–102.

THE GENITALIA

The genitalia of both boys and girls are swollen in the newborn period, since they respond to maternal hormones. Boys will have a swollen, enlarged scrotum, while girls will have enlarged genital lips and an enlarged clitoris. The swelling should subside within several weeks. Vaginal bleeding and discharges occur frequently. They are discussed in Problem 91.

THE FEET

An infant's feet assume many unusual positions. It is easy to understand why if you think of the cramped quarters in which the infant has recently been living. Most babies have feet that are turned in with the soles facing each other; the feet will assume a more normal position within a few months. Parents can check the normality of the feet by wiggling them about. It should be possible to wiggle an infant's foot into all of the positions that your own foot will assume.

There are undoubtedly things that you will notice about your newborn that have not been covered in this brief discussion. Most physicians are more than willing to sit down and explain the concerns that parents have over their babies. Very often, however, parents forget to ask about a small item because of the excitement of having their child and because of the chaos of the hospital ward. We suggest that you write down any questions about your baby and make sure that you get a satisfactory answer to each one.

FEEDING

The feeding of infants and children is more than just satisfying the hunger urge. The first goal is to meet the nutritional requirements of children so that they can grow adequately. The second goal is to help children to develop muscle and coordination skills. As infants become older, they learn to feed themselves. This process requires complicated skills such as the tongue reaching around a spoon, grasping the spoon, and eventually coordinating movement of the spoon with its portion of food into the mouth. The third goal of feeding is to assist infants and children in developing social skills. Eating is a social activity that involves interaction with other family members.

Techniques of Breast Feeding

With proper guidance and encouragement, most mothers can master the technique of breast feeding. Some mothers, through no fault of their own, will be unable to breast feed. An individual mother stands the best chance of success with supportive help. Many physicians are supportive but few have had the experience to be truly helpful. Often the maternity nurses are helpful in early instructions. The best source of help in breast feeding is a friend or neighbor who has successfully breast fed her baby. The LaLeche League or the local Nursing Mothers Association are also good sources for advice on techniques.

Do not let anyone undermine your desire to breast feed. Also, do not let anyone push you into nursing longer than you want. Rely on your own judgment after you have listened to advice. You know what is best for you and your baby. Judge for yourself how long you want to breast feed. Two weeks, two months, and two years are all acceptable choices.

Recommendations vary widely as to the proper preparation of the breast for breast feeding. By and large, we do not feel that very much preparation before birth is necessary. We suggest a common-sense approach. During the last few months, the breast should be washed with a damp washcloth without the use of any soap preparations. Most creams and lotions should be avoided, although the use of lanolin on the areola (the dark area around the nipple) is acceptable. Exposure to air or massage of the nipples several months before birth sometimes helps. The purchase of several supportive nursing bras is a good investment for most mothers.

Infants can be put to breast within moments of birth. For the first several feedings, the breasts produce a material known as colostrum. The colostrum is rich in antibodies that serve to protect the child against infections in the coming months. There is no need to worry about the number of calories in your milk in the first several days, since infants are born with an excess of weight that will tide them over until the high-calorie milk comes in. Between the third and fifth day milk begins to come in abundantly.

Nursing can be accomplished lying on your side or sitting up. Leaning forward a little in the sitting position helps. Placing the nipple near the baby's mouth will stimulate a reflex, the rooting reflex, which will help the baby find the nipple. Don't nudge him or her with your finger or the baby will root toward the finger. You may need to use your finger to hold the top part of your breast away from the infant's nose to allow breathing. Babies will let you know if they are having trouble breathing by pushing off the breast or opening their mouths and crying.

Feeding a small, premature baby can present special problems, but they can often be overcome. Indeed, many nurseries feel that breast milk is more important for the premature infant than for the full-term baby. Special bottles with "premature" nipples are available. Until the premature child is strong enough to suck and control the flow of milk, you can pump your breasts and bottle-feed with these small nipples.

Mothers also have reflexes that assist them in breast feeding. The sight of their child, hearing their child cry, or even another child's cry will begin the flow of milk. Besides the rooting reflexes that help them find the nipple, infants have sucking reflexes that form the basis for their feeding. After an infant has been sucking for a while, a vacuum is created and a tight seal is formed by the mouth around the nipple. Irritation to the nipples can be avoided by breaking the vacuum by inserting your finger between the infant's gums before removing the infant from your breast. Newborns will require feeding every two to three hours. (Every four hours is unusual!) Frequent, prolonged feedings may help to prevent engorgement. You should begin by allowing the child to suck several minutes on each breast and gradually build up to about 15 minutes on each breast by the third day of life. Infants will reject a partially full breast because the taste of the milk changes somewhat during feeding. They should be allowed to reject the breast and go on to the other one. If your breast is so full that the infant is having difficulty grasping the nipple, express some milk by using your thumb and index finger to compress the breast at the areola.

As the child becomes older, the interval between feedings can become greater. Infants often begin to sleep through the night at a weight of about 12 pounds. Many mothers who breast feed find that the father can begin giving a supplemental bottle within the first two months. The father should usually give the supplemental bottle at the same time each day, although this is not a rigid rule. To prevent breast engorgement, mothers may pump their breasts when the father will be giving the supplemental bottle. Some parents prefer to have the mother pump her breasts and have the father bottle-feed the breast milk. Other women find that their breasts adjust within a short period of time to the uneven schedule that is created by the father's feeding.

Although you may have heard that the iron content in breast milk is low, the amount of iron in breast milk is absorbed so well by the baby's intestines that supplemental iron drops are seldom necessary.

Babies have their own style of eating. Some are ravenous eaters, others are picky, while still others seem to fall asleep shortly after they begin nursing. Your baby will let you know his or her style early; they will all feed differently but will all thrive beautifully.

For further reading on breast-feeding techniques, see *Nursing Your Baby* by Karen Pryor (New York: Pocket Books, 1975) and *The Womanly Art of Breastfeeding*, La Leche League Tandem (London, 1971) (somewhat judgmental but good technical advice).

The following helpful hints are from mothers who have breast fed and enjoyed their experiences.

The more relaxed you are about it, the easier it is. In the early weeks there is bound to be some tension, but it can be minimized and with it the process becomes natural and easy. Try to find a comfortable place in the house where you will have the things you need close by and won't have to get up to interrupt the feeding. Either having the telephone within reach or taking it off the hook is helpful.

Mother of one

Set the feeding time aside for you and the baby to relax together. Keep interruptions and distractions to a minimum (this may be hard if you have other children). It is a good time to listen to music, watch TV, or read. It may be your only chance to sit and do these things. It is important to realize that it is okay to say to friends you are feeding the baby and excuse yourself from the demands of the phone, doorbell, and visitors until you are finished.

Mother of two

Authors' note: The above is also good advice for mothers who choose to bottle feed.

Wear loose clothing, especially things you can pull up from the bottom which will give you more privacy in public than things that button and zip up in front. You can also take along a small blanket or shawl to shield you and the baby.

Mother of two

Lying down is a very comfortable position for the mother especially in the early weeks and during late night and early morning feedings.

Mother of one

By hand-expressing a little milk or putting the baby to breast you can relieve some of the pressure of engorgement. If it really becomes bad, hot compresses work. But take heart; generally it will occur only the first month or two until you and the baby are synchronized. At some point in time, it is important to stop the middle-of-the-night feeding. This is important for the mother's health (and sleep). Letting the baby cry and not getting up for him usually will cause him to give up feedings within three or four nights. He will cry a lot (15 minutes) the first night, but gradually the crying will decrease over the next few nights.

Mother of two

Bottle Feeding

Whole or skim cow's milk has too much calcium and phosphorus for infants and should not be given before the fourth month. Evaporated milk (not to be confused with condensed milk, which is sweetened) is the cheapest commercially available formula. One can (or 13 ounces) of evaporated milk is added to 17 ounces of water. One tablespoon of sugar or Karo syrup is then added to provide additional calories and to prevent the constipation that frequently results without its use. Should you choose not to add sugar or syrup, add only 15 to 16 ounces of water rather than 17 ounces to the evaporated milk.

Prepared formulas include Similac, Enfamil, and SMA. They are essentially the same and your decision should be determined by prices in your local area. The most economical way to prepare the formula is to use the powdered form (generally, two scoops of formula to four ounces of water). While mixing the concentrated liquid requires less shaking, it also requires more money. Care should be taken to mix the formula according to instructions; using too little water can cause serious problems for the infant. The temperature of the formula need not be higher than body temperature; room temperature is fine.

Children who are bottle-fed need an iron supplement. Most commercial formulas are available with or without supplemental iron. The child, however, should not be on an exclusive diet of whole cow's milk, or that child will become moderately iron-deficient by the age of one year. Iron is present in a variety of other food sources, especially cereals, meats, and many vegetables.

The newborn needs about 50 calories for each pound of weight (or 110 calories per kilogram) daily. Requirements drop to about 45 calories per pound by a year. Formulas and breast milk provide 20 calories per ounce; thus, a seven-pound newborn needs about 350 calories (7×50) each day or 17½ ounces ($350 \div 20$) of milk. Such calculations are seldom necessary, since infants will let you know when they are hungry or full.

How Much Food and How Often?

Most newborns will not take more than three ounces at one time and hence require about six feedings a day. Every-four-hour feedings are seldom achievable. Your child will let you know when he or she is hungry. Don't be surprised if feedings are as frequent as every two hours or if the time interval varies daily. As infants become older, they can eat more and be fed less often. The middle-of-the-night feeding usually falls by the wayside, when the infant begins sleeping through the night by about the fourth month. By one year of age, most infants will be satisfied with three meals and an occasional snack.

Solid Foods

Fruit juices, especially orange juice, can be served within the first two to three weeks of age. However, physicians and nutritionists disagree about the best age for beginning solid feedings. Almost all infants are capable of digesting whole foods at birth, but lack of appropriate tongue coordination may interfere with feeding. Most nutritionists and physicians feel that there is no need to begin solids until three to four months of age. Many parents, however, claim that children sleep through the night better if given a solid feeding late in the evening. Children with a strong family tendency toward allergic disorders may do better if the addition of solid foods is deferred until four months of age. If the baby doesn't seem satisfied with milk alone, it is possible to add rice cereal to the milk in order to thicken the consistency; rice cereal is highly unlikely to produce any allergies.

Infants generally do well on most strained foods or baby foods between three and six months of age. These foods tend to be expensive, and generally have a fair amount of added water, so there has been recent interest in the home preparation of baby foods. (To make baby foods that will be acceptable to your child, consult one of the many books available. There are also a number of machines available that help in preparing baby foods.) Between six and nine months of age, many children are given "junior" foods. Finally, between nine and twelve months of age, most children are capable of eating finger foods or table foods.

The best guideline for feeding your child after the first year is to feed the child small portions of everything you eat. Foods from all of the basic food groups should be included. These include the milk and cheese group, the meat-fish-chicken group or their protein equivalent in either eggs, cheese, or beans, the fruit group, the yellow-and-green vegetable groups, and the bread, potatoes, and cereal group.

Feeding Ability

Most children have a vigorous sucking action at birth, although many do not perfect this skill until they are four weeks of age. At four months of age, tongue control begins to develop, but children cannot yet remove food from a spoon. At this age, the infant will swallow a fair amount of air and burping will be necessary periodically. At four months, the infant begins to show signs of waiting for food. The child's arm will often move at the sight of food. Tongue protrusion begins developing to the point where the tongue will project out after the spoon. At this stage, food should be placed well back on the tongue; as more control develops, the child will become able to remove the food with the tongue. Between five and six months, lip control develops and the lips can be brought to a cup. Hand development is improving by this age and the child can grab a bottle with both hands. Soon the hands can be brought to the mouth, and the ability to grasp a spoon with the hand begins to develop.

Between six and nine months of age, the child learns to remove food from the spoon and is finally able to drink from a cup. The child learns to eat a cracker without any assistance. Between nine and twelve months of age, the infant achieves better finger control and is able to use fingers to obtain small pieces of food. He or she will try to use a spoon alone, but more often than not the spoon is still a better toy than a feeding instrument. A cup can be held, but the contents will be easily spilled. During this age the child first begins to become choosy about food. Many myths have developed about the tastes of children. While infant taste buds are quite developed, infants are more sensitive to food texture than to taste and are likely to reject a food because of texture.

The period between 12 and 15 months of age is one of the more trying times for the parents. Children begin throwing food and utensils and become more assertive in the eating and rejecting of certain foods. Between 15 and 18 months of age, the muscle skills become more sophisticated and a cup full of liquid can be handled without spilling. Between 18 months and two years of age, the child handles a cup well and can drink through a straw. The social aspects of feeding become more evident at this age as the child begins to say "eat," begins to name certain foods, and also knows when food is "all gone." At least half of a child's first six words are usually related to food. At this age, children begin feeding their favorite stuffed animals or dolls. By three years of age, a child should not be spilling too much, and is able to coordinate talking and eating.

Social Eating

Feeding is an integral part of a child's social development. During mealtime children learn how to interact with family, and they learn how to choose their foods. Although it may seem unbelievable to many parents, nine-month-old children have been shown to select a nutritionally balanced meal when presented with a wide variety of foods, and these children did not become either overweight or underweight. It was learned that a child's taste differs from day to day. A food rejected one day may make an entire meal the next. We are not fond of the practice of using foods, such as desserts, to reward children, and feel that a child should not be forced to eat a disliked food as a punishment.

Feeding time can become a battleground. Some of these battles may be avoided if parents realize that nutritional requirements change dramatically at one year of age. Infants gain about two pounds a month in the first six months of life and about one pound a month in the next six months, but then only four to five pounds a year up to the age of six. It is easier to tolerate a child's pickiness knowing that nutritional needs are being met. Children won't leave the table hungry; their appetite is a good guide.

As children become older, the dinner hour becomes the one time when all family members are assembled in one spot. This is an important social time.

Watching television or reading during the dinner hour is wasting time that could be better spent with the family. Good communication during the dinner hour is an important measure for promoting mental as well as nutritional health.

Common Food Concerns

Junk food is an all-encompassing term that generally refers to candies, snacks, sodas, and the products of fast food houses. The nutritional value of items called "junk food" varies tremendously. Some are quite nutritious and some are nearly devoid of nutritional value. All are expensive. Use your common sense, read the labels, and do not use junk foods as rewards. Food can mold a child's behavior and parents should not encourage the use of expensive food with minimal nutritional benefits. Parents are often concerned that their children seem to eat only junk food. However, children do not do the shopping and it is usually within a parent's power to control consumption of these items.

Dry cereals range from products that are of exceptional value to products that are nearly worthless. The sugar content of dry cereals varies from 7% to 70%. The composition of dry cereals is printed on the package box and you should read before you buy.

There are over 2700 known *additives* to the foods we consume. Two-thirds of these are of no known benefit; they include food colorings and artificial flavorings. The harm from useless additives is unknown, but is potentially unlimited. While some food additives, such as preservatives, are necessary, the majority are not. Since any foreign substance can cause an allergic response in a sensitive individual, there are undoubtedly many allergic reactions that are caused by these additives. Research is presently under way to determine whether food additives are responsible for behavioral problems as well as allergic problems. Evidence is suggestive, but not conclusive, that food additives may affect behavior in some children.

Chapter

4

Growth and Development

One of the most pleasurable rewards of being a parent is watching your children grow. The excitement of witnessing your child's first steps or hearing your child's first words is difficult to exaggerate. As the years roll by, scrapbooks become as important to parents as the writings of their favorite author. Home movies are in a league above and beyond this year's Academy Award winners. Your favorite Van Gogh is no more priceless than your favorite crayon creation.

Parents with no interest or ability in history suddenly become meticulous historians of their child's life. The precise timing of the first step, the first word, the first birthday party, and the first date is remembered after the date of the Magna Carta has long been forgotten. As other historians do, they remember battles—the battle of the bottle, the battle of the toilet. Momentous pacts and treaties also have their day. Parents also grow. They learn to deal with the trauma of beheaded toy bears, bogie men in the dark, departing friends, and illnesses in brothers, sisters, and pets. In just a few years, parents watch their children grow from complete dependence to total independence.

Watching children grow is fun, but sometimes it is worrisome. Parents are easily and naturally concerned that their children are not developing properly, and sometimes parents worry unnecessarily. As a society we often seem preoccupied with predicting the future success of our offspring. A child throwing a ball at an early age should prompt excitement, but not necessarily anticipation of a career in sports. And children who read at an early age may be destined for mechanical or artistic interests rather than headed toward a scholarly life.

Much of the work on child development of decades ago is still being used to predict a child's future performance. There are no crystal balls. We discuss patterns of growth and development in this chapter, as well as some of the tools used to measure and predict this process. Part of the purpose of this chapter is to point out the limitations of these tools.

YOUR CHILD'S WEIGHT

The physical growth of infants is remarkable. They usually double their weight in the first six months of life and triple their weight by the time they are one year of age. These are average weight gains. There are wide variations that are normal. Their height increases by a full 50 percent by the end of the first year. At birth, a child's head size is already nearly 60 percent of the adult size, and by the age of three years the head size will be nearly 90 percent of its adult size. Except in cases of rare diseases, physical growth is determined by two factors: proper nutrition and heredity.

Proper nutrition begins during pregnancy and continues throughout infancy, childhood, and adult life. The measure of growth that is most sensitive to nutrition is, of course, weight. Children largely make up their own minds about when and what to eat. So there are periods when children will refuse to eat a great deal of food. Remember that if your child will not eat carrots or spinach today, it will have no effect on his or her weight, and certainly will have no effect on height or brain growth. Prolonged periods of not eating will eventually affect weight, and then height, and ultimately brain growth, but malnutrition of this severity is extremely uncommon in this country.

The eating habits of children concern most parents. In discussing feeding problems with parents, we have found that all children either eat too much or too little and not enough of the right kind of food. It is hard for children to eat too little if presented with food. Hunger cravings are biologically determined and the survival instinct is strong. Normal children always eat enough.

More often, the problem is that children eat too much. A child in the first year who eats too much gets chubby, but also undergoes several invisible changes. An excess number of fat cells develop within his or her body. Once these fat cells have multiplied, they send out messages that help to determine appetite cravings. Although losing weight in the future will decrease the *size* of these fat cells, the *number* of fat cells will remain the same. So a lifetime of strong appetite cravings sometimes can be traced to the overfed infant. Excessive eating also can stretch the size of the stomach. Hunger pains are caused when the walls of the stomach contract against one another. Stomachs that are large and stretched require more food to decrease the empty feeling of hunger. Other factors appear to determine eating patterns. For example, thin people seem to be able to tell precisely when they have had enough and will not eat any additional food. Fat people, on the other hand, tend to continue eating even beyond the point when hunger has been satisfied.

Children learn eating patterns from their parents and proper weight is partly culturally determined. In some countries, being heavy is considered a sign of prosperity, and the same holds for some subcultures in the United States. A wide range of weights must be considered as normal. Being ten pounds overweight or ten pounds underweight for your height, when compared with the average weight, makes little health difference. But as you get beyond a few pounds overweight, you must pay a price. That price is poorer health.

YOUR CHILD'S HEIGHT

The genetic factors important to physical growth are reflected in the height of the parents. Tall parents tend to have tall children and short parents tend to have short children; it is as simple as that. However, an interesting phenomenon called "regression toward the mean" has been observed. Tall parents have children that are taller than average, but shorter than the parents. Shorter-than-average parents will have children who are shorter than average, but who tend to be taller than the parents.

The upward growth trend is not a steady trend. For long periods of time children may not grow at all, and at other periods they may exhibit rapid growth spurts.

Your physician will record the growth of your child on a growth chart similar to the charts shown in Part III of this book. After recording a series of heights and weights at different ages, you can visualize the growth of the child. If growth is extremely fast or stops for a long period, it will show up on the graph and be noted much more easily than with the traditional marks on the closet wall. Instructions for using those charts are given in Part III, together with charts for your children. Don't worry too much about how your child compares to the "normal" lines. At some time during growth and development, most children will be very high or very low in something, because of growth spurts or lags. Usually the growth rate is roughly parallel to the lines on the growth chart and does not deviate more than two or three lines from the original. A prolonged period of delayed growth requires investigation. The charts will help you with Problems 67 (Overweight) and 68 (Underweight).

We are pleased that tall women are no longer considered "unusual." Height has always seemed a trivial characteristic by which to judge any person. Unfortunately, many tall women can remember being teased because of their height when they were younger. This attitude is no longer common but many parents understandably wish to protect their daughters from such experiences. Other parents have been concerned that their daughter's height might interfere with a ballet career. Hormones that will prematurely stop bone growth are available but they are dangerous and have numerous side effects. To be effective they are best given before puberty when career decisions about ballet are seldom seriously made. Once growth is stopped, it cannot be restarted. Except for *very* unusual circumstances, we do not recommend the use of these hormones.

Many parents are concerned that their child will be handicapped because he or she is too short in a culture that places a value on being tall. Some have heard that *growth hormone* is a drug for increasing height. Growth hormone is produced by the pituitary gland and enhances growth, but this hormone is only effective in children who have a deficiency of growth hormone, and this is extremely rare. It is of no use to a child with a normal pituitary gland, and in fact may be harmful.

GROWTH AT PUBERTY

Initially, growth is controlled by two hormones: growth hormone and thyroid hormone. During puberty additional hormones are responsible for growth.

These hormones are also responsible for the development of sexual characteristics in boys and girls. While hormones are primarily responsible for sexual behavior in animals, they play only a minor role in human beings; sexual behavior in adolescents and adults is far more a psychological than a hormonal response. Even in most animals, mature sexual behavior requires far more than the presence of hormones.

As an adolescent reaches puberty, the pituitary gland increases the secretion of a hormone called follicle stimulating hormone (FSH). FSH in women stimulates the ovaries to produce estrogen (female hormone), and stimulates the development of sperm in men. In males, another pituitary hormone stimulates the increase in testosterone (male hormone) from the testicles. Testosterone can also be produced by the adrenal glands in men and women.

In boys there is no single dramatic event that makes it clear that puberty is on its way. There is a typical sequence of changes, however. These changes may not be immediately obvious since they tend to occur over a fairly long period of time. These changes usually begin between the ages of 9½ and 14, but some of the changes are so subtle that they may not be noticed until a later age.

In most boys, enlargement of the testicles begins at about age 11 and continues until about age 18. Penis enlargement usually begins about a year later and continues until about age 16. Pubic hair generally does not begin to appear until about age 13½, although some 11-year-old boys show signs of early pubic hair. If there are signs of pubic hair development before age 10, a call to the physician is in order. Testosterone, which is responsible for the enlargement of the penis, testicles, and pubic hair is also responsible for the development of axillary and facial hair, voice changes, adult body odor, acne, and increasing muscle mass at about age 15.

Half of all boys will experience some enlargement of one or both breasts. Commonly there may be a lump or tenderness under one or both nipples. While this can be easily explained on the basis of hormonal changes, it is often very embarrassing. Your son will need your help and support without having undue attention drawn to this condition. Obesity may accentuate this problem by giving the appearance of very large breasts while at the same time making the penis and testes appear small. Occasionally breast enlargement may be so great and so prolonged that you and your son may wish to discuss the possibility of cosmetic surgery with your physician. Usually, however, the condition resolves itself within a year.

The process of sexual maturation in women usually starts about two years before the first menstrual period. The first sign of puberty can be seen as early as age eight or nine and still be perfectly normal. Signs of pubertal development before the age of eight requires an evaluation by your physician. While the ages at which changes occur vary widely, their sequence is pretty much the same. Breast development begins at age 11 and is followed shortly by the appearance of pubic hair. Hair under the arms begins to increase at age 12. Between ages 12 and 13, a growth spurt results in a noticeable gain in height. Menstrual periods begin around age 12½. Over this entire period there is some change in the way fat is distributed over the body, particularly in the hips and buttocks. Widening of the hips, as well as development of the uterus, vagina, and external genital organs, also occurs. Problems associated with menstrual irregularity and vaginal bleeding are discussed in Problem 91.

Variation in breast development is often a cause for concern. Breasts usually begin to develop one or two years before the first period, but this may not occur for as long as two years after the onset of menstruation. Often one breast develops more rapidly than the other so that temporarily the breasts may be of unequal size. Frequently this is of concern and embarrassing, but most breasts reach nearly equal size by age 18. Sometimes there is worry that the areola (the dark area surrounding the nipples) may be elevated too much or not enough. In about 75 percent of women the areola is elevated, while in the remainder it is not; both patterns are perfectly normal. Inverted nipples are another condition that is not a problem and needs no treatment other than reassurance.

Finally, there are the inevitable concerns over the size of the breasts. We are happy to note the decline in emphasis on huge breasts as the ultimate sign of sex appeal. Still, every girl worries about being flat-chested, while virtually none of them will be. Mostly, the problem is one of timing. Remember that the breasts may not begin to develop until two years after menstruation has begun, and may not be fully developed until age 19 or 20. It is perfectly possible for one 13- or 14-year-old to have undergone very little or no breast development, while most of her friends will be well into breast development and some will essentially have completed their development. Your reassurance is a most important factor in easing your daughter's anxiety. Efforts at stimulating breast development artificially have no place in the developing child or mature woman. Oral or topical estrogens are potent drugs that should not be used to promote cosmetic changes.

Excessively large breasts are also of concern. Emotional support from parents as well as physical support from a good brassiere is important during adolescence. Surgical procedures are available for cosmetic reduction, and this procedure can be considered by older adolescents and their parents.

YOUR CHILD'S DEVELOPMENT

Watching your child grow in size is only part of the fun. Development of coordination is even more exciting, and infants quickly acquire a variety of skills. They acquire muscle abilities, which give them mobility and allow them to explore. They develop extremely fine motor abilities, which enable them to accomplish complex tasks such as playing a musical instrument. They develop the ability to convey anger, disappointment, or love by use of facial expressions. Language develops in order to express needs. These needs are simple at first, but gradually these language abilities become more sophisticated until children are finally able to use words to express feelings. Social skills provide early rewards for children. Smiling begins very early, often in the delivery room. Soon this smiling becomes more specific; infants are soon able to recognize their parents and recognize that parents are exhibiting warm feelings toward them. Gradually, children learn how to play games with others. Soon afterward, they learn how to share things and ultimately they develop the capacity to love. Learning is one of the more complicated skills, and progresses from primitive basic memory to abstraction, moral judgment, and creativity.

The development of skills progresses in an orderly rather than a haphazard fashion. Pediatric and psychologic research has focused on this sequence, and has been helpful in establishing the expected order of events and the limits of "normal." Attempts to correlate the age at which something happens with future capabilities have not been very successful. This sequence is, in fact, a logical building of increasingly complicated skills. As an example, let us look at the sequence required for a child to use a pencil.

The first stage in the sequence is reflex control. You may remember that your infant kept his hands clasped in a fist for most of the first few months of life. All infants have what is known as a grasp reflex. They will grab and hold on to any object placed in their palm, such as a finger or a pencil. Physicians may demonstrate the strength of an infant by allowing him or her to clasp each of the doctor's index fingers, and then lifting the child off the table. The infant demonstrates his or her strength admirably, but this is not a sophisticated use of the hand; there is no control over this reflex and anything in the palm will be clutched.

As the nervous system develops, the grasp reflex is overcome, usually by about three months. The infant is now ready to use the hands in a different fashion. By about four months, the infant's hands are held open and can hold onto objects placed in them. Although vision is good, coordination is not sophisticated enough to reach for an object and retrieve it. The infant will usually overshoot the object.

At five months, retrieval abilities get better. The process known as raking is begun; objects are brought closer by use of the entire hand. At nine months or so, the infant achieves control of thumb and forefinger and can bring them together so as to pick up tiny objects. Soon, small objects, such as raisins, pennies, and pills, are picked up, looked at, and ultimately placed in the infant's greatest exploratorium, the mouth. Development of this finger-to-thumb pinching motion is unique to humans; unfortunately, this ability also places the infant at risk for stuffing nose, mouth, and ear full of "goodies and baddies."

By now, the infant is able to let go of items voluntarily. The ability to release items in a projectile fashion—better known as throwing your food on the floor—begins after the child's first birthday.

After a year, things progress rapidly. Hands that were first able to release toys voluntarily only a few months earlier are now gentle enough to release one block precisely on top of another. By age two, the budding engineer can create a tower of six stories (or blocks) high. Like any engineer pleased with a building, our growing child feels the need to leave records of building successes, and the ability to draw develops. At first, the child draws with crayon in fist, but before the third year begins, the crayon is held like the adult holds it. Pencils are somewhat trickier than crayons, but this skill is also soon mastered.

Finally, the apprentice learning skills needs help from the master craftsman. A child cannot develop artistic skills without paintbrush and paper. A child needs raw materials with which to practice. Encouragement is also required. Children are social beings; a smile or kind word lets the child know you are pleased with the progress on the product.

This evolutionary sequence is illustrative of most other processes in child development, like walking. First, involuntary reflexes must be overcome in order for a child to have voluntary control. Second, there is a logical progression; cruder movements always precede finer movements. Third, coordination of several senses is necessary for skill development. For example, the child relies on sight, depth perception, and balance to build a tower of blocks. Fourth, a skill can develop only when the nervous system is mature enough. Building a tower of blocks is impossible for a six-month-old, no matter how much exposure to blocks the child has had.

The growth of every individual is unique; this is the most important point of this chapter. Even identical twins brought up in similar fashion grow differently and ultimately do different things with their lives. Children are all very different and will demonstrate their unique tastes, even for music, at an early age. The infant, as well as the parents, is important in determining the family environment. Babies quickly learn how to manipulate their parents. A child soon learns that jabbering will, as if by magic, produce parents. Parents sometimes substitute a favorite teddy bear when the child cries or jabbers, rather than spend time with the child. Or a parent may comfort the child vocally when physically occupied with other tasks. The infant quickly decides whether these responses are sufficient. For a time, they may suffice, and then the game begins again as the infant discovers a new way of drawing attention. Quieter infants may use smiling or eye contact, rather than voice, to make their demands known. In short, the infant is an active participant in creating his or her own environment.

TOILET TRAINING

Toilet training is an important developmental milestone both for toddlers and their parents. The skills required for bowel and bladder control are similar. Because these skills are acquired at slightly different ages, we will be discussing them separately. These skills are the culmination of a long series of accomplishments, and parents play an important role by recognizing, reacting to, and rewarding each accomplishment.

Bowel Control

Young infants have a reflex known as the gastro-colic reflex. About 20 minutes after eating, the infant will have a reflex bowel movement. This reflex, like other early reflexes, will gradually diminish, usually by 12 to 15 months of age. Willful control of bowel elimination can only develop after the child has overcome this reflex.

Many parents recognize this happening, and will begin toilet training by capitalizing on the reflex. We have all heard stories of children being toilet trained by the age of six months. These children were, of course, not really toilet trained, but were passing stools in a regular pattern determined by the gastro-colic reflex. Some parents have confused the natural disappearance of this reflex with a conscious decision by their 12-month-old to be uncooperative. This is far from the truth; a 12-month-old is still much too young to toilet train. Other skills must first develop and mature.

The child must first be able to sense that a bowel movement is occurring; most children acquire this knowledge after one year of age. (Parents can often recognize that their child is producing stool by facial expressions or other gestures.) Initiation of bowel control is often begun at this time, and is most often begun unconsciously. You will often mention "BM" or some other word when the child is having a bowel movement. The association between act and language will have begun. But the final act of this complex learning task will not be accomplished for another year or two.

After the child is able to detect the sensation of a bowel movement, he or she becomes able to sense the presence of fecal material in the rectum before it passes. Following this, the child begins to achieve some muscular control over the passage of the stool. Newborn infants have no muscular control at the anus; this muscular coordination develops at different ages in different children. Some children develop it early in the second year of life; others not until the end of the third year. The rare child with a neurological condition may develop this control much later or not at all.

The length of time that a child can use muscular control to withhold the stool gradually increases. In the middle of the second year, the child may be able to tell you that a bowel movement is on the way, but the movement will probably have occurred before you reach the toilet.

Children should not be "rushed" to the toilet. Frantic activity can be a frightening experience for some children, who might associate normal body functions with dirt and disgrace. Of course, many households have such a high level of activity that rushing may be normal. In short, the speed with which you take your child should be similar to the speed with which you do other things with your child.

Once your child begins to inform you of an impending bowel movement, you can begin taking the child to the toilet. Most children will be able to do this when they are two or three years old. Introducing your child to the toilet ("potty") should be a relaxed affair. Initially, there is no need to even remove the child's pants. A word of caution about the first approach being a "bare-bottom" one: The child's potty is often on the floor where cold tends to concentrate. Sitting on a cold seat can be a shocker to anyone, and especially so to a two-year-old. Merely associating the bowel movement with the potty is enough at first; staying too long should be avoided. The energy level of two-year-olds is such that they will not wish to remain on the potty too long anyway.

A major accomplishment during the long process of development is the ability to put things off, or the ability to delay pleasure. Learning to postpone urges can take months or years. (Indeed, the postponement of some urges remains difficult for many adults.) Having a bowel movement is biologically a pleasurable experience; a child learns to delay this pleasure in order to receive something equally pleasurable—a parent's reward. The child is beginning to make decisions about the pleasures that social behavior can bring. The child of two is becoming more social and appreciates the social interaction with Mom and Dad. Smiles and praises, not overdone, should accompany potty sitting. Praises can be more laudatory when a bowel movement is produced, but they should also accompany nonproductive sittings. You should not keep your child sitting on the potty until a bowel movement is produced. Children take time to learn and there will be many dry runs. Persisting will frustrate both you and your child. When your child is tired of sitting, time is up.

The second year is a period of negativism. The child will frequently say "no." This negativism is an important developmental milestone for the child, for he or she is developing an individual personality that is not a part of mother or father. The drive toward independence will eventually motivate the two-and-one-half or three-year-old child to control bowel eliminations. However, the early part of this struggle for independence may mean a struggle over who will make decisions about bowel movements. It does not pay to engage in battles about bowel movements. Reward, or disengagement, is the key. Punishment will only intensify the opposition and prolong the struggle.

Some pointers about introducing potties and toilets. Potties that sit on the floor generally seem more secure than toilet seats placed way up high on that big toilet. It is also easier to push with feet on the ground. These portable potties can easily be taken on trips and they become the individual possession of the child. Initially, when the child produces a stool, it should be allowed to remain in the potty for a while. Your child will be pleased with the product and may be disappointed when it is taken away. One friend, confronted with a shocked two-year-old noticing her missing bowel movement, invented the "B.M. birdy" who needed the stools. His daughter was satisfied with the explanation and loved to talk about the birdy. Remember also that the roar of the toilet can be frightening; seeing this roaring monster consume a stool can upset and frighten a two-year-old; it may thrill a three-year-old.

Bladder Training

Bladder control in children follows the same developmental sequence as bowel control, and lags behind bowel control in most children. At birth, infants urinate by reflex when their bladder is stretched to a certain point. As they get older, they can hold larger and larger amounts of urine.

By 18 months, children can sense when they are urinating. The muscular ability to hold urine in the bladder is usually acquired between the ages of two-and-one-half and three-and-one-half years. Usually by the age of two-and-one-half years the child is well on the way to learning bowel control, and bladder control is often learned soon afterward. Many toddlers are very much concerned about being in control and learn quickly to hold on to their urine. They are training themselves by holding their urine longer so that they may spend more time at play or gain the social rewards offered by their parents.

Because calling mom or dad for assistance in going to the potty is a handy way of getting attention, parents can expect some dry runs. Accidents should be expected since a child at this age can become easily preoccupied or forget.

Daytime bladder control is achieved by age three in 85 percent of children and by age four in over 95 percent of children. Occasional accidents will occur. Often, older children with the "giggles" will have accidents even in school. Children will usually learn quicker when their older brothers or sisters are around to help and demonstrate.

Bed-wetting

Nighttime dryness takes longer to achieve. Nearly 20 percent of five-year-olds are still subject to frequent nighttime wettings and more than 10 percent of six-year-olds still wet the bed. On the other hand, some three-year-olds, if taken for a late-night trip to the bathroom, will make it through the night just fine. Expect an occasional accident, but avoid any sort of punishment. Children should not be kept in overnight diapers until they are 100 percent dry; these do not encourage the child to develop his or her own control. (See Problem 65, Bed-wetting.)

Since bladder control, like bowel control, is the culmination of a maturational sequence of sensory, muscular, learning, and social development, all these areas will be investigated by a competent medical professional. Medication may occasionally be necessary. Surgery is virtually never needed. Most therapy will focus on the social aspects of changing this behavior. Frequently, improvement will occur when the child makes the decision that a dry bed is important, such as when visiting with a friend or relative.

Relying on a drug to increase urinary retention through increased muscular control, or an alarm to modify behavior through negative reinforcement, is a narrow approach to a complex phenomenon. They have a very small role, and then only as part of a therapeutic process involving coordination of efforts with child, parents, and professionals. Don't buy the devices advertised with coupons on the back of magazines.

WHAT IS NORMAL DEVELOPMENT?

Is my child normal? Why is Johnny so short? Why does George wet the bed still? He is almost 8! Why didn't my second child start to walk as early as my first? Our society seems preoccupied with the prediction of the future success of children, creating a natural environment for parents to worry. The spirit of competitiveness lives in all of us. We worry unnecessarily about such things as whether Suzie will walk before the little girl across the street does.

While children are constantly developing in all areas, certain areas can develop more rapidly because of the individual needs of the child. As an example, consider a child growing up in a large family. The daily event known as dinner, in a large family, is often the experience that most of us have only at Thanksgiving or at large picnics. In short, it is fun but chaotic. The relative chaos tends to produce two types of children, the quick and the hungry. In order to survive, the youngest child in a large family must develop quick hands. Some of these children will develop hand skills at an early age. But later in childhood, the child from the smaller home will catch up. Both are normal.

The opposite seems to occur in the development of walking ability. With many other feet belonging to larger bodies running about, the small child in a large family is likely to be knocked over frequently. It is not uncommon to see late walking in children from large families. These children, however, do have the need to explore and discover new things, and they develop other means of locomotion. Some are clever enough to get their older brothers and sisters to carry, push, or pull them about. Others develop a pattern of extremely rapid creeping or scooting. Children are constantly developing and adapting to their environment. They are adapting in the way that is best for them, and *not* according to printed schedules in textbooks.

An important consideration in interpreting the limits of "normal" is the concept of variability, which describes the outside limits of age at which a given skill should develop. For example, most children begin to smile by about three to four weeks of age, but some children begin on the first day of life, and other children don't begin until they are seven to eight weeks of age. We say that the average child smiles at one month, but the variability is either a month earlier or a month later. As tasks become more and more complicated, the variability always increases. Most children sit at about six months, but the variability is between four and eight months. Most children walk at one year, but some begin as early as nine months of age, and still others may not walk until 16 months or even later. Verbal ability has even greater variability. Some children say three words (other than mama and dada) before a year of age; others may be almost two before this is accomplished. While Beethoven was said to be composing and playing at the age of three, adults ten times that age have difficulties with these tasks. Variability limits are far more meaningful than single "normal" values in interpreting whether a given milestone has occurred on schedule or not. In other words, a child who does not walk at the average one year of age is still normal if walking at 16 months. However, the child would be considered abnormal if not walking by the age of three years.

Normality in one area of development does not guarantee normality in all others, and abnormality in one area does not signify abnormality in others. Consider a child who, for whatever reason, has acquired an injury that affects muscle (motor) development. This child may lag considerably in sitting, walking, and the more sophisticated locomotion skills, while acquiring language, social, and other skills at the appropriate age.

A common misconception is that a child's intelligence can be predicted by observing how rapidly he or she develops in the first years of life. Except for rare cases of severe retardation, development rates offer very little help in predicting ultimate intelligence, let alone whether or not that person will use intelligence creatively, productively, or not at all.

Experts can only put a fuzzy border around what is normal and what is abnormal. Nobody can say what your child will be like in the future. A child who is developing slowly at first may develop rapidly later on. Other children may develop very rapidly initially and then slow down. Most usual are periods of alternating rapid, slow, and average development in response to changes in season, changes in family composition, and other changes not yet determined.

ADDITIONAL READING

Brazelton, T. Berry, M.D. *Infants and Mothers: Differences in Development.* New York: Dell, 1969.

Brazelton, T. Berry, M.D. *Toddlers and Parents: A Declaration of Independence.* New York: Dell, 1974.

Chapter

5

Personality Development

The complexity of human personality development eludes discussion in a single volume, let alone in a single chapter. Freud, Piaget, Erickson, Sears, Maccoby, and hundreds of others have devoted their entire lives and thousands of volumes to expanding our knowledge in this area. In this section, we will provide a framework for personality development that can help you to understand better some of the common problems that you may encounter.

INFANCY: BIRTH TO ONE YEAR

Each infant is born with an individual personality. Theories that a child's personality is dependent only on environmental factors are now felt to be untrue; infants are individuals from the very start. Some come out active and screaming and remain at a high level of activity throughout life. Other children are very mellow at birth and continue with this personality trait.

We now know that infants exert a strong influence over their parents' behavior toward them. An active child will quickly learn how to attract his or her parents' attention. These active children with their high levels of demands will force parents to interact with them more often and will often encourage parents to provide them with more play objects. Quieter children may show the greatest pleasure while being held or merely looking at a parent. Quiet activity pleases this type of child the most, and parents, sensing this pleasure, respond with the level of activity that the child enjoys the most. Often children will interact differently with mom or dad.

When infants have quiet times, they are listening, learning smells, judging distances, and developing intellectually. During active times they are moving and discovering limbs, exercising muscles, and developing coordination.

The newborn quickly learns how to obtain food. While babies are born with reflexes that enable them to suck vigorously and locate the nipple on the breast by rooting, they must learn how to make the milk appear. Crying most often serves this function. Parents influence this behavior by modifying feeding schedules to their own preferences. Development progresses quickly and infants develop an interest in their environment. They soon learn that toys can be manipulated by kicking and reaching; hence they begin to control their surroundings.

Within the first few weeks of life, children are already becoming social and beginning to smile. Smiling is clearly an expression of joy. From birth to six months, infants will often smile at anything and all persons that please them. By the age of six months, many children can recognize the faces of their principal caretakers. Faces other than those may bring anxiety, terror, and screaming. Children raised in households with many people may not experience as much anxiety.

Crying

Crying is a normal activity of all infants and serves many functions. In a newborn infant it helps the lungs in adjusting from the fluid-filled amniotic sac to an air-filled world. Infants cry in response to their needs. They cry when they are hungry, wet, cold, or, on occasion, in pain. This crying is a way of communicating with their parents and is effective, since the necessary response—the parent to alleviate the need—is usually produced. Parents quickly become adept at distinguishing different types of cries: the cry of hunger, pain, boredom, or anger.

Some crying is not due to a specific need of the infant. With this type of crying, neither hunger, wetness, nor pain is responsible. The infant is merely fussy. Holding and rocking does not always relieve this type of crying and parents need not be concerned about this fussiness.

Several years ago Dr. T. Berry Brazelton did a study on healthy infants, which revealed that two to three hours of fussiness per day in the first few months of life was to be expected. Some infants were fussy for as much as four hours a day. The crying increased gradually, becoming most prolonged by six weeks of age, and declined thereafter. By three to four months, most infants were fussy less than one-and-a-half hours daily. Most of the crying seemed to occur between the hours of 6 P.M. and 10 P.M. Unfortunately, this crying occurs at a time in the day when parents are becoming tired and the irritability is harder to tolerate. In the young infant sleeping on the stomach can cut down on the amount of fussiness, prolong sleep, and produce more regular sleeping patterns.

Crying may also occur as a result of being frightened by a loud noise or a sudden movement. Other infants may cry in response to lights being turned on or being turned off.

As the infant becomes older, crying becomes less frequent. Children can delay a need for gratification longer and longer. Older infants, however, begin to miss their parents and will cry when they are lonely. By six months of age the child recognizes his or her parents and consequently recognizes their absence. Some people recommend that the infant be held if loneliness is the cause of the crying. Others warn that cuddling the child after crying will spoil the child. We believe in a common-sense approach. A few whimpers when a child wakes up at night and is lonely need not be attended to. Frequently playthings in the crib will serve to comfort the child. If the whimpering persists, often the voice of the parent is enough to quiet the child. If crying becomes intense and prolonged, the child should be held and comforted.

Beyond one year of age, crying is often a product of the child's frustration at not being able to control his or her surroundings. This is, of course, a healthy sign of personality development but can be disruptive to the family. It is better tolerated if it is better understood.

As children become older, crying can be triggered by emotions. It is helpful for parents to teach a child to be able to say that he or she is angry or frustrated rather than to continuously demonstrate this feeling by crying. Sadness and separation are also frequently accompanied by crying.

Crying can, of course, also be a sign of pain, especially in a young child who cannot verbalize the presence of a headache, stomachache, earache, or sore throat. If illness is causing the pain that is producing crying, other symptoms will usually be present as well.

TODDLERS

Toddlers are moving from a period when they have been totally dependent on their parents to a time when they are trying to control themselves and their universe. They begin to discover their individuality and try to determine how much power they have as individuals. This is an age of daring for toddlers; it is an age of exploration. They will climb ladders far too high, attempt to run much too far away, and attempt to eat dangerous things. Parents of children in this age group must set limits without overprotecting the child. The child must learn what is too high, what is too hot, what is too sharp.

Children are very negative during this period. Because of the child's extreme inquisitiveness, parents find they often must say "no." The child, on the other hand, is driven by a burning desire to explore and to control anyone who would interfere with these explorations. The constant "no, no, no" of the child is meant to ensure the autonomy of this explorer. Children will often say "no" when in fact they have every intention of doing what the parents ask. Again, this is their way of telling you who is in charge. They will say "no" to the parent and really mean, "No, I'm not going to do it because you want me to do it, but I will do it because I feel like it and because I am in charge here." Parents would do very well to study some of the tactics of diplomats. Every diplomat knows how important it is for the opponent to be able to save face. Parents will do well to allow the child to protest "no" while at the same time making sure that the child does what is expected.

Like the "no" syndrome, temper tantrums in toddlers are often a reaction to a world they cannot control. It is their way of reacting to parents whom they perceive as trying to interfere with their autonomy. The tantrums are a sign of their frustration. They are frustrated not only with parents and the world, but also at their inability to communicate their frustration. As children become more verbal and are more able to express their own anger, temper tantrums become far less frequent. A parent can be most helpful by encouraging children to communicate their feelings directly rather than to use tantrums or other aggressive acts. Try not to let tantrums become a successful tactic for the infant to obtain a goal.

Despite the first steps toward independence, the child still requires a tremendous amount of holding and touching, which are important for personality development in this age group.

It is not easy being a parent of a two-year-old. For that matter, it's not easy being a two-year-old. This period often creates the greatest amount of anxiety for parents and it has been dubbed as the "terrible twos." The "terrible twos" may not seem so terrible if the parents have some basic understanding of what is going on. The task of a toddler's parents is to aid the child in becoming independent. This requires not only tremendous affection and more patience than at any other stage of development, but also a thorough understanding of what the child is going through. We recommend Selma Fraiberg's excellent book, *The Magic Years* (New York: Scribner, 1968) for a better understanding of this period.

Temper Tantrums

Temper tantrums are common in children between 15 months and 4 years of age, and tantrums almost invariably arise when there is conflict between parent and child. The pattern of the tantrums is familiar to many parents of toddlers. A child is asked to do something—put down a toy, come in for a nap—and returns a few "nos" in response. As the child realizes he or she is not going to be indulged, an outburst begins. There may be kicking, crying, shouting, rolling on the floor, fist banging, shouting, and spitting. As often as not, these displays are put on in public. If a tantrum occurs in public, you will probably feel embarrassed and want to beat a hasty retreat with your child. If the tantrum is at home, you are also tempted to pursue an evasive course of action.

A good approach to temper tantrums is to ignore them as much as is humanly possible. It is especially important that your child not get his or her own way after a tantrum. Punishing the child briefly and then indulging the child ensures repetition of the tantrums. You are then essentially teaching your child that temper tantrums are effective in getting what is desired. Giving in even occasionally will prolong the persistence of these outbursts.

The best approach to temper tantrums is to try to prevent them. Understanding of a child's personality development, consistency in discipline, and a common-sense approach as to what demands and restrictions are reasonable for your child are all helpful. As children grow older, parents should teach them to verbalize, rather than demonstrate, their feelings. It is better for a child to say "That makes me mad" or "I'm frustrated" than to display anger through physical acts of violence. It will also be easier for you to deal rationally with verbal, rather than physical, protests.

All parents become frustrated and angry with their children. These are natural human feelings. While we all accept anger as a normal part of everyday living, there are many ways of dealing with anger that are unacceptable.

There are many indications that children are often the ones to suffer most, often physically, when family relationships are strained and anger flairs. Abuse of children is becoming an increasing societal problem. Recent films, such as *Small Change* by François Truffaut, are helpful in bringing this problem out of the closet.

We learn how to handle our emotions from our own parents. It is not uncommon for us to encounter three-year-olds who will throw a puzzle to the floor and shout "oh damn." Our temperament clearly has its foundation in the temperament of our parents. It is highly likely that if you remember your parents being impatient with you or having difficulty controlling their temper, some of this may have worn off on you. At the end of a long and hectic day, we all deserve to sit down to a peaceful dinner. But more often than not, dinner with a one-year-old child will be punctuated with shouts, tossed spoons, and thrown food. On the wrong day at the wrong time, this can be unnerving. Becoming exasperated and angry is likely. However, it is important to remember that your one-year-old is behaving exactly as a one-year-old should. If it were a ten-year-old throwing food and utensils, punishment, such as being sent from the table, might be in order. However, it is inappropriate to punish a one-year-old who is exhibiting appropriate behavior. What would you do in this situation? Would you start shaking your child violently? How would you control your temper? If you felt you were going to explode, who could you turn to, who could you talk to in order to prevent this explosion?

The problem of extreme anger with accompanying potential abuse can be dealt with most easily once people accept that it is a problem of being human and therefore not a problem to be ashamed of. However, it is difficult for most of us to admit that we have a problem that may require help. Asking for help is difficult. Often the first person to turn to is your husband or wife. Neighbors can sometimes help. While it is often difficult for us to pry deeply into or expose extensively personal problems, a true friendship should give you license to talk openly with friends about your or their temper problem. Your physician is another possible contact. If there is no close person to talk with, it is possible to call the parental stress hotlines that many communities have organized. The presence of so many hotlines is an admission by most communities that we all become angry and it is important for us to keep this anger from harming our children.

The solution of a complex problem is seldom simple. While most communities have services available to help parents and children involved in severe abuse, services geared to preventing abuse are only in the earliest developmental stages. Many childbirth preparation classes now spend time focusing on preparing expectant couples and individuals for parenthood. Other courses deal specifically with the problems of becoming a parent.

Very often we do not know what to expect when we become parents. Parenting involves more than just adding a family member. It involves the readjustment of relationships between the existing family members. Some parents will find it easier than others to readjust. However, none will find it easy. The time that parents once had to unwind at the end of a day or to talk out problems between themselves may no longer exist once a child is added to the family. And yet, this time is important.

We should all be working to make resources available to our neighbors in need of help. If you feel that programs in your community are inadequate, you should contact your physician, county department of social services, or members of the local American Academy of Pediatrics in order to inquire about the development of such programs.

Breath-holding Spells

The factors that may precipitate a temper tantrum—conflict, frustration, anger, a contest of wills—are also responsible for breath-holding spells in some children. Breath-holding spells also occur as a result of pain in some children. The spells are most common around the first year of life, but occur anywhere from a few months to five years.

Usually a child will begin to cry and suddenly will hold his or her breath at the end of a cry. After a few seconds the child becomes blue, and then relaxes and recovers. In moderate cases, the child prolongs the breath-holding period even longer, becomes blue, and then temporarily becomes limp and unconscious. As soon as the child becomes unconscious, the reflex system that controls breathing quickly resumes the normal breathing pattern. It is this reflex system that the child has overcome in the process of the outburst. On rare occasions a breath-holding spell can lead to a seizure. In seizures that are due to other causes, it is unusual for a crying episode and blueness to precede the seizure; in febrile seizures and in epilepsy the blueness follows the seizure.

The approach to breath-holding spells is exactly the same as the approach to temper tantrums. Although these episodes are extremely frightening, damage is quite rare. Breath-holding spells almost invariably resolve by the age of five.

Thumb Sucking and Pacifiers

All newborn infants are born with a sucking reflex. Because of this reflex they will suck on a fist, finger, nipple, or anything else that comes in contact with their mouth. The sucking is, of course, necessary for feeding; hence the infant soon associates sucking with a feeling of satisfaction and security. As the child grows older it is normal to suck on fingers, pacifiers, or favorite objects. Often the child will hold a favorite object in one hand and suck the thumb of the other, or will suck a thumb and insert a corner of a blanket or teddy bear's ear in the mouth as well.

Sucking activities increase when the child is anxious, tired, hungry, or stressed. The sucking of objects, in addition to thumb sucking, most frequently occurs between the ages of one and two-and-a-half. There is no need for concern about these sucking activities. They are perfectly normal and demonstrate resourcefulness in finding a way to deal with stress and anxiety.

Several words of caution. Pacifiers should not be sweetened, since this can encourage development of dental cavities. Pacifiers should be of hard rubber and should have a sufficiently large "skirt" to protect the infant from suffocating on the pacifier; several deaths have been reported from a pacifier with a small skirt lodging inside the infant's mouth. These pacifiers have skirts less than four centimeters (1½ inches) in diameter and have a clown, bear, horse, or sailor's head. Some liquid pacifiers have been found to be contaminated with bacteria. Pacifiers with strings attached should have the strings removed, since strangulation can occur.

Children will generally outgrow thumb sucking by the age of five. Parents should not make an issue over thumb sucking, since this will heighten anxiety and hence increase the need for an object that can pacify. Persistent thumb sucking beyond age five should be discussed during a regular medical visit.

Sleeping

Individual sleep patterns and requirements vary tremendously. The average infant sleeps approximately 16 hours a day, with some infants sleeping as little as 10 hours and others sleeping as many as 22 or even 23 hours. As children get older, the sleep requirements gradually decline. By one month of age, children sleep only about 14 hours. By four years of age they sleep an average of 12 hours and by age 8 an average of 9, but as few as 6 and as many as 13 hours a day.

Newborn infants have as many as five or six sleep cycles throughout the day. By one year of age most children have just two sleep cycles, the afternoon nap and evening sleep. Most children outgrow their need for an afternoon nap by the time they are five years of age, but even many adults choose to take an afternoon nap whenever possible.

Many of the sleep problems of childhood are based on the fact that children's sleep patterns are different from those of adults. Many parents would prefer that their children would go to bed at 7:30 or 8:00 in the evening and awaken shortly after the parents arise. These wishes do not, of course, correspond to the needs of the children. We feel there are some sleep problems that can be avoided by careful planning. Children get to sleep most easily when there is a pre-established, predictable routine. If children are highly wound up because of exercise or vigorous play, it will be difficult for them to go to bed; ordering a child into bed at such a time is futile. A good wind-down routine consists of a nighttime bath, brushing of teeth, and a nighttime story when in bed. These periods serve to calm the child down and to provide a time for parents and children to enjoy each other.

Young children often do best with night-lights in their room and these should be provided when necessary. You can also expect your toddler to spend some time in the room talking or playing after you have left; it is unnecessary to interrupt this type of activity. Some children may begin whimpering after the parents have left their bedroom for the night and common sense as well as the age of the child should dictate your approach to this problem. Further discussion is provided in the section on crying.

It is common for children to waken between 5:00 or 6:00 in the morning. Here again, younger infants may prefer to spend time in bed babbling and playing with toys, and toys can be provided in the bed for this period. Toddlers generally rush off to their parents' room upon awakening. Depending on the hour, some parents prefer to bring the toddler in bed with them in order for them to get an extra hour of sleep. We feel this approach is entirely a matter of parental choice. Sometimes three- and four-year-olds will go through periods of trying to sleep in their parents' bed. While there is, of course, no harm in permitting this activity occasionally, we do not encourage children to sleep with their parents for prolonged periods of time.

Fear of the dark and nightmares are so common that we should probably not even consider them as problems. The best approach to fear of the dark is the use of a night-light. Nightmares occur commonly in children of preschool age, and generally they can be handled with a few moments of cuddling and reassurance. Rarely, children experience something called night terrors, which are quite distinct from nightmares. Night terrors occur in a different stage of sleep than nightmares do and the child is generally hysterical and cannot be comforted. Persistent night terrors will require medical help.

A frequent cause of sleep disturbances is the use of medications. This is particularly true with antihistamines and decongestants, which can interfere with the child's normal sleep pattern. If your child is having sleep problems and is simultaneously taking a medication, you should consult your physician about the possibility that the problem is linked to the medication.

Another cause for concern is the use of a milk bottle to get children to sleep. Children who are put to bed with milk bottles are subject to increased numbers of dental problems and increased numbers of earaches. Children can be given a bottle of milk before being put to bed, but the milk should be drunk in the upright position and the milk should not be allowed to remain in contact with the teeth for a long period of time.

THE PRESCHOOL YEARS

The use of language is perhaps the most dramatic development at this age. Children progress in a few years from the use of two-word phrases to the ability to tell stories and describe fantasies. They begin grasping concepts such as size, numbers, orientation in space, and time.

Play begins to occupy a great deal of their time. Play in this age group accomplishes many things. Children learn many fine motor skills and concepts through play. In the early preschool years, children will most often be seen playing independently and exploring their toys. If placed with other children, they will not interact. As children become older, they begin to play together, although the sharing of toys is not always accomplished easily. Besides aiding intellectual and social growth, play is also a way in which three- and four-year-olds, who seem to have enough energy to run for 36 hours every day, can divert this energy into activities that are less socially distracting to parents. Fantasy friends and stories are common at this age. Fantasy at this age is not fibbing; it is a way of learning.

This is an age of further emotional development. Parents can provide a tremendous service by beginning to teach children to discuss their feelings. Three- and four-year-olds are sometimes able to tell their parents that they are grumpy or angry or sad. When children can talk about these feelings, it is easier for parents to help them through hard parts of the day. Inability to recognize one's own feelings can lead to problems in later life; we encourage parents to assist their children in developing a sense of their own feelings. This is also an age of sexual exploration, which we discuss later in this chapter.

Many children attend day-care centers or nursery schools at this age. The activities there aid in socialization and help prepare for the activities of formal schooling. Children who do not go to day-care or nursery schools still hear a great deal about school from other children or older siblings. Most children are therefore socially ready for schooling at the time that they enter.

THE EARLY SCHOOL YEARS (6–11)

During the school years, children make the transition from being members of a family to being members of both a family and society. A teacher becomes an extremely important figure in the child's life. Playmates, however, remain the most significant persons in a schoolchild's society.

This is a period of organized games, which tend to stress competitiveness as well as cooperativeness. Psychology texts often stress that this period is one of sexual identity, where eight- to eleven-year-old boys associate chiefly with boys, and similarly aged girls associate chiefly with girls. With new societal attitudes toward the dichotomy of sexual roles, we expect some of this polarization to diminish. Indeed, the degree of polarization between boys and girls varies greatly, depending on the circumstances of the moment. For example, ball games may require full participation of girls and boys in order to provide the necessary number of players as well as the necessary equipment. Balls are frequently lost down drains and the greater the number of balls, the greater the chances of completing the game. In addition, jumprope, jacks, potsy (hop-scotch), and other games are frequently played by both sexes.

Because of the importance of friends in this age range, parents must be sensitive to their children's needs if a move is planned. A promise of a bigger house, a room of your own, or a swimming pool is negligible when compared with the loss of friends. Fortunately, new friends are made, but the parents must be supportive during this period.

Children in the school years are also developing their own code of justice, their own code of what is right and wrong. Moral judgment begins at about the age of six or seven, when children begin looking at the circumstances surrounding an event in order to decide whether the event was right or wrong. Piaget has written extensively on this subject in *The Moral Judgment of the Child* (New York: Free Press, 1932). The moral codes of seven- and eight-year-olds come chiefly from their parents and other members of the adult world. Between the ages of eight and twelve, children begin to talk more with friends and evolve their own code of justice. Stealing is frequently a problem in this age group. Some of this stealing is merely the child's testing of boundaries in order to determine what proper limits are, and most children who steal during these years have a sense of guilt. Occasionally, children may steal as a group act or be forced to steal as an initiation rite. While it is a parent's role to maintain the limits demanded by society and parents should define the limits clearly, they should not overreact to such actions. Stealing by a child is a profound disappointment to the parents, but does not often herald the beginning of a life of crime. Let your child know firmly, but with love, that certain behavior is not acceptable. Your child is essentially saying, "Here's what society says, but is society right? How do I really feel about this action? The only way I can really tell how I feel is to test it." The ability to question society's values is important. The right to question should be encouraged. Mature reaction to the discovery of stealing by your child can be a learning experience for both parent and child, can establish the limits of acceptable behavior, and can teach the child the relationship between actions and consequences.

Schooling accomplishes many things for our children. Children acquire academic skills and learn about the nature of our universe. In addition to knowledge, schools foster the ability to function within society. Students discover how to work with other children, and begin to appreciate what will be required of them. Often, especially in large classes, it is easy for children to be denied individual attention. In order for a teacher to deal with 30 children, a tremendous amount of order and uniformity of action is a necessity. However, socialization can be detrimental to the extent that it denies an individual the ability to think or act differently; this is clearly undesirable to mature development, and creativity can be stifled. Children require an atmosphere that allows learning for all at the same time, yet encourages each child's development as a unique individual.

All school systems are under perpetual attack for fostering either too much competition or not enough. We are enthusiastic about the development of alternative schools. We are anxious, however, about schools that see their *only* role as developing individuality or creativity. Preparing children either for the rugged individualism necessary in a pioneer society or for cooperativeness that calls for complete submission to the needs of society can potentially produce children who are historical or cultural misfits. Children must learn a combination of competition, cooperation, and creativity from their parents and from schools. The parent must understand the school program and complement it so that the child is prepared for a world that is not always fair and not always good.

ADOLESCENTS

"The trouble with today's youth is . . . ." How many times have you heard that expression? How many times have you heard the same tired cliches: "They are irresponsible, hung up on sex, never show any respect, only interested in drugs, cars, etc"? Youths and adolescents have suffered from countless dehumanizing generalizations and oversimplifications. By lumping all teenagers together, we essentially deny youth the freedom to be individuals by *expecting* certain adverse behavior. When this expected behavior occurs, the media leap upon it and we all nod our heads knowingly and feed our own prejudices.

It is interesting to see how the media portrays adolescents. For instance, in the 1950s adolescents were portrayed as angry young rebels. Marlon Brando in "The Wild Ones" and James Dean in "Rebel Without a Cause" rose to fame in roles portraying youth at odds with the world. Now that the youth of that era control the media, they portray the black leather jacket-wearing youth, such as Henry Winkler or "the Fonz," as polite, well-groomed, respectful, superheros. The good old days of today were the terrible times of yesterday.

Some authors have portrayed adolescents as the conscience of our country. Others view youths as passive and merely reflecting the common value system of our society. The truth lies in between.

Studies of adolescents have revealed several interesting facts. Most adolescents have attitudes and values that closely reflect the attitudes and values of society as a whole. Their political orientation is usually that of their parents. The majority of adolescents approve of their parents' attitudes toward discipline, although they, of course, would not be expected to enjoy being subject to the discipline. Most adolescents feel their parents understand them and most feel that the communication lines to their parents are open. There is, of course, a wide spectrum here, since many adolescents are at odds with their parents. No individual can be expected to agree with a parent, spouse, or friends all of the time. Disagreements will produce tension and because of their unpleasant nature will often be remembered. A thousand productive acts are often forgotten in the wake of one heated argument.

Adolescence is often a difficult period because of the many complex tasks required of young people and their parents. The adolescent is defining his or her identity and at the same time rapidly moving toward legal, economic, and psychological independence. Legal independence is coming at an earlier age than ever. The ancient custom of legal majority at the age of 21 is nearly extinct and most states now recognize the age of 18. Youths are recognized to be at the age of majority for health care at an even younger age in many states. Emancipated minors or youths living by independent means away from home are also recognized as having achieved the age of majority.

Economic independence means that young people must learn to plan for the future, an ability that develops during adolescence. This planning includes assessing the educational tasks that must be accomplished to reach economic goals. Work-study plans are available in many communities. Vocational counseling is very important at this age. Goals that are unrealistic or unclear are difficult to achieve and can lead to lifelong frustration. Many adolescents do not have clear-cut goals. Some do not develop goals until they are in their twenties. Parents can offer support but statements of what adolescents "should" do are not helpful. Maturation is complex and occurs at different ages.

Psychological independence is, by far, the most important and most difficult part of adolescence. This is a period in which individuals develop abstract thinking and begin to develop a theoretical framework by which they will live. This involves developing a way to deal with the contradictory values of society, as well as developing ethical and moral values for the adolescent's personal life. During this time our children first begin to recognize the contradictory values with which we all must deal on an everyday basis. The grey zone between black and white is a supremely disturbing discovery. Contradictions about war, pollution, exploitations, and class differences are difficult enough for anyone, and even worse if you have been raised by parents and teachers to believe in peace, love of fellow humans, and equality. How do the idealistic teachings of parents and teachers measure up to the reality of how the world is truly constructed? This contradiction is extremely difficult for young people to resolve.

Adolescents also come to realize that they must soon move away and separate from their parents. While many adolescents talk enthusiastically about leaving home, this is a major source of anxiety. At the same time, adolescents are developing their own personal value system. Most of these developments have something to do with how they relate to other people. Friendships are extremely intense, and very often these friendships are with members of the same sex. Best friends often become inseparable in early adolescence. Younger adolescents will sometimes deal with their sexuality by homosexual encounters. This can be frightening to adolescents and even more so to their parents. However, it is a normal developmental phase for many adolescents. Younger adolescents are vulnerable to sexually exploitative homosexual or heterosexual acts. These acts are far more significant than the transient homosexual episodes more commonly encountered.

Finally, the task of learning how to develop meaningful interpersonal relationships must be accomplished. Learning how to deal with sexuality is only one aspect of developing meaningful relationships. The sexual drives that adolescents experience cannot be denied; they provide a learning experience, requiring the youth to decide on a set of actions that are consistent with his or her own evolving system of values.

The availability of methods of contraception has become a double-edged sword. While it has allowed many adolescents to test their sexuality in a mature and responsible way, it often leaves some young persons without an "excuse" for not engaging in sexual activity. Adolescents need support from parents and sometimes from professionals in sorting out the path of action that is best for them. Good sexual education programs stress the importance of mature choice, as well as the mechanics of contraception. It is important to stress the maturity of most adolescents toward sexuality. The vast majority of sexually active adolescents have one partner. The level of promiscuity among adolescents seems to be less than that of adults.

One of the best ways in which parents can assist adolescents is to encourage them to make a personal choice for their medical care. We feel that the best way to encourage good health through life is to encourage responsible decision making about health and illness. Pediatricians and family doctors are often viewed by adolescents as persons that their parents have chosen for them, and this lack of control in choosing their doctor can discourage the development of mature medical behavior. An important issue in the adolescent's right to select his or her own health professional is the right to privacy and confidentiality. Although very few physicians would violate an adolescent's confidentiality, the fear that a physician might do so may interfere with the seeking of necessary medical services.

The development of the free clinic movement, primarily serving youths, is a testimony to the desire of adolescents to seek medical care in confidence. Because no bills are sent home by these clinics, confidentiality is closely maintained. Most adolescents with good pathways of communication to their parents will wish to discuss their medical concerns with the parents. But they should be allowed to decide when. Responsible approaches to medical problems will develop more quickly in youths who are treated as mature individuals capable of rational choices. We encourage parents to begin fostering independent medical decision making in young children, and to allow adolescents their individual choice of medical provider. We feel the best care can be given by the physician who has been seeing the adolescent throughout the years. We therefore encourage parents to permit a "letting go" of the old parent-child-physician relationship and consent to confidential communication between physician and adolescent.

How can parents best support their children through this intense and often emotional process of adolescence? It's not easy. You are actively involved in gradually granting more independence, yet you are often uncertain about how much independence is appropriate. Your children may be becoming very independent in one area, while still showing youthful tendencies in another. For their part, youths often become anxious about their own independence. They look forward to becoming an adult on the one hand, and yet many of the freedoms of childhood are also appealing. You can help by providing support and by helping them to acquire the best information possible in matters such as health, education, employment, and sexuality.

What should be done when problems arise? Many people adopt the attitude that problems of adolescence are temporary and will disappear with time. However, the percentage of adolescents who are emotionally impaired corresponds rather precisely to the number of adults who are similarly impaired. While many of the minor turmoils of adolescence give way to the different but nonetheless tumultuous problems of adulthood, the severe ones do not go away by themselves. Severe emotional impairment in adolescents or adults is a problem requiring help from doctors, social workers, or counselors. The six-year-old who cannot function in school, the 16-year-old in trouble, and the 36-year-old who cannot hold down a job all need help.

SEXUALITY

Like all other aspects of human development, sexual development begins at birth and continues in a logical progressive order throughout life. This process includes the development of sex roles as well as the development of sexuality.

The concept of sex roles is formed early and reinforced continuously throughout life. A child's sexual identity begins in the nursery when pink or blue cards are used to identify girls or boys. Little boys are handled in a much different manner than little girls are, even in the first few weeks of life. A close friend of ours, firmly committed to sexual equality in raising children of both sexes, began calling her newborn boy "little tiger," a term she had never used for her daughter. This subtle and not-so-subtle discrimination of sex roles that begins in the nursery is reinforced by families and schools, and continues throughout an individual's life.

A child's sexuality begins within the first few moments of life. Achieving pleasure through genital stimulation is only one small part. Affection and fondling of the newborn infant is a natural thing, affording pleasure to both parent and child; this is probably the first sexual interaction.

Parents often notice that newborn boys have erections. These erections are controlled through the nervous system and can occur spontaneously or in response to a number of different stimuli. There is no reason to believe that infant boys do not feel pleasure during these periods. Certainly by one year of age, both boys and girls are able to reach their genitalia and notice that rubbing will produce a pleasurable sensation. At this age, most parents recognize that their children are merely exploring their bodies and are not concerned about genital manipulation. The infant is more concerned with other stimuli. In the first year of life the infant derives more pleasure through the oral gratification of feeding and sucking.

As the infant moves into toddlerhood, pleasure continues to be derived from many other areas, including interactions with parents, food, toys, and eventually the ability to control bowel movements. However, when a child is three and four years of age, there is often renewed interest in genital manipulation, and masturbation occurs in both sexes. Masturbation to orgasm is common in this age group. Parents often have questions about how to deal with masturbation in young children. Certainly, this natural experience is not to be condemned in children. However, parents may wish to talk to their children about when and where it is appropriate to masturbate. Teaching children how to control their sexual impulses should not be regarded any differently than teaching them not to talk loudly in church.

Children between the ages of three and six have a great deal of curiosity about their genitalia and are frequently anxious to compare theirs to those of their parents and to those of children of the opposite sex. Questions should be answered openly and frankly. Detailed explanation of precise anatomical differences is not what is required. Little girls concerned about why they do not have a penis should be told that they have a clitoris instead, and may be told that they have a vagina in addition. Focus on what the girl has instead of why she does not have something that the boy does have. It is more satisfactory to have something else than to have something missing. This is also the age of questioning about how children are born. Explanations appropriate to the level of the child's understanding are important. Again, detailed anatomic dissertations certainly are not what the child wants. Answering a single question at a time is better than a confusing full discussion.

These are also the years in which children like to examine the genitalia of their playmates, especially those of the opposite sex; these activities sometimes lead to conflict with parents of neighboring children. Although you will probably want to acknowledge to neighbors that you are sorry that they are upset, there is no need to apologize for the activity of your child. This is especially true in the presence of the child, for the child may begin to think that he or she has done something terrible. Convey to your children *your* feelings on appropriate behavior, as opposed to what Mr. and Mrs. Jones feel is appropriate behavior.

As children reach the age of five or six, they often will play "house" or "doctor" with children of the opposite sex. Often these games are played where the children may be discovered. Children are often wondering whether this type of activity is right or wrong. Often they have guilt feelings and need reassurance from their parents that they will not be rejected. An acceptable parental attitude is again to acknowledge the activity without encouraging it in inappropriate social situations and without punishing the child for it.

Between the ages of six and twelve, children are occupied chiefly with tasks of learning, developing, and making friendships. These activities take precedence over all others. Genital manipulation does persist throughout this stage although it is less visible and important than at other ages. Although parents may feel that the Boy Scouts, the Girl Scouts, and school projects are molding their child's development, this is also a period when children learn a great deal about sexual relationships. At this age, children have a certain "street knowledge" about the mechanical aspects of sexual intercourse. All school children have their repertoire of "dirty" jokes. In rural areas children often see farm animals and dogs copulating. We doubt that anyone learns very much from the birds or the bees.

Children at this age are also astute observers of parental as well as male-female interaction in general. The most significant impression a child will form about how men and women interact is by observing his or her parents. Parents must provide as good a model in this area of development as they do in others. It is important for children to witness affection between parents. Naturally, parental battles will occur; when they do, you should explain to your children that they are not responsible. Children can adjust to a spectrum of emotions between their parents. They are apt to suffer, however, if they are witness *only* to fights or hostile interactions.

Between the ages of ten and twelve, most parents attempt a discussion of "the facts of life" with their children. Parents should recognize that their childrens' education in these matters has been ongoing for many years. The "facts of life" are often presented differently for girls and boys. Girls tend to be taught about the biology of ovulation and menstruation and the importance of preventing pregnancy. If a girl's mother has been having menstrual difficulties, often the daughter will be apprehensive about her coming periods. Very often children form early impressions about the pain of menstruation. In young children, blood is a sign of pain. Therefore, finding a tampon soaked with blood or witnessing their mother changing a blood-filled tampon or napkin may suggest to the child that mother is being hurt. Explain to children what is going on.

Boys, on the other hand, often receive a discussion about how to acceptably channel their developing drives toward sexual intercourse. In other words, boys are talked to about masturbation, whereas girls are not. We do not feel that discussions that deny the pleasurable parts of sexual activity are helpful. It's important to acknowledge that sexual activity, including masturbation or intercourse, can convey a great amount of pleasure. However, you will probably also want to discuss the personal, emotional, and ethical aspects of sexual activity. Emphasize the long-term benefits that mature interpersonal interaction and sexuality can afford, and discuss how much more pleasurable sexual activity can be if accompanied by affection, intimacy, and love.

During adolescence, interest in the opposite sex increases, sometimes to almost intolerable levels. During this period, hormonal influences add some impetus to psychosexual development.

There is currently controversy about the "sexual revolution" in the United States. While many have proclaimed the existence of this revolution, many others have not been able to find it. It seems that if there is a sexual revolution in the United States, it has been a revolution in the attitudes of the citizens. There now is an openness about sexuality, but behavior may have changed little. Recent studies have pointed out that the number of adolescent males having sexual intercourse has changed very little over the past 50 years, although more adolescent women are having intercourse now than 50 years ago. The trends over the past ten years have not shown dramatic changes in either sex. Estimates now suggest that from 30 to 60 percent of women have adolescent sexual experiences and that 50 to 75 percent of men do.

Perhaps there is a sexual revolution, if one considers the decrease in the double standard. No longer is adolescent male sexuality condoned while adolescent female sexuality is condemned. The number of women actively having sexual experiences is approaching that of their male counterparts. This has created, however, new stresses for many women. In the past, women were made to feel guilty if they had a premarital sexual experience. Today, however, many women feel that, rather than being pressured into celibacy, they are being pressured into sexual activity. Both men and women at this age need support from parents in dealing with these complex sexual issues. They need information, but they also need to be able to discuss their feelings with adults who will understand the difficult decisions they must make and who will encourage responsible actions on their part.

Finally, it is important to remember that you are the cornerstone of your child's personality development. You are required to provide constant love and yet set limits. Children sometimes must be punished, but it is important to make clear that a specific behavior, and not the child, is being chastised. Parents should teach their children to be sensitive to and to respond to feelings. They can help children to talk about their feelings, to be able to say "I am frustrated," "I am sad," "I am depressed." Sadness, depression, joy, and affection are emotions of young children as well as adults. And it is important to state in capital letters that WE ALL MAKE MISTAKES. Making mistakes is part of being human. We are all faced with uncertainty many times. There is no certain approach to all problems and we must all make decisions in the face of uncertainty. We all do the best we can, we all do things differently, our children all grow up differently, and that's the way things will always be.

ADDITIONAL READING

Brazelton, T. Berry, M.D. *Infants and Mothers.* New York: Dell, 1969.

Brazelton, T. Berry, M.D. *Toddlers and Parents: A Declaration of Independence.* New York: Dell, 1974.

Fraiberg, Selma H. *The Magic Years.* New York: Scribners, 1959.

Gersh, Marvin J., and Iris Litt. *The Handbook of Adolescence.* New York: Dell, 1974.

Chapter
6

School Days

School is a critical factor in the growth and development of your child. Not only does it teach a child the necessary academic skills for functioning in an adult world, but it also attempts to teach social skills. To help your child get the most out of this experience, you need to understand and complement the experiences that your child has in school. In this chapter, we will briefly discuss some of the common concerns that parents have about the academic and social aspects of school.

DAY-CARE CENTERS

The day-care concept is not a new one. Over 100 years ago, day-care centers functioned chiefly as a storehouse for children with working mothers whose fathers had left the home. By the end of the nineteenth century, however, Maria Montessori began teaching three-, four-, and five-year-olds in such day-care centers, beginning a movement of preschool education that is still popular today.

There are valid reasons for children to spend time away from home in a day-care facility. For a single parent, this may be a necessity; more than one half of single mothers are working. For many families, it is economically imperative that both mother and father work; more than one third of all mothers of preschool children are working a few hours away from home daily. Children also benefit from the new experiences encountered in day-care centers.

Adequate facilities can be found for children of all ages. Infants and toddlers require more attention and should have at least one staff person for *every four* children. By the age of three, most children have moved beyond the period of independent or parallel play and are ready to begin playing with other children. This is a good age to start children in day-care centers where there are fewer staff members.

Besides enjoying the company of others, three- and four-year-olds usually have a fair language ability as well as some control of their bowels and bladders. Children in day-care centers learn at a rapid rate. They also learn to cope with separation from their parents by spending part of the day away from home. To help ease the shock of this separation, parents should introduce their children to the day-care center gradually. Spending a few hours a day there and gradually decreasing this time often helps. A second child usually has much less trouble if an older brother or sister is already there. Many parents participate regularly by helping out and teaching at the day-care center; this lessens the burden of separation. Children who learn to accept this separation from their parents in day-care and nursery school will generally make a smooth transition to the full-day separation that the first grade demands.

Day-care centers today take a variety of forms. A day-care facility may be in a neighbor's home or in a new elaborate institution. Licensing requirements for formal day-care centers vary from state to state. Before deciding on a particular day-care center, parents should assess the needs of their child. Is the child able to communicate needs to others? Is the child toilet trained? Does the child have any feeding difficulties? What are the child's sleeping patterns?

Day-care centers should be able to meet the individual needs of your child. Most children at this age require an afternoon nap, and the facilities should provide for this. The staff members should be willing to sit down with you and discuss the needs of your child. There should be a balance between play with children and interaction with adults. Meals and snacks should be suitable and familiar to the child. And, there should be some place where children can play independently. Facilities should, of course, be safe. Equipment and toys should be appropriate to the child's age level, and supervisory staff should be accustomed to children of your child's age. Discuss in advance how potential discipline problems might be handled; it may avoid conflict later on. Some parents find out much too late that staff members have completely different attitudes in child rearing from their own. Observing children's behavior in the day-care center will give you a good idea of how it is run. After choosing a day-care center, plan on frequent conversations with the teachers to ensure that your child's needs are being met.

Many parents are concerned about the possibility of frequent illnesses that often go along with increased exposure to other children. Children attending day-care centers are every bit as healthy as children who remain at home. These children do become exposed to more viral infections earlier in life, but the majority of these infections never produce any illness. In addition, some evidence suggests that viral infections are better handled earlier in life and provide immunity in later life when the illness might be more severe.

SCHOOL READINESS

Children mature at different rates; hence there is no particular age at which it is best for all children to begin school. Some children are ready at age four; others may not be ready until age seven or later. Having a child begin school too early may lead to frustration and early school failure and may hamper the child's future school experiences.

Many things are important for success in school. For example, good general health is required. Children with serious diseases will be under medical supervision long before school begins. Knowing that your child can see and hear adequately are important prerequisites for entry. In addition, most states require that immunizations be up to date for entering children.

Social skills are important for doing well in school; sitting in one place all day is not easy. Most children should be able to play well with other children, separate easily from parents, get dressed alone (except shoe tying), have daytime bowel and bladder control, and enjoy games.

Language ability is, of course, very important. Children with severe speech defects will require additional help.

Interest in learning is also an advantage. It helps if the child likes books, is curious about things, knows colors, can repeat a few numbers, can hold a crayon, and can draw a square. Many children will demonstrate ability to grasp complex concepts before they have entered school. They may know about the difference between summer and winter, and understand concepts such as "over" and "under." They may even be able to tell you the color of grass and the sky without looking at them directly. Children also must be able to follow a series of commands such as "go to the closet, select a puzzle, and return with it to your seat."

If your child is able to do many of the above tasks, there should be no problem in beginning school. However, if you are concerned about your child's inability to profit from school because of any one of a number of factors, you should consider a conference with school or medical professionals before enrolling your child.

FAILING IN SCHOOL

Children learn at their own rate. The best learning is an active process involving an exchange between the teacher and the student. This one-on-one type of learning experience can best be done by parents. The active exchange that takes place when an adult is reading to a child and the child is questioning is an extraordinary learning experience; this experience is not matched by the slickest educational television program. While we applaud some of the excellent television education programs, they are a supplement and not a substitute for other types of learning. They are a passive technique and not an active exchange. The feelings that children acquire when interacting aid their emotional development as well as their mental development.

Many problems can impede a child's learning; some are so complex that it is impossible to deal with them here. *Dyslexia* is a term that means inability to read. It is not a single diagnosis; there are literally hundreds of reasons why children may be unable to read. There are just as many reasons why learning in other areas may be impaired. Below we have listed a few factors that may interfere with your child's learning. If you suspect any of the following, a professional should be consulted.

- *Visual problems.* Vision testing is simple in children over four years of age. Strabismus or "lazy eye" can be detected in children over the age of two years.

- *Hearing problems.* Children must not only be able to hear sounds, they must also be able to identify fine differences in sounds such as "p" and "b." Hearing and complex language disabilities should be suspected if there is excessive nonsense verbalization after 18 months, if the child is not talking at all by age two, if the child began talking and then stopped, if the child is not using sentences at all by age three, or if there is no verbal communication of the child's wants.

- *Coordination problems.* These can, of course, interfere with performance in school. Much of the time in the first grade is devoted to writing and drawing. Children who develop coordination skills slightly later are at somewhat of a disadvantage. This, however, may be merely a maturational lag and is not necessarily something to be concerned about.

- *Visual motor ability.* The child's ability to see an object and then copy it involves coordination of eyes and hands. Inability to copy designs may be a sign that visual motor ability is lacking.

- *Auditory perception.* Hearing sound accurately is not enough. The child hearing the word "boat" must be able to picture a boat in his or her mind and recall what a boat looks like and what a boat does. Furthermore, the child must be able to respond to describe the images that have been evoked.

- *Attentional problem.* Some children have difficulties concentrating on the task at hand. They may become easily distracted. It may be difficult for them to concentrate if there is a distracting sound or sight going on. Other children may dwell on a task for an unusually long period of time.

- *Maturational lag.* Children mature differently. Not all six-year-olds are capable of learning in the same way. Some need a few months more before they are developmentally *capable* of learning normally. This delay does not mean that these children will always be behind. It is similar to the case of the child who does not walk until the age of eighteen months. Nobody can tell this child from the child who walked at age nine months when they are both five years old.

- Children from homes where the *primary language is not English* are at a disadvantage when beginning an English-language school. These children generally catch up very quickly but ostracism in the first few months of school (by either classmates or teachers) can seriously hamper a child's confidence and development. We favor bilingual education programs in areas where there are numbers of students who speak Spanish or other languages in the home. Bilingual ability is extremely advantageous for the child where the primary language at home is not that of the overall society. These programs are also excellent opportunities for English-speaking students.

■ Children who *change schools frequently* may encounter school problems. Some of this may be due to differences in curriculum, but much of it is due to the child's need to readjust after losing friends and familiar surroundings.

■ Special types of *seizure disorders*, known as "petit mal," generally cause short periods in which the child does not respond to the environment. The periods may last only two to three seconds, but children may have up to several hundreds of these in an hour. During these periods, the child is unaware of the surroundings and will not be learning. This is a very unusual reason for a learning problem but can be treated effectively, which is why we mention it here.

■ Children with *physical defects* are often teased by classmates. While the deformity may not interfere with the child's ability to learn, the feeling of being an outsider certainly does.

■ *Lack of sleep* can also interfere with the child's learning ability. Many children now have television sets in their rooms, a practice we deplore, and so stay up quite late at night; inadequate sleep can hamper their learning abilities. In addition, children who are often tired in the morning should be suspected of the "reading the comic book with the flashlight under the blanket" syndrome.

■ *Physical size* may also interfere with learning. Surprisingly, this generally affects taller children. A tall seven-year-old who looks like a nine-year-old will be expected to act like a nine-year-old. The discrepancy between the adult expectations and the child's ability creates the problem for the child. Remember, a child should be judged by his or her chronological and developmental age, and not by how old he or she looks.

■ *Hyperactivity* is an extremely overworked complaint. Often one parent will think a child overly active and the other will think not. Hyperactivity is often first noticed by a teacher and brought to the attention of parents. Some extremely curious children who are learning at a rapid rate appear to be overactive. Other children's overactivity interferes with learning. It is important to focus on the quality of the child's activity and not just the quantity. If hyperactivity is noticed at school and not at home, a learning problem should be suspected. We all are bored by lectures that we do not understand. Children who are having difficulty learning become uninterested in what is going on in the classroom and consequently find something else to do. Some children have difficulty adjusting to the different standards of behavior at school than at home. Children who speak little English in an English-only classroom can be expected to find something to do other than sitting in a seat listening to a language they do not understand. Finally, many medications, including the antihistamines in common cold preparations, can cause hyperactivity responses. See Problem 64 (Hyperactivity) for further discussion.

Investigating Learning Problems

The child with serious learning or school problems needs thorough evaluation; these problems are best handled early. The number of teenagers who are unable to read is distressingly high and is partially a reflection of the failure to intervene appropriately at an early age. While some children have school problems because their nervous system development is temporarily behind their age group, many children have causes other than maturational lag. Parents should be told that their child will "grow out of this phase" only after a thorough evaluation. Below is what we feel constitutes an adequate evaluation for a learning problem.

The medical history will focus on the pregnancy, labor, and delivery. Early health and early functioning, such as feeding, activity levels, and behavioral problems, will be discussed. The child's early development will be assessed. This will include questions about the child's coordination, language development, and social development. A school history will include questions about day-care, preschool, kindergarten, school failures, and school successes. If a physician is performing the evaluation, the physician may request a copy of the teacher's reports as well as any achievement or psychological testing performed at school. An evaluation of a school problem cannot be conducted by a physician without cooperation from the school. The physician may spend considerable time discussing the child's behavior and how certain types of behavior are rewarded and punished. Finally, a physician will perform an extensive physical examination, an extensive neurological examination, and a developmental examination. He or she will be checking for the impediments described in the previous section on learning problems. Depending on the results of the history and physical examination, additional tests and psychological testing may be advised. Treatment of a school or learning problem necessitates cooperation between physician, both parents, and the school.

INTELLIGENCE TESTING (I.Q.)

Intelligence testing is more than seventy years old, and was originally designed to predict school failures. Instruments of prediction, whether they be crystal balls or intelligence tests, are never completely accurate. Group testing, most often done in schools, is much less accurate than individual testing. Group tests depend greatly on the child's ability to read in order to assess intelligence. A bright child who may be lagging in reading abilities will perform poorly on these tests, and will be falsely labeled as having a low intelligence.

Individually administered tests are far more accurate. They usually test both a child's verbal and performance abilities. It is easier to take into account a child's poor performance due to a cold, sleepiness, or nonapplication if an individual is working with only one child.

Verbal skills tested include vocabulary, general information, understanding, and arithmetic. Performance tests evaluate picture completions, block designs, and mechanical skills. A separate verbal and performance score, along with a total score, is obtained.

The term I.Q. stands for intelligence quotient. In most tests a number, such as 105, is the result. This number is derived by dividing the child's mental equivalent age by the child's actual age. If a five-year-old scored as well as the average six-year-old, the fraction 6/5 would be formed and multiplied by 100 to give the score 120. A five-year-old scoring as well as the average five-year-old would have a score of 100.

Tests of younger children are far less predictive than tests of older children. Group tests are often grossly inaccurate, and all tests are inappropriate if they do not match the child's previous experiences. Black children have different experiences from the children of a Mexican-American migrant farm worker, who in turn have little in common with children living in a New York suburb.

Parents should be aware of the frailties of intelligence tests. Your child's I.Q. is not an indelible number that will be carried throughout life to grant or deny access to schools, jobs, and success. While there are some who would use the I.Q. for this purpose, the most responsible use of I.Q. tests is to help design an educational program most suitable for your child. Children who do poorly on group I.Q. testing often do not do well in the standard group teaching of our school systems. They may be fully capable of learning but often require a different teaching approach. A child who does poorly on a group I.Q. test should have an individually administered intelligence test. Many low I.Q.'s disappear quickly when this is done. Remember, a group I.Q. test measures how interested your child happens to be in taking that test at that particular time. It does not measure accurately your child's intelligence or potential success.

SCHOOL AVOIDANCE

Tom Sawyer and Huckleberry Finn led a glamorous life by avoiding school. There is scarcely a woman or man alive today who has not at some time thought of repeating the adventures of these two folk heroes. Almost everyone at some time or another has considered staying home from school or has actually played hooky for a day or two. These feelings are especially common after a child has returned from vacation or recovered from an illness. However, while thinking about avoiding school may be considered innocent, actually avoiding school is another matter.

Most children who avoid school state that they like school and that they actually want to go. However, a morning headache, a morning stomachache, morning weakness, morning nausea, or other symptoms conspire to keep them from going to school. There is always an excuse; it is a question of threshold. Most children have a runny nose much of the time; as we have stressed earlier, runny noses and colds are really not illnesses in children. A minor cold is not a reason for a child to stay home.

Avoiding school is really a symptom. The cause is not very often a terrible teacher, although this is the reason often given. Sometimes a teaching program that is suitable for most children may not meet the needs of an individual child. More often, the child may be experiencing a learning problem, a problem with friends, a physical problem such as being too small or too tall, or a problem at home. Often parents feel guilty during periods of stress at home and want their children to stay home so that they can demonstrate that they still care about them.

School avoidance is a complex problem with multiple roots. It must not be treated lightly. Children who are missing more than five percent of their school days because of problems not accompanied by a fever should be considered to be avoiding school. A program to return the child to school will involve the cooperation of a physician, the teacher, and both parents.

CHILDHOOD ATHLETICS

Children have been running, throwing, climbing, and swimming for thousands of years; there are tremendous benefits to a child from athletics. Children learn new skills and how to control these skills. The exercise that is part of athletics is important for conditioning; adults who follow a regular exercise program are less likely to succumb to a cardiovascular catastrophe. Children and adults who are in good physical condition generally feel good about themselves.

Learning how to play a sport is a learning exercise that is as useful to a child's development as other learning experiences are. There are beneficial socializing aspects. The competition that children impose upon themselves is also potentially beneficial. Most of us can fondly remember that some of the best moments of our lives occurred during pick-up games of stickball or basketball or hide-and-seek. Athletics for all children of all abilities should be encouraged. Unfortunately, there are many aspects of athletics that are sorely in need of improvement. Here is the way we see it.

First, most of the sports glorified in our culture, and consequently of great importance to children, are sports in which adults have little opportunity to participate. These include football, baseball, basketball, hockey, and others requiring a number of players. Sports such as running, skating, biking, rowing, and tennis can be enjoyed on a lifelong basis. We favor programs that emphasize sports with long-range benefits; we want healthy children to become healthy, fit adults.

Second, the sports that receive the most glory are often the most violent, and therefore the most hazardous, to a child's health. We prefer sports emphasizing speed, skill, and coordination to those emphasizing violence and mayhem.

Third, competitive sports for adults should be clearly separated from competitive sports for children. The sets of rules that govern professional athletics should not be the model for childhood athletics. Children often have a difficult time dealing with failure. When children interpret their parent's love as being dependent on their winning a game, a psychologically dangerous situation exists.

Fourth, children need to develop in many areas. To the extent that competitive sports, or any other single skill, precludes their intellectual, social, and emotional development, that sport or skill is to be condemned. A full day of practice for a mature adult making a conscious decision to do so is a different situation than a twelve-year-old practicing for the same amount of time because of pressure from school or parent or coach. We do not believe in pressuring any child to practice any sport for long hours daily.

Fifth, school athletic programs spend large sums of money on interscholastic football, basketball, and baseball. The most money is spent on the best athletes, that is, on the children who need it least. Physical education, as all education, should recognize the principle of equity.

We are supportive of competitive sports, but we do not feel competitive sports are for all children, just as we do not believe violin lessons are for all children. Your child must make the decision about the extent of his or her participation and you should be supportive of your child's decision.

Is Your Child Ready for a Sport?

You should ask yourself the following questions.

- Does my child have the coordination for the sport? The hand and eye coordination necessary for some sports such as tennis and baseball requires an older child.

- Is my child the proper size for the sport? There have been several 5′ 6″ college All-American basketball players, but no 100-pound college football tackles. Children mature at different rates and ages. Children who enter puberty late can be physically injured if matched with opponents of greater weight. Forcing competition with younger opponents of the same weight can hurt their ego almost as badly. Varsity "lightweight" programs should be encouraged in the schools.

- Is my child in proper condition for the sport? Size is not everything. A child wishing to join a team in mid-year may have the size and coordination but not the stamina to play successfully.

- Does my child have any medical conditions that might be limiting? Many schools have rules that prohibit children with certain problems from playing contact sports (football, baseball, basketball, wrestling, hockey, lacrosse, boxing, soccer, rugby). Often these children can participate in noncontact sports.

Conditions that often disqualify children from contact sports include:

- Brain concussion

- Head injury with residual skull defects

- Absence of an eye

- Detached retina

- Glaucoma

- Lung infection (tuberculosis, pneumonia)

- Certain heart rhythm disturbances

- Severe heart defects

- Severe or recent heart inflammation

- Certain types of undescended testes

- Missing kidney

- Bone infection

- Hemorrhagic blood disease

(A physician may sometimes permit participation with some of these problems.)

Temporary conditions that often disqualify students from formal sports competition include:

- Active infections
- Perforated ear drum
- Hepatitis or enlarged liver or spleen
- Healing fracture
- Injured growth plate of bone
- Pregnancy

Conditions that may disqualify some students from sports, and for which individual decisions are most appropriate, include:

- Physical immaturity
- Diabetes
- Severe visual handicap
- Hearing loss
- Asthma
- High blood pressure
- Absent testicle
- Seizure disorders (epilepsy)

Sports Safety

Children should be taught safety as a basic skill continually; this is the best insurance against serious injury. Supervising adults should be prepared to deal with common emergencies. In interscholastic competition, where risks of injury are high, professional help should be nearby. The following are some often forgotten problems.

Contact lenses. We do not feel that contact lenses are necessary for all those participating in high school sports. Safety lenses in steel frames with safety straps are often a less costly alternative. The safety record of soft contact lenses is excellent and recommended by many for older competitive athletes. Wearing hard contact lenses is not advisable.

Heat exhaustion and stroke. Workouts should not restrict water from athletes. Loss of water and salt from the body through prolonged sweating can cause heat exhaustion. Under severe conditions, heat stroke can occur, resulting in markedly elevated body temperatures, and can be fatal. Salt and water should be replaced.

Weight loss. Losing weight to place into a certain weight category should be restricted to loss of fat. Weight reduction of more than two-and-one-half pounds per week should be discouraged. Weight loss by attempts at dehydration are dangerous and can compromise a child's strength. A substandard diet to maintain a weight category deprives a growing child of food necessary to grow normally.

Have fun, that's what sports are for. If taken too seriously, they may not be healthy. That's the important message.

Chapter
7

The Medical Encounter

In the normal course of growing up, your child will need various kinds of medical attention—from physical examinations to laboratory tests to surgical operations. In this chapter, we discuss some of the encounters that your child will have with medical professionals and provide guidelines to help you choose a doctor or other health worker to meet the needs of your family.

FINDING SOMEONE TO CARE

A variety of professionals provide medical services to children and their parents. *Pediatricians* are physicians who have spent at least three years after medical school in formal training for the management of childhood and adolescent problems. The pediatrician is no longer a "baby doctor"; many treat a large number of adolescents. In fact, adolescent medicine has been a field developed almost exclusively by pediatricians. *Family practitioners* (general practitioners) are physicians who spend part of their formal medical training in the management of children's problems, and who are trained to treat the whole family. Those who have become family practitioners recently have had training in the psychological as well as medical aspects of family interactions. *Internists* (specialists in internal medicine), while not trained in the care of children, are familiar with many diseases that occur not only in adults but in children as well, and see many children referred by general practitioners.

Several new types of practitioners have recently appeared who are also capable of dealing competently with the common problems of children. *Child health associates*, trained at a Colorado school, undertake a four-year training program after graduation from college. They have not attended medical school but have had more exposure to childhood problems than most physicians except pediatricians. *Nurse practitioners* have an R. N. degree and in addition have attended a program (usually from six months to a year and a half in length) that gives them further training in the management of common medical problems. Some nurse practitioners spend their entire time with children; others, family nurse practitioners, spend part of their time with the problems of childhood. In addition, *MEDEX's* and *physician's assistants* have graduated from a one- or two-year training course, enabling them to work alongside physicians in the management of common problems.

The most important factor in selection of a medical care provider is your confidence in the individual. Confidence develops with time and experience; be careful about first impressions. Initially, you may do best to ask friends for their opinion of local providers.

Look for the following attributes; they are hallmarks of good medical and pediatric care.

- Does the practitioner listen to you? He or she must perceive the same problems that you do.

- Does the practitioner encourage questions? Are your questions taken seriously?

- Do you receive satisfactory answers to your questions? The quick phrase ''She'll grow out of it'' may not always be enough explanation.

- Does the practitioner take an appropriate medical history? Be wary of practitioners who listen for only a few seconds before deciding on a course of action; actions taken on a partial story are often in error. Injuries and simple problems may not require many questions by the provider, but a complicated illness requires more.

- Does the practitioner do a careful examination before ordering laboratory tests? Some practitioners will hear that a child has fallen off a bicycle and order a whole series of X-rays before performing an examination; with some severe injuries, sending the child for X-ray examination can be dangerous. A good medical history and physical examination will suggest most diagnoses to most competent practitioners. Laboratory tests should be used only when necessary to confirm the diagnosis. The test-oriented practitioner will not only waste your money; dangerous side reactions or radiation exposure may result from many tests.

- Does the practitioner try to solve the underlying problems, or does he or she merely make sure that there is no biological illness? Being told that your child does not have meningitis, sinusitis, or a seizure disorder may ease anxiety, but if your child is having headaches three times a week and is missing school because of it, the practitioner's job is not yet done.

- Is your practitioner concerned about the child's development and about safety matters? About preventing illness, or just treating it?

- Is there a back-up person available when the practitioner is out of town on vacation or at educational meetings?

- Does the practitioner take throat and other cultures or does he or she give antibiotics carelessly?

Feel free to seek additional opinions where your child's health is concerned. However, remember that you can always find a number of different opinions about any given problem. Much has yet to be learned about illness, and there are many different ways of interpreting what is already known. Two explanations for the same phenomenon may sound totally different to you. We recommend a "second opinion" strongly if your purpose is to ensure the correctness of a serious decision. On the other hand, if you are merely trying to find agreement with your own opinion about how to manage a problem, you are playing a dangerous game. There may well be some practitioner who will agree with your interpretation of a given problem. But the real question is which solution is best for the child!

Finally, some advice from a mother: "The doctor is such a mixed blessing . . . you have this kid whom you know so intimately . . . you know him as nobody else does . . . and then there is this guy who has all this medical knowledge who knows things about your kid that you don't know, and there can be a subtle something in this relationship between the mother and the physician that can undermine altogether her confidence in herself and her mother role . . . and at the same time the support can be terrific . . . someone else is there especially in the crisis times . . . someone who takes part in the decision making . . . pick the doctor with care and don't accept an autocrat . . . ."

WELL-BABY EXAMINATIONS

Well-baby visits provide an opportunity for parents to question the practitioner about *any* concerns including feeding, safety, learning, etc. Many parents have their first contact with their child's physician before the baby is born. This visit is an excellent opportunity to discuss early concerns. The visits also provide a check on the growth and development of young children. The first visit generally occurs within the first two weeks after birth. By now, parents have come to know some of the unique characteristics of their baby and often have many questions. In addition to this initial visit, at least three more visits in the first year and two in the second will be required. Immunizations will be given during these visits. There is nothing magical about well-baby visits. The purpose of the visits is to help you and your child, so schedule additional visits periodically when and if you have concerns.

Besides a check on development, the most important parts of the examination are the simple measurements of the infant's height, weight, and head circumference. Head measurements are important because there are several correctable problems in development of the skull and of the brain that may be detected during the first few months of life. One of these is an early fusion of the bones of the skull preventing further growth of the skull, known as *craniosynos-*

tosis. Another is obstruction of the fluid system bathing the brain, known as *hydrocephalus.* Both of these problems are detectable by careful head circumference measurements. Periodic measurements of height and weight should be carried out throughout childhood. These measurements are useful in detecting nutritional problems and in detecting metabolic or glandular growth disturbances.

Examination of the hips is especially important in infant girls. Detection of dislocated hips is difficult at birth and this examination should be repeated after a month or so. Congenitally dislocated hips are very easily treated in the first few months merely by the use of extra-thick diapers. Failure to detect this condition until later may require surgery or casting.

The feet should also be examined carefully in newborn infants and during the first few months of life. Foot abnormalities such as *metatarsus adductus,* when detected early, can be corrected simply with a few weeks of casting. Metatarsus adductus causes an exaggerated curving of the outside of the child's foot. Children often have a certain degree of toeing-in, and this is normal until the age of two. Toeing-in may also result from the twisting of one of the bones in the lower leg or rotation of the thigh bone at the hip joint. Careful practitioners will examine the child's feet and legs and assure you of their proper development.

Periodic examination of your child's eyes is also necessary. Infants are capable of seeing at birth, and their eyes can follow you around the room. Infants begin focusing clearly at about six weeks of age, and at this time the wandering of their eyes starts diminishing. A wandering eye, also known as strabismus or a weak eye, is not normal in two- or three-year-olds. You can check for strabismus by having the child focus on any bright object and alternately covering and uncovering one of the child's eyes. When the eye is uncovered, the child's eye should not move; any movement is a sign of a weakened eye muscle and should be checked out. Untreated strabismus can result in blindness of the weak eye.

Hearing disturbances can also interfere with the child's development. Newborns will startle after hearing a sound, and later turn to locate the sound. Although elaborate methods have been devised for testing the hearing of infants, the best way to assess hearing ability is to assess the ability to talk clearly. You don't learn to talk if you can't hear. Thus, more precise hearing can be most readily tested after 12 months of age. Parents are usually the first to suspect hearing problems. If you are concerned, be sure to have a satisfactory evaluation done.

Blood pressure measurements are not hard to do in older children and should be done at least once.

A word about heart murmurs: The casual statement by a physician that a child has a heart murmur is enough to strike terror into the heart of many parents; some perspective is needed. Certain heart murmurs are *normal* in children! A murmur is just the sound of blood rushing through the heart. In fact, during a fever, during excitement, or after exercise, a heart murmur can be heard in almost any child; this does *not* mean heart disease. Such murmurs occur in the part of the heart cycle known as systole, and are frequently called "innocent" murmurs, "benign" murmurs, or "functional" murmurs. They will usually disappear as the child gets older, although many adults have these murmurs as well. Don't worry about them. If your physician hears a murmur in the diastolic part of the cardiac cycle, or if the child is growing poorly or is blue (cyanotic) or short of breath, then further evaluation will be required and your physician will explain this situation to you. If you are in doubt, ask the doctor if it is an innocent murmur. We have seen serious problems in family interactions develop from a misunderstanding of the statement that a child has a murmur.

Genital examinations are also important. Boys should be checked for undescended testicles and foreskin problems. Girls should be checked for problems with the external genitals. We feel that regular external examination of girls will make the first internal (pelvic) exam seem somewhat less frightening.

There are many other aspects of well-child examinations; almost anything can be noted for the first time at such an examination. Most important problems, however, are noted at home first.

THE FIRST PELVIC EXAMINATION

While hearing and vision are the most important parts of routine childhood examinations, the pelvic examination in girls arouses much concern because of its social and sexual connotations. When should the first pelvic examination be performed? How often are such examinations necessary? Briefly, here are some of the considerations to be taken in reaching this decision.

Pelvic examinations are performed in adult women to detect problems, such as cancer, before they cause symptoms. These problems are so rare in childhood and adolescence that routine pelvic examinations are seldom necessary. There are two exceptions: The first is if the child's mother received a drug called diethylstilbestrol during pregnancy. This drug was used until 1971 fairly widely to help prevent miscarriages. Female children of such pregnancies have occasionally developed cancer of the vagina as early as age eight or nine. The present standard medical recommendation is for yearly pelvic examinations after age eight in these few children. Second, girls who have regular sexual activity at an early age should also begin regular pelvic examinations. Moderate to heavy sexual activity, especially with multiple partners, has been shown to increase the possibility of venereal disease and possibly cancer of the cervix (mouth of the womb).

We feel that the routine of a mature woman should be assumed when regular sexual activity begins. The opportunity to express fears and worries about sex is at least as important as the possibility of detecting disease. We suggest Pap smears every few years until age 25, and more regularly thereafter. If a Pap smear is totally normal, a five-year interval is not unreasonable. If minor abnormalities are noted on a Pap smear, do not exceed two-year intervals. And, if the Pap smear is suspicious of early cancer, follow the recommendations of your doctor closely. Pap smears do *not* detect venereal disease; a special culture is needed.

If a child requires a pelvic examination prior to adolescence, the procedure should be done by the family physician or pediatrician with the mother present.

Returning to the family doctor eliminates the necessity of an introduction to a strange physician and a strange office. Only occasionally will a gynecologist be necessary.

During adolescence, the decision about which doctor to use is more difficult. Some adolescents view their pediatrician as a "baby doctor" and feel that they should go to a gynecologist, internist, or family physician. Of course, many pediatricians spend a great deal of time practicing adolescent gynecology; but the choice should always be left to the young woman. Whoever the doctor is, confidentiality is extremely important. The mother should *not* be present during the examination or during discussions between the doctor and the adolescent, unless requested by the adolescent. Do not demand that either the doctor or your daughter tell you exactly what happened; these are adult problems and conversations and must be treated as such.

You can help the most by providing an explanation of the procedure *before* you get to the doctor's office. Discuss the reasons for the examination and the purpose of each one of its steps. Make it clear that there may be some discomfort, but that there will be no cutting or severe pain. If the procedures are not understood, then fantasies and fears of damage to sexual organs may be aroused. Not only do these make the examination more difficult, but they may result in psychological harm.

The pelvic examination is usually performed by a doctor with a nurse in attendance. Amenities are important. The metal "stirrups" on which the heels rest can be wrapped, and the speculum to be used can be warm. A sheet will usually be placed as a drape over the knees so that the patient feels less exposed.

The full examination consists of inspection of the outside genital parts, palpation (feeling) of the internal organs, inspection of the inside of the vagina, and the taking of a Pap smear, not always in that order. There should be no douche for the preceding 24 hours, as it may make diagnosis of some conditions impossible. Inspection of the outside parts includes the genital lips, the clitoris, and the anal opening. Rashes, sores, small growths, or other problems may be identified.

Palpation of internal organs includes the vagina, the mouth of the womb (cervix), the womb (uterus) itself, and the ovaries. Usually, this is performed with two gloved fingers inserted into the vagina. It can be uncomfortable, but is not painful unless a serious infection is present. Much of the same information can be gained by palpating with a single gloved finger in the rectum, and this may be done in virginal patients. Or, a "bimanual" examination may be performed, with one finger in the rectum and one in the vagina. Uncomfortable, and somewhat undignified, but not painful.

Internal inspection requires a light and a speculum. The speculum is metal or plastic, and gently spreads the walls of the vagina so that the inside may be seen. The speculum is not a clamp, and will not pinch or hurt. It will be lubricated with water or a vaseline-type lubricant so that insertion is easier. Speculums come in several sizes, and smaller ones will be used with young girls or virgins. The procedure should always be performed gently, with all actions explained in advance. The patient can assist by relaxing as much as possible and by taking slow deep breaths.

The Pap smear is performed through the speculum, with a stick similar to a narrow tongue blade. It does not hurt. Some of the secretions are collected on the tip of the stick and examined under a microscope by a pathologist, who classifies the cells seen as normal or malignant. Sometimes a culture will be taken as well. This is a very similar painless procedure except that a cotton swab is used instead of a stick and the secretions are cultured so that any germs present may be identified.

In some parts of the country women are performing their own pelvic examinations in self-help clinics. Medically, this practice seems to work out well, and it is a matter of personal preference.

The manner in which the examination is performed will help you judge the quality of care that you are receiving. The examiner who is abrupt, rough, or doesn't explain is insensitive to a fault. Pelvic examinations are medically essential in many situations, but the examiner who is not sensitive to the complex psychological and human dignity considerations that are involved cannot be giving good medical care.

ROUTINE LABORATORY TESTS FOR CHILDREN

Eye tests and hearing tests are the most important screening examinations for your children. Some of the more common laboratory examinations are discussed below. Except for tuberculosis screening, we do not feel that these tests need to be done routinely for all children; they are needed only for particular children.

Tuberculosis screening. Tuberculosis is still common in some parts of the country, particularly in low-income inner-city areas, and we believe that children in such areas should be routinely screened on an annual basis. Children known to have contacted a person with active tuberculosis should, of course, be immediately evaluated. The current screening test for tuberculosis (the Tine test) is relatively inexpensive, and most pediatricians recommend routine screening every two to three years.

Anemia screening. The best way to screen a child for the most common form of anemia, iron deficiency anemia, is to ask what the child is eating. Children fed a nutritionally balanced diet are almost never iron-deficient. We see iron deficiency anemia most commonly in children about one year old whose diet consists mainly of milk. Milk is low in iron; by one year of age the child should be eating lots of different things. Detection of most other types of anemia at an early age does not help since there are no treatments that need to be started. Hemoglobin is a measure of the amount of protein that carries oxygen in red blood cells. Hematocrit is the percentage of your blood that is composed of red blood cells.

Sickle-cell screening. Sickle-cell *anemia* is a severe genetic blood disease occurring almost entirely in blacks. For a child to have sickle-cell (anemia) *disease*, a sickle gene must have come from each parent; two genes are required. Someone with a single sickle gene is a "carrier" and is referred to as having sickle *trait*; he or she does *not* have anemia. The two-gene disease causes anemia, infections, and other problems; the one-gene trait does not cause any problems and appears to protect the individual from malaria. We believe that sickle-cell screening should be available to adults planning pregnancy who would like to know whether or not they are carriers of a single sickle cell (trait) gene. Sickle-cell disease causes problems in children and it would be most unusual for an adult to have sickle-cell disease without knowing it. Routine screening of children for sickle trait is *not* appropriate since it is not a medical problem. However, parents with known sickle-cell trait (carriers) should have their infants screened since this may result in early detection and treatment of children with sickle-cell disease; we repeat that this disease can occur only if *both* parents have sickle-cell trait. Unnecessary concerns raised by detection of the carrier (trait) individual in mass screening programs have outweighed any benefits of these programs, since there is no need to treat these individuals. Any screening program must have an associated educational component to ensure that anything learned from the program is correctly interpreted by the individual.

Urine screening. Controversy currently surrounds the question of routine urine examinations to detect bacterial infections that are not causing symptoms, especially in girls. Some studies suggest that treatment of these asymptomatic problems is of benefit. Others refute this. We should like to see further studies before making a recommendation. In general, treatment of "diseases" that are not causing trouble often does more harm than good. For children who have had urinary tract infections in the past, a periodic analysis of the urine may well be in order.

Screening for diabetes. Juvenile diabetes mellitus is a different disease from adult-onset diabetes mellitus, and cannot be detected by screening examinations. The first episode will bring the child to the doctor with increased urinary frequency, excessive thirst, nausea and vomiting, shortness of breath, or coma; prior to this time the screening tests are negative.

Rubella (German measles) screening. We recommend rubella screening, once, for preadolescent or adolescent girls who have not received rubella vaccine or had a documented case of rubella. If the test is negative, we recommend rubella immunization.

Cholesterol screening. The blood cholesterol level and heart disease are linked, but an elevated cholesterol is only one of many factors that contribute to heart problems. Children should not be routinely screened for cholesterol. If one of the parents has had a heart attack in his or her thirties, a comprehensive approach to the family will be required. This will include discussions about exercise, cholesterol, diet, stress, and anxieties. We believe that attention to these factors, including a diet moderately low in saturated fats, is indicated for everyone, regardless of the cholesterol level. (See further discussion in Chapter 8.)

All children contract a large number of colds (upper respiratory infections) in the process of growing up. We do not like to consider these episodes as sickness or illness. Many parents are surprised that we would call a three-day episode of a temperature of 100°F, runny nose, and slight cough anything but an illness. The point that we are trying to make is that respiratory infections are a normal part of growing up and actually provide benefits to the child. We regard common respiratory infections in children as a type of immunization. Like other immunizations, viral infections may have side effects, such as fever, runny nose, and cough. And, like most immunizations, many viruses produce no symptoms at all and yet afford lifelong protection against the virus. Children usually fare better with a given viral respiratory illness than adults do.

In careful studies conducted at several university medical centers, infants and young children have been found to develop between six and nine viral infections per year. The older the child, the fewer the number of infections, but even first graders average about six viral episodes per year. We are not usually disturbed by a child who has nine viral infections a year unless these interfere with the child's daily routine or are causing slowing of growth or maturation. Two bouts of pneumonia or two bouts of skin abscesses are more significant medically than nine colds are. In a child who is having frequent illnesses, the question is not so much how frequent, but how serious. (For a further explanation, see the decision chart and discussion in Problem 74, Frequent Illnesses.)

Don't be afraid to send your child to school with the sniffles if he or she feels like going. For most illnesses, the period when the child is most contagious is the period *before* he or she gets sick. It is regrettable that children are often sent home from school at the first sign of a cold; the cold can serve to immunize the other children against that virus. Here's a good general rule: fever, home; no fever, school.

SURGERY

Any recommendation for surgery for your child should be thoroughly discussed with your family physician. You should understand why the operation is being done and the possible implications and complications. In this section, we will discuss some of the more common operations performed on children.

After circumcisions, tonsillectomies and adenoidectomies are the most frequently performed operations in the United States today. Because they are operations on separate organs and because they are done for different reasons, they will be discussed separately.

Tonsillectomy

The tonsils are located on both sides of the back of the throat, and can be seen quite easily when your child's mouth is open. Tonsils consist of lymphoid tissue, which is useful in fighting infections. Because children between the ages of four to seven develop so many colds (upper respiratory infections), the tonsils are largest in this age group. It is important to remember that large tonsils are a natural process; they are enlarged because they are busy fighting infection. Occasionally, the tonsils themselves may become infected, but only when there is an infection of the entire throat.

Removing a child's tonsils does *not* reduce a child's chances of developing a sore throat. Nor does it reduce a child's chances of developing a cold. Nor does it reduce a child's chances of developing an ear infection. Then why are so many tonsillectomies done in this country? This is indeed a difficult question to answer, since every carefully performed study in the past 45 years has demonstrated the futility of removing tonsils to eliminate sore throats or any of the consequences of sore throats. And several hundred children die each year as a result of tonsillectomies.

There are, of course, some indications for tonsillectomy. If the tonsils are so large that they are interfering with the child's breathing, the tonsils should be removed; this condition is, however, exceedingly rare. When such airway blockage occurs, it is the heart and lungs that are put under stress and the problem is detected by evaluation of the heart and lungs. Merely looking at the tonsils will not reveal obstruction to breathing; many normal tonsils nearly touch in the midline of the throat. Although we have never seen it occur, it is conceivable that very large tonsils may interfere with eating or swallowing; this may also require their removal. In addition, if a serious abscess occurs in one of the tonsils, it is likely that this abscess will recur; this may be prevented by a tonsillectomy.

Adenoidectomy

Tonsillectomies have been traditionally accompanied by adenoidectomies. So long as a patient was going to be placed under anesthesia, the physician often decided to remove the adenoids as well. The adenoids, however, are located in a different region and have their own functions. Adenoids can create problems and there are indications for removing adenoids. However, removal of adenoids when only a tonsillectomy is indicated will increase the risks of a bad result from the operation. In addition, removing adenoids can lead to ear problems in certain children.

The adenoids also contain lymphoid tissue. They cannot be seen by looking at the throat; they are in the back of the nose above the palate and near the opening of the (eustachian) tube that drains the middle-ear secretions into the nasal passages. Adenoids enlarge as they fight infection in the upper respiratory tract. If they become too large, they can block the opening of the eustachian tube and increase the likelihood of an ear infection.

An adenoidectomy may be considered in a child who has had frequent bouts of ear infections. If the ear infections are caused by allergy, children generally do not profit from an adenoidectomy. Children who may potentially profit can be identified by X-ray studies, and all children who are being considered for an adenoidectomy, in our opinion, should have such studies done beforehand. Some children will actually be made worse by an adenoidectomy and it is sometimes possible to identify these children before the operation.

Severe obstruction of breathing or interference with speech may also be indications for considering removal of the adenoids.

Again, if an adenoidectomy is indicated, there is no need to remove the tonsils during the operation.

Ear Tubes

Ear tubes are small plastic tubes that are inserted through the child's eardrums. They are placed in children who have frequent bouts of earaches in order to provide adequate drainage of the middle-ear chamber. Drainage aids the healing process and prevents the middle-ear chamber from becoming sealed off; an ear infection cannot develop unless the normal drainage is blocked.

The placement of ear tubes is a very simple procedure and is done in the office without anesthesia, usually after the summer season is over. Indications for ear tubes include (1) recurrent ear infections that have not responded to medical therapy including prophylactic sulfisoxazole (Gantrisin), and (2) presence in the middle-ear chamber of material too thick to drain under normal conditions.

Repair of Umbilical Hernia

An umbilical hernia results from the failure of stomach muscles to grow together in the area surrounding the belly button. Umbilical hernias are very common in black children, but do not pose any risk. Generally, the hernia disappears within the first few years of life, and most others slowly heal themselves by the time the child is of school age. Since these hernias are of no risk to the patient and since they usually heal by themselves, we do not advocate surgical repair except in rare cases where cosmetic improvement is psychologically important. In general, time is a better and safer healer than a scalpel.

Undescended Testicles

It is not uncommon to find that one or both of your boy's testicles are not in the scrotal sac. The testicles are often in the inguinal canal, located just above the scrotal sac. One of the most common reasons for the testicles to find their way *out* of the scrotal sac is because of the presence of an examiner's cold hands. Occasionally, the testicles may withdraw all the way into the abdominal cavity. (This is a feat that can also be accomplished voluntarily by some Japanese wrestlers.)

Testicles that are permanently located within the abdominal cavity should be brought down surgically. Physicians differ as to their recommendations for the best time for operation, but the procedure should be done somewhere between five and eight years of age.

It is of the utmost importance to determine whether the testicles can or cannot descend into the scrotal sac normally. The best way to decide this is to have your child sit with legs crossed (the Buddha or lotus position) and check for presence of the testicles within the scrotal sac in that position. We do not recommend hormonal treatment for bringing testicles into the scrotal sac; usually it doesn't help and may have side effects.

Hydrocele or Hernia

Hydroceles and inguinal hernias both cause swelling of the scrotal sac in boys. It is difficult to tell the two apart, and a physician's visit will be necessary.

A hydrocele is a fluid sac within the scrotal sac and is often present in newborn boys. The fluid does not create any problem for the child and will be reabsorbed in time. Some physicians prefer to remove the fluid from the scrotal sac with a needle. Nature will work just as well, though not as quickly.

An inguinal hernia will also cause a swelling in the scrotal sac. Hernias generally first appear *after* the newborn period and often following a vigorous bout of crying. Severe problems can result from inguinal hernias, because a hernia is a small portion of the child's bowel that has found its way through the canal and into the scrotal sac. Unlike inguinal hernias in adults, which physicians are able to feel on examination, hernias in children can only be evaluated when the scrotal sac is swollen, and the child should be seen by a physician at a time when the sac is swollen.

Appendectomy

Appendicitis is discussed in Problem 84, Acute Abdominal Pain.

Circumcision

Circumcision is discussed in Chapter 2 (see pp. 28–29).

Chapter

8

Staying Healthy

This chapter presents, as simply and clearly as possible, the groundwork for a healthy life. Some of this information you already know, and much of it you have heard before. We realize that most of our readers will rely heavily on Part II of this book, in order to respond promptly and appropriately to new medical problems and to save time and money. This chapter is less dramatic. But overall, the measures recommended here are the most important health investment that you can make. We believe that the best approach to dealing with serious problems is to prevent them. This chapter discusses four major problem areas in which prevention is essential: accidents, immunizations, dental care, and the diseases of adult life.

ACCIDENTS

Accidents are the number-one threat to your child's health. More children are seriously injured or die as a result of accidents than the combined attacks of cancer, infectious diseases, and birth defects. In adolescents, accidents and other violence (homicide and suicide) account for more than 70 percent of the deaths in this age group.

Young children spend most of their time at home; this provides them with the greatest opportunity for getting into mischief. Here is a checklist to help you evaluate the safety of your home. You should review this important list every year. Remember that as children grow the opportunities for accidents increase. You must keep one step ahead of your child at all times. Before you know it, crawlers become climbers and they will be able to get up to that previously unreachable cabinet.

The Kitchen

- Are oven cleaners and other caustic materials, such as drain cleaners, locked or placed out of reach?

- Are pot handles routinely kept away from the edges of the stove?

- Are the electric cord extenders on appliances such as coffee makers removed from the socket immediately after use?

- Are ant poisons and insect sprays out of reach?

- Are electric irons kept away from children?

The Bathroom

- Are razor blades discarded safely?

- Are all medicines kept locked or out of reach?

- Are all prescription drugs left over from an illness flushed down the toilet?

- Are bathroom cleansers locked up or out of reach?

The Living Room

- Are electric cords in good repair?

- Is the fireplace adequately screened?

- Are containers that hold combustible liquid used in the fireplace kept out of reach?

- Are fire extinguishers appropriately located in the house and ready to use?

- Is there a fire alarm system?

- Are electric sockets not in use covered?

- Is there a guardrail around space heaters, Franklin stoves, and similar devices?

- Are children instructed in a fire exit plan?

- Beware of poisonous plants such as poinsetta leaves, daffodil bulbs, and castor beans.

The Nursery

- Does the crib have no more than two and one-half inches between slats so that the baby's head cannot become wedged between them?

- Are all cords (from Venetian blinds, mobiles, etc.) that could become tangled around the baby's neck kept away from the area of the crib?

- Are crib mattresses and bumpers of the correct size and fastened so that the baby's head cannot be wedged between them and the crib frame?

The Bedroom

- Are cosmetics and perfumes kept out of the reach of children?

- Is shoe polish kept out of reach?

The Dining Room

- Are children kept away from dangling tablecloths when a hot meal is on the table?

The Children's Room

- Do toys have sharp edges?

- Do toys have small parts that can easily be removed and swallowed by young children? Have old broken toys been discarded?

- Are windows in rooms above the ground floor closed or protected so that children cannot fall?

- Is there a fire escape from which children can easily fall?

- Is model glue kept away from toddlers?

The Yard and Garage

- Are children kept away from rotary lawnmowers when in use?

- Do rotary lawnmowers have protective shields?

- Are solvents in the garage kept away from children's reach?

- Are pesticides, fertilizers, and snail bait stored away from children?

- Are turpentine and paint products stored away from children and in their original containers? (*Caution*: Never use soda bottles.)

- Is your yard free from poisonous plants (such as oleander, scotch broom, etc.)? Your local nursery will generally be glad to help you out with plant identification and safety if you have any questions.

- Is there an old refrigerator or freezer in which children could play?

Although the child spends the most time within the home, there can be an increased risk of accidents away from home. The surroundings are unfamiliar, and families without children or with older children often have hazards not present in homes with young children.

While it is important to make your child's environment as safe as possible, it is also important for the child to gain experience with his or her environment and to learn to make personal safety decisions. This requires a testing of the environment and some painful experiences. The adult world is not totally safe, and there are perils in both underprotection and overprotection. Common sense is the best guide.

Automobiles

Automobile accidents are the number-one killers of children. There is absolutely nothing more important for your child's health than protection in the automobile. Drive prudently and use seat belts or safety restraints. The average infant or child seat costs just a bit more than the average physician's office visit, and can be used for years for many children and then passed on to a friend or relative. It is the number-one health bargain of all time.

In selecting an infant or child seat be sure that you understand how it must be installed. Many require anchoring that will involve placing a bolt through the floor. Seats that require anchoring are ineffective if installed improperly. It is also important to consider convenience. Some parents have found highly recommended seats so complicated to use that they were forced to buy a different seat. Remember, the best seat will not protect your child if it is not used. Be sure you understand proper usage before buying any restraining seat.

Currently recommended infant seats (for children under a year) are as follows.

- *The General Motors Infant Love Seat.* This is a very convenient seat. It can easily be removed from the car to double as a home infant seat without waking a sleeping baby.

- *The Petersen Safety Shell.* This is convertible for older children. However, since most families have more than one child, the Petersen shell requires the purchase of another seat later. Some parents have found this seat inconvenient.

Currently recommended children's seats are as follows. *The Strolee Wee Care Car Seat 597S* is the children's seat recommended by *Consumer Reports*. It can also be converted into an infant carrier but *Consumer Reports* tested the seat for its use as a child carrier. The next highest rated group of child safety restraints (in alphabetical order) are the *Century Motor-toter, General Motors Child Love Seat, Swyngomatic American Safety Seat 300,* and *Teddy Tot Astroseat V.*

Harnesses, seat belts, and shoulder straps can be used for older children. Children over 40 pounds can use seat belts. Children under four-and-a-half feet tall should not use shoulder straps since they can cause neck injuries. Place the strap behind the child. The best way to teach a child to use a seat belt is to use one yourself; the child will quickly learn that when you enter a car, you automatically put on a seat belt.

Additional information can be obtained from the June 1977 issue of *Consumer Reports* which can be ordered from Consumers Union, 256 Washington Street, Mount Vernon, New York 10550 ($1.00 each). Additional groups concerned with child automobile safety who have helpful information include Physicians for Automotive Safety, 50 Union Avenue, Irvington, New Jersey 07111; and The Action for Child Transportation Safety, 400 Central Park West, Room 15P, New York, N.Y. 10025.

Finally, an extra word of caution must be added about leaving small children in cars during shopping trips. Families who would never leave pills or solvents in reach of children at home often leave them unattended in cars with shopping bags full of these same dangerous products. Although safety caps on both pills and solvents have decreased the risk, children display remarkable ingenuity in removing these "childproof" caps. In addition, remember that children can suffocate in an enclosed car. NEVER LEAVE SMALL CHILDREN ALONE IN A CAR!

Bicycles

A bicycle is a friend, companion, horse, source of transportation, and source of exercise. With the recent bicycle boom, bicycles have become a means of transportation and exercise for many adults as well. For the past several years, bicycles have outsold automobiles in this country. It is important that a child learn the basic principles of bicycle safety. Here again, the principles that a child learns with a bicycle will provide lifelong benefits for general and automotive safety as well.

There are many excellent books about bicycle safety that can be purchased for children. However, parents' lessons are the ones that are best remembered, and books should be used in order to supplement, not substitute for, parents' teaching. You will want to teach your children the following: How fast can the bicycle be ridden safely? How fast is too fast going down a hill? How quickly can the bicycle stop when the brakes are applied? Remember, bicycles traveling at faster speeds require a much greater distance in order to stop. Can the child interpret and obey traffic signs and signals? Is the bicycle ready to ride? Children should be taught to check the handlebars, the tires, and the brakes before beginning a ride. Do children ride on streets where it is safe? If they ride on the sidewalk, are they careful of adults and other small children? Are they careful about riding near automobiles where doors may suddenly open? Are they careful when riding around small children and animals?

As parents, you will be familiar with the local hazards of your neighborhood. Teaching a child how to balance a bicycle is not enough. You must also teach the child how to safely maneuver the bicycle. And you teach a child to stop at stop signs by doing so yourself.

Even with good safety preparation, bicycle accidents will occur. "Spider" bicycles with small front wheels and big handlebars are notorious for children flying over the handlebars and hitting their heads. We discourage the purchase of such bicycles. First bicycles should be simple and sturdy; the flashy accessories won't last long anyway. Many parents move the child to sophisticated multi-speed bicycles far too early. Only after the child has learned to care for a simple bike and is ready for a permanent adult-size bicycle do we think that this investment should be made.

Adult bicyclists who carry children on their bicycles should use a rear-mounted child seat with a safety strap and side panels. Wheel covers will prevent foot-in-spoke injuries.

Drowning

Children and water are a natural combination. The beach, swimming pool, bathtub, and lake offer more opportunities for fun than all the toys ever invented. However, water tragedies are all too common.

Young children must be watched carefully near water. It is easy for parents to fall asleep while lying on a beach or at poolside, and fatal consequences for children have followed even short lapses in supervision. More and more classes are being offered in infant swimming for children as young as six months of age.

While these classes do not actually teach infants how to swim, they do teach them to kick sufficiently to get to the surface. This will help if a child falls into the far side of the pool with the parent watching. The infant can reach the surface and kick long enough for the parent to reach the child. Drownings also occur frequently in bathtubs. Use your common sense in deciding when your child is old enough to be left alone in the tub.

It is important for all children to learn how to swim. The local YMCA, the local Red Cross, and many other organizations provide these services either free or at minimal cost. If you yourself are a competent swimmer, you will enjoy the time spent in teaching your child how to swim. Water safety is as important as bicycle or automotive safety. Children should be taught never to swim by themselves and never to go too far from the shore without at least one experienced adult swimmer.

We prefer to talk about prevention. Yet it is important to know what to do if you are first on the scene at a drowning. The techniques for resuscitation of a drowned child cannot be learned by reading a few pages in a book. The Red Cross, in all parts of the country, offers an eight-hour multimedia safety course that we recommend highly to all individuals interested in being able to deal with emergency situations themselves.

Pets

Every year, thousands of children are bitten, sometimes severely, by dogs. Very few of these dog bites are by vicious dogs or dogs with rabies. Most often the bite comes from the friendly old dog next door, Phred, who hadn't done anything more energetic in the past few years than wag his tail while lying on his back. The friendliest dogs bite children. It is not because the dog is having a grumpy day. Almost invariably it is because the dog has been threatened by the child in some fashion.

Children and their parents are too often unaware of what constitutes good pet safety. It is natural for small children to be afraid of dogs. Even medium-sized dogs tower over toddlers and weigh as much as seven- or eight-year-olds. It is the parent's responsibility to teach a child how to act around dogs, even if the family does not own one, since all children come in frequent contact with dogs. Here are some hints to help prevent bites.

Explain to children that they should not squeal in loud, high squeeky voices around dogs. Dogs have sensitive ears to high tones and loud squeeky noises will often terrify dogs, who then react in order to protect themselves. Teach children not to make sudden moves around dogs. These may be interpreted as attacks and dogs may react to defend themselves. At other times, a dog will respond to a quick move in a playful fashion. Dogs, when playing with each other, can be seen to nip at each other in fun. (Parents and children do not consider dog nipping as much fun. This is a cultural difference between dogs and humans.) Obviously, children should not wave sticks or throw stones around dogs. Again, the dog may feel an attack is imminent or may try to retrieve the stick out of the hands of the child. Children should be cautious about running behind lying or sitting dogs. Most dogs have their tails stepped on too frequently and may react to protect them. Children should be taught how to approach a dog. The child should approach the dog slowly, allow the dog to sniff his or her hand for a few seconds while talking calmly, and then proceed to pet the dog gently.

Finally, let's protect the puppies too. Small children often love puppies, and because the child is bigger, most parents consider this a safe relationship. However, children of two, three, and even four often delight in swinging a puppy by the tail and throwing it. This type of puppy abuse may produce a very nervous or even vicious older dog. Remember also that since dogs grow more quickly than children do, the abused puppy may become a vicious adult dog in several short months, and the child will suffer. In general, we feel that five should be considered a minimal age for a child to get his or her own puppy. Children should be old enough to demonstrate responsibility in keeping up with the routines of feeding, grooming, and cleaning up after their pets before being given the responsibility of caring for them. Parents remember the joys of their own childhood pet and tend to rush into getting pets for their own children too early. This can convert a joyous situation into a troublesome one.

IMMUNIZATIONS

Infectious diseases were historically the most significant wasters of human life, but now have been controlled by many methods including improved nutrition of the population, improved sanitation, improved housing, and, more recently, the development of immunizations and antibiotics. Immunizations are undoubtedly the most significant contribution of science to the control of disease. Smallpox has virtually been eliminated from the face of the earth in the past decade by the worldwide campaign of the World Health Organization. Polio, which used to cripple 20,000 a year in the early 1950s, now affects only a handful of children a year in this country, thanks to immunization campaigns.

We are now in a critical period in this nation's history with regard to immunizations. Many people have become complacent about immunization because of the rarity of the diseases that immunizations have aided in eliminating. In addition, the recent swine influenza controversy has undermined the confidence of many in immunizations and raised questions in the minds of many parents. There have always been problems in the use of immunizations. However, the risks of the vaccines are usually minimal when compared with the risks of the disease. Because we feel immunizations are so vital to the health of children, we have chosen to elaborate on the issues rather fully in the following pages.

Avoiding an illness often presents many practical problems. Since the bacteria and viruses responsible for causing infectious illnesses may be spread by contact with people, with animals, or with airborne droplets, avoidance is often impossible. On the other hand, protection by the use of immunizations is a practical solution.

The principle of immunization is to develop your body's defense system to a point where it is capable of foiling any attack by a particular agent. To accomplish this, a small dose of the modified infectious agent is given. For some immunizations, the virus has been modified in a laboratory so that it causes a very mild infection. Other immunizations use a dead virus that is chemically the same but cannot infect. Others inject just a part of the viral organism. The body's defense system builds up an immunity to this part, which in effect creates an immunity to the whole infecting agent. Still another method of immunizing involves substituting a related virus, which causes a much milder infection. This technique is used for smallpox, where the individual is inoculated with cow pox in order to prevent infection with smallpox.

The practice of immunization dates back several thousand years to attempts by a Chinese monk to prevent smallpox. Immunization methods were developed long before the nature of the infecting agents was known. Jenner, who is credited with the modern development of immunization in the late eighteenth century, borrowed the idea from English farmers who had been utilizing cow pox to protect themselves from smallpox for centuries. Jenner merely performed a study validating what the farmers had been doing for years.

Immunizations have been developed to combat some of the most devastating illnesses affecting human life. Remember, however, that immunizations are only one of the ways of defending against illness. Persons in good health are less likely to be devastated by infectious disease than persons in poor health. Many diseases, such as tuberculosis, have been steadily decreasing in frequency because of improved nutrition, sanitation, and medical care.

Modern virological techniques allow the manufacture of vaccines effective against many illnesses. But all immunizations carry with them the possibility of side effects due to the immunization itself. No immunization is 100-percent effective or 100-percent safe.

If you have questions about a particular immunization, your physician or health department should be willing to explain in detail the current risks, benefits, and recommendations for that immunization. If you are not satisfied with the explanation, you may turn to any of the following groups: (1) The Academy of Pediatrics, Committee on Infectious Diseases, Evanston, Illinois; (2) The United States Department of Health, Education and Welfare, Public Health Service, Center for Disease Control, Atlanta, Georgia 30333; (3) Advisory Committee on Immunization Practices, United States Public Health Service; (4) Council on Environmental Health, American Medical Association, Chicago, Illinois.

Questions you may have about a particular immunization include: (1) How effective is this immunization? (2) What are the possible side effects? (3) Who is likely to experience a side effect? (4) Will persons in contact with the immunized person also become immunized? (5) How long does the immunity last? (6) Is the immunization safe for pregnant mothers? (7) Is the immunization safe to give children if their mother is pregnant? (8) Is the immunizing agent free of contaminating substances?

The DPT or Three-In-One Shot

The DPT shot is a single injection that gives immunity against diphtheria, pertussis (whooping cough), and tetanus. The combination injection works as effectively as three separate shots and hurts less. We will discuss them separately.

Diphtheria

Nature of the illness. At this time, there are about 300 reported cases of diphtheria each year in the United States and probably far more than that are not reported. Diphtheria affects the throat, nose, and skin and is contagious. Complications of diphtheria include paralysis (in approximately 20 percent of patients) and heart damage (in approximately 50 percent). Diphtheria can be treated by a combination of penicillin and serum injections. However, despite treatment, approximately 10 percent of persons who acquire diphtheria will die from it. Only immunization can successfully prevent diphtheria.

Nature of the immunization. Diphtheria immunization has been available since 1920. A portion of the toxin (the chemical product of the bacteria that causes damage) is altered with formalin to render it harmless. This modified toxin, known as a toxoid, stimulates the body's defense system to produce an antitoxin. Immunity persists for many years after several inoculations. Although the person may come in contact with bacteria and even become infected with it, the toxin will be neutralized by the antitoxin within the person's body and the infection will cause no harm.

Reactions to diphtheria toxoid are extremely uncommon. Generally, they are limited to a slight swelling at the injection site. This reaction can be decreased in older children and adults by giving lower concentrations of toxoid, known as "adult-type" diphtheria toxoid.

Diphtheria toxoid should be begun (in combination with pertussis and tetanus) at the age of two months. The primary schedule consists of three immunizations given several months apart in the first year of life. A booster shot should be given one year later. An additional booster shot should be given when the child enters school and every ten years thereafter.

Pertussis (Whooping Cough)

Nature of the illness. Pertussis is a bacterial infection with a high mortality among infants. It causes extremely long and severe bouts of coughing. The prolonged coughing so robs the child of air that the child breathes in violently, causing a whooping sound. Pertussis is contagious. It can be treated with antibiotics with some success.

Nature of the immunization. Pertussis vaccine has been administered for the past 30 years. The vaccine consists of killed pertussis bacteria. There have been recent changes in the vaccine that may increase its effectiveness. There is some controversy about the pertussis vaccine because of the frequency of side effects. The concern over the safety of the vaccine stems from reported neurological side effects, described for more than 40 years and consisting primarily of convulsions. The risk of a convulsion is small and ranges from 1 in 6000 to 1 in 100,000. However, there are numerous reasons for convulsions in children within the first six months of life, and some of the convulsions attributed to pertussis vaccine have occurred days to months later. But many convulsions occur within 24 hours after immunization and many experts feel that convulsions occurring within several days must be considered at least in part due to the vaccine.

We feel that pertussis is an effective though not an ideal vaccine. We advise parents to go ahead with pertussis vaccinations, after discussion with their own physician, and to follow future reports on the safety and effectiveness of this vaccine. Children who develop high temperatures (greater than 103°F) or convulsions or extreme somnolence (sleepiness) after one pertussis vaccination should not have any more. Such children should receive the DT immunization without the P. Some physicians now question the use of pertussis boosters in older children.

Tetanus (Lockjaw)

Nature of the illness. Tetanus is a dangerous illness. The tetanus bacteria and its spores are found everywhere; they are present in dust, soil, pastures, and human and animal waste. Symptoms consist of severe muscle spasm, often of the neck and jaw muscles, causing lockjaw. The symptoms are caused by toxin produced by the bacteria. The tetanus bacteria grows only in the absence of air, so wounds that are created by punctures or sharp objects, possibly introducing bacteria underneath the skin, are the wounds with the greatest likelihood of causing tetanus. After tetanus develops, it may be treated with antibiotics and tetanus immune globulin, but mortality may still be as high as 40 percent. Tetanus can and should be prevented by immunization.

Nature of the immunization. Tetanus is one of our best immunizations. The tetanus immunization is a toxin that is produced by the tetanus bacterium and modified in the laboratory so that it has very little of its toxic potential. Of all the vaccines available, tetanus comes closest to 100-percent effectiveness after the initial series of shots. Local reactions are rare and usually cause only mild discomfort for a short time. Severe local reactions can occur if too many shots are received; this phenomenon was frequently seen in military recruits who received unneeded immunizations. Tetanus shots are needed only every ten years unless a particularly dirty wound is suffered. (See Problem 5, Tetanus Shots.) Maintain your own records of your child's immunizations; do not rely solely on the physician, health department, or clinic where the immunizations are given.

Reactions to the DPT shot

Reactions sometimes occur. There may be slight swelling at the injection site. Other symptoms such as fussiness, loss of appetite, mild irritability, and slight fever commonly occur several hours after the injection. Acetaminophen or aspirin can offer relief; convulsions are very rare and should be reported immediately.

Polio

Nature of the illness. Polio is a contagious viral illness and a devastating disease that was familiar to almost everyone a few years ago. Besides the paralytic form, which crippled tens of thousands as recently as the 1950s and caused more than 1000 deaths annually, polio also causes meningitis and respiratory infections. There are no antibiotics that are effective against polio. The only way to prevent polio is through immunization.

Nature of the immunization. In 1956, Dr. Jonas Salk introduced the inactivated polio virus vaccine (IPV). This injected vaccine caused a dramatic decline in the frequency of polio in this country. In 1961, the Sabin vaccine was introduced, in which live polio virus was prepared in such a way as to markedly weaken it. This live polio virus vaccine is known as the oral polio virus vaccine (OPV) because it can be taken by mouth. It was initially felt to be preferable because it activated the body's defense system in the upper respiratory tract and reduced the chances of an immunized person spreading a live virus.

There are other advantages to the oral polio virus vaccine. Longer-lasting immunity eliminates the need for repeated booster doses once the basic series is completed. And the record of the oral polio virus vaccine is outstanding. In this country, in 1975, only eight cases of polio were reported.

The problem with oral polio virus vaccine is its rare side effects. One or two persons out of 10 million will develop paralytic polio. With present knowledge, the injected polio virus vaccine does not cause paralytic polio. But many of the people who developed paralytic polio after the oral vaccine had rare diseases that predisposed them to developing the infection. A recent court decision finding the vaccine manufacturer liable for damage caused to a recipient will undoubtedly have a future policy impact. It is possible that the injected polio vaccine will be brought back, and that parents will be given a choice of vaccine for their children. The American Academy of Pediatrics has recently revised its recommendations, which listed oral polio virus vaccine as the only acceptable vaccine, and now regards either vaccine as acceptable. Breast feeding does not interfere with the oral polio vaccine.

Have your child vaccinated against polio. The risks of either vaccine are small compared with the risks of the disease.

Measles

Nature of the illness. Measles is one of the "usual" childhood diseases, but is potentially much more serious than the others. It is by no means a mild disease to be passed off as a ritual of childhood. Before the 1966 introduction of an improved measles vaccination, there were 400 deaths annually due to measles. Far more often than causing death, measles causes devastating complications such as brain infection, pneumonia, convulsions, and blindness. In 1976, there were 37,000 reported cases of measles in this country and undoubtedly many more unreported cases. This is extremely disturbing, since it represents a 60-percent increase over 1975 figures when less than 25,000 cases were reported. And the increase continues.

Even uncomplicated cases of measles can be serious (see Problem 54, Measles). Fortunately, most infants are protected against measles during the first few months of life because of antibodies that they received from their mother's blood, if the mother has had measles. This immunity wears off by the fourth month of life.

Nature of the immunization. The first measles virus vaccine became available in 1963. This vaccine contained a dead virus, but the weakened live virus vaccine introduced in 1966 is far more effective. Reactions to measles virus vaccine have been minimal, and may not appear for five to ten days. Symptoms generally consist of fever, mild irritability, or rash.

Measles vaccinations have been suspected of causing exacerbation of tuberculosis. Ideally, a tuberculosis skin test should be done prior to a measles vaccination. This is usually not done in practice because many physicians question this finding and because tuberculosis is very rare in a young child. The most widely used vaccine today is the Schwarz strain, which causes a rash in an estimated 5 percent of children and fever in an estimated 15 percent of children. Although there has been concern over the possibility of allergic reactions in children allergic to eggs, no adverse effects have yet been reported.

The vaccine is most effective when given after the first year of life. Previous recommendations were to vaccinate at twelve months; approximately 90 percent of one-year-old children receiving vaccine will be adequately protected. Current recommendations are to immunize children later, at age 15 months, when the percentage protected is even higher. During epidemics, younger children should be vaccinated against measles. Protective antibody is developed within seven days and the incubation period of measles is 10 days, so that children brought to the physician immediately after exposure to a case of measles will be afforded protection by immunization. Children known to have been exposed several days earlier can still be given passive immunization in the form of measles immune globulin. Children who receive immunizations before the age of one year should be reimmunized after the age of 15 months. Children who were immunized before 1966 were immunized with the inactivated strain and may still be susceptible to measles. These children should be revaccinated with the live attenuated strain.

Rubella (German Measles)

Nature of the illness. Rubella, as well as rubella immunization, provides us with a set of very difficult decisions. Rubella is a mild illness, usually with a mild fever and a mild rash. Many people do not even know they have had the illness. The danger from rubella lies in the risk to a developing fetus during early pregnancy.

In 1964, during the last rubella epidemic in this country, more than 20,000 children were born with deformities caused by the rubella virus. The deformities included heart defects, blindness, and deafness. While many fetuses escape these devastating effects, the huge number who have suffered greatly make efforts at eliminating this disease worthwhile.

Nature of the immunization. The purpose of a rubella immunization program is to prevent pregnant women from becoming infected. Before rubella immunization became possible in 1969, over 80 percent of women had already been infected and therefore were not at risk of producing an infant deformed by rubella. Women who have had rubella infections can become reinfected with rubella the second, third, or even fourth time, but it is doubtful that these reinfections pose any threat to the fetus. It is presently assumed, though not proven, that only the initial infection with rubella can damage the fetus.

A rubella immunization program was undertaken in this country in 1969 for several reasons. The most compelling reason was that rubella epidemics run in seven- to ten-year cycles and the next epidemic was expected soon. In order to avert the epidemic, widespread community compaigns were conducted. By immunizing at least two thirds of the population, it was hoped that the entire population would be protected (so-called herd immunity). Unfortunately, even in communities in which 95 percent of the population has been immunized, introduction of the virus has been shown to result in infection of the remaining five percent.

It was decided to immunize children over the age of one year, hoping that the mothers would be protected by immunizing the children. This was a unique policy in the annals of immunization practice; for the first time, individuals were being exposed to vaccination and its complications in order to protect other individuals. This may or may not have been a reasonable policy. Supporters point to the fact that the expected epidemic did not occur. However, we are currently not certain how long the protective level of the immunizations will last. Some studies indicate that immunity may eventually be lost. If the protection does not remain sufficiently high to interfere with the production of deformities, then we may be producing a generation of women who will be susceptible at childbearing ages. Remember that in the past, more than 80 percent of the population was immune at childbearing age. Is it possible that the next epidemic will be even more devastating because a larger number of women will be susceptible?

Other countries have adopted a different policy and only vaccinate teenage girls who are shown by blood test to have no protection against rubella. Vaccination of males doesn't seem to make much sense, since "herd" immunity does not work. The policy of vaccinating teenage women diminishes the chance that the immunity will fall to such a low level that it will not be protective in the childbearing years.

But there are problems with adopting a policy of late immunization. Side effects from the immunization are much more common at this age. Particularly troublesome are the joint pains that occur in over ten percent of women receiving the vaccination during adolescence or later. Some of these women have had arthritis for as long as 24 months following immunization. In addition, a few women (between 1 in 500 and 1 in 10,000) experience a peripheral neuropathy (a sensation of tingling created by an inflammation in the nerves of the hands).

An additional risk in administering the vaccine in older women is the possibility of pregnancy at the time of vaccination. Although none have occurred yet, rubella vaccine may possibly cause birth defects if given to pregnant women! Thus far, no congenital anomalies have been reported in women whose *children* were given rubella vaccine. It is probably safe to immunize the children of pregnant women, although it is not advised. A policy of immunizing women of childbearing age requires adequate contraception for two to four months following immunization.

Fortunately, a major rubella outbreak has not occurred since 1964. This has been a worldwide phenomenon both in countries immunizing infants and in countries immunizing only teenage females. We assume that the predicted epidemic has in part been avoided by the use of rubella immunization. We recommend the continued immunization of women before pregnancy, if a blood test shows no antibodies. We also recommend carefully following future information on rubella immunizations.

Mumps

Nature of the illness. Mumps is a contagious viral illness. It infects and causes swelling of the salivary glands. Swelling can be on one or both sides and is often painful. Meningo-encephalitis (inflammation of the brain and its coverings) occurs but is far less frequent and less serious than with measles. The greatest concern about mumps is the possibility of inflammation of the testes in males and of the ovaries in females. Inflammation of the ovaries is far less frequent than inflammation of the testes. Inflammation of the testes is usually one-sided, and although it is commonly believed that it can result in sterility, this is very seldom the case.

Nature of the immunization. The mumps vaccine is a live weakened virus and is one of the most recently developed immunizations. Its long-term effects are not known. Exposure to the mumps virus usually gives two types of protection. One type of protection is carried by the blood serum, and the other type is carried by the white blood cells. It is too early to tell whether the mumps immunization will provide long-lasting protection of both types. The possibility exists that the white cell immunity will persist while serum immunity will not, and that reexposure to mumps virus may produce a more severe form of the disease.

It seems reasonable to immunize only those at greatest risk for serious consequences of the illness—that is, adolescent males and females who never had mumps, where the potential for testicular or ovarian inflammation exists, and even this is optional. At this time, we do not advocate immunizing all children for mumps. Many health departments do not charge for DPT shots, oral polio virus vaccine, and measles and rubella shots, but mumps immunizations usually cost because of these uncertainties.

Smallpox

Smallpox, a disease that has killed millions of people over the centuries, is about to become an illness discussed only in history books.

Nature of the immunization. Smallpox vaccinations are no longer given in the United States. The recommendation to discontinue smallpox vaccinations was made more than five years ago for several reasons. First, smallpox has not been introduced in this country for more than 20 years. Second, the last cases of smallpox, introduced in the city of New York, were quickly controlled without any spread of the disease. Third, the risks of the vaccination are significant and children have developed severe skin lesions, blindness, and even death following smallpox vaccination.

Smallpox vaccinations are not required for travel in most countries. They are not required for travel anywhere in North America. Small pockets of smallpox remain only in Ethiopia. However, several countries still do require smallpox vaccinations, and you should consult the United States Public Health Service, local health department, consulates of the countries you intend to visit, or the World Health Organization for travel recommendations.

Influenza

Nature of the illness. Influenza is a respiratory tract infection caused by the influenza virus that produces severe muscular symptoms as well. There are many illnesses that may mimic influenza, and the term influenza is applied liberally to many syndromes involving cough, cold, and muscle aches.

Nature of the immunization. Influenza virus vaccines are live weakened viral vaccines. They are recommended only for children who have chronic illnesses, particularly respiratory and cardiac diseases.

One of the long-term benefits of the media coverage of the swine influenza controversy of 1976 will be to sensitize the public to the complexities involved in making rational medical decisions. On the other hand, it is our hope that individuals will not be dissuaded from obtaining vaccines with a long history of demonstrated safety and effectiveness in preventing serious illness.

Rabies

Nature of the illness. Rabies is a viral illness that is transmitted in the saliva of wild and domestic animals with rabies; it is fatal if not treated. Animals known to be significant carriers of rabies include skunks, bats, and foxes. Rabies in dogs and cats does occur but has become rare. Rabies is rare in rodents such as squirrels, chipmunks, mice, and rats. Fortunately, there are only one or two cases of rabies in humans reported in this country each year. See Problem 3 (Animal Bites).

Nature of the immunization. Both attenuated rabies vaccine and antirabies serum are available. The complex methods of administering these vaccines will not be discussed here. Immediate cleansing of any animal wound is the first line of defense. Bites from wild animals or unknown domestic animals should be reported to a physician immediately.

Immunization Schedule

Those are the details; here is the bottom line. Below is the current immunization schedule that we recommend.

Age			
2 months	DPT (diphtheria, pertussis, tetanus)	and	Oral polio virus
4 months	DPT	and	Oral polio virus
6 months	DPT	and	Oral polio virus
15 months	Measles		
18 months	DPT	and	Oral polio virus
4–6 years	DT	and	Oral polio virus
10–12 years	Rubella (only for females with rubella hemagglutination test negative or less than 1:16)		
Every 10 years	T(d) (Adult tetanus, diphtheria)		

DENTAL CARE

Children's teeth begin forming early during the fetal stage. The mother's diet provides the essential nutrients for tooth development. Calcium and phosphorus are the basic building blocks of teeth and are found abundantly in milk and dairy products. Vitamins C and D are also important, as are small amounts of the element fluoride. Drugs, especially tetracycline, should be avoided during pregnancy partly because of their capability for staining and weakening teeth.

Most children begin teething actions several months before the eruption of the first tooth. The first tooth usually appears on the lower jaw and is one of the front teeth, known as incisors. These incisors appear in most children by the age of eight months, but may begin as early as four months or as late as thirteen months. Usually, the two lower central incisors come first, followed by the four upper incisors. Many children will have these six teeth in place shortly after their first birthday. The next teeth, appearing between 18 and 24 months, are the first four molars and the remaining two bottom incisors. Before the child's second birthday, the pointed teeth, also known as the canine teeth, usually appear between the incisors and the molars. After the child is two, the remainder of the first set of teeth, the last four molar teeth, appear.

The eruption of teeth and the practice of teething has led to many folk tales. Some are true, but there are common misconceptions. For example, teething does *not* usually cause high fever. Children experience many mild viral infections within the first three years of life, and some of these viral infections will occur simultaneously with the eruption of teeth and during periods of increased teething activity. Teething hurts; however, it is not the cause of high fever, extreme irritability, or a marked change in your child's daily activities.

Teething is important and necessary, and can be done on almost any hard rubber object. Certain pacifiers, such as the Nuk pacifier, can be used in teething infants and may have the advantage of ensuring proper tongue thrust for proper jaw development. Parents should be careful about allowing children to teethe on plastic objects, as splintering has resulted in injuries. *Children should never be allowed to teethe on a bottle full of milk.* Milk is for the feeding of young infants and not for pacification or teething. Major problems may be caused by allowing an infant to fall asleep with a bottle of milk in his or her mouth. The milk remains in constant contact with the teeth, providing an ideal setup for tooth decay. And studies have proven that children who lie flat in bed with a bottle in their mouths drain some milk into their eustachian tubes and consequently experience a higher incidence of ear infections.

Tooth Decay

Although dental problems are less dramatic than some other health problems, they nonetheless remain the most frequent health problem in children. Virtually every child in this country will need dental work at some point. More than 25 million adults in this country have no teeth at all. Dental cavities (caries) and, more important, gum disease can be prevented.

Genetics is one important factor in the development of cavities. There are people who have never had a cavity; they should in part thank their parents. More important than what we acquire from our parents, however, is what we do to ourselves. Food! If our teeth never came in contact with food, our teeth would never develop cavities. Given that all of us do eat, it is important to know the components of food that cause tooth damage: sugar and starch. Normal mouth bacteria require sugar and starch in order to survive. An excess number of these bacteria can lead to rapid decay. These bacteria produce an acid that is capable of eating through the hard enamel that covers our teeth. Once the bacteria have eaten through the enamel, they then set up housekeeping inside the soft portion of the tooth. These bacteria are extremely resourceful and can live quite well in the absence of air. But they still need sugar and starch in order to survive. Their food supply now has to come to them. Only sugar and starch in extremely minute, dissolved form can enter a small hole in the surface of the enamel. This is why highly refined sugar is such a problem in fostering tooth decay. We now eat more than fifteen times the amount of refined sugar as a century ago. A lost tooth of childhood, placed in a glass of cola, will dissolve almost overnight! A certain amount of the acid that mouth bacteria produce is neutralized by the saliva; this is why our teeth do not rot quite as quickly from drinking cola as they do when allowed to sit and dissolve overnight.

A sound program of cleaning teeth, in order to remove trapped particles of food, is critical. This includes brushing, dental floss, and water jets. Finally, a diet that is high in roughage provides us with a natural toothbrush. It is the custom in many European countries to have salad at the end of the meal. This makes a good deal of sense, since the salad is an extremely rough part of our diet, serves as a natural toothbrush, and clears away the sugars.

Brushing Your Child's Teeth

Brushing should begin when your child is ready to begin. Most children will enjoy brushing their teeth with their parents during their imitative years (from age two on). A two-year-old will not be very proficient yet at brushing teeth and will need help from mom or dad. However, by the age of 3½ children have acquired the fine skills necessary for doing a good job by themselves. Parents can help by encouraging brushing as a family activity and regarding tooth care as a pleasurable experience and not a chore.

Choice of toothpaste. Several toothpastes have been recommended by the American Dental Association for their effectiveness in preventing cavities. The potential for preventing cavities lies in the fluoride content of these toothpastes. The fluoride content of our foods and water supplies is slowly increasing and the importance of using the right toothpaste is slowly diminishing. We continue to recommend a toothpaste that is ADA approved. So-called "glamor" toothpastes may contain caustic materials that may gradually wear out the tooth enamel. Your child should enjoy the taste of the toothpaste being used in order to reinforce brushing as a pleasurable experience. Regular nonfluoride brushing is better than sporadic fluoride brushing, but regular fluoride brushing is best. Soft toothbrushes are as good as hard ones, and the direction of the brushing is not nearly as important as the thoroughness of the brushing.

Dental Flossing

The use of dental floss is an excellent method of removing particles from between the teeth and encouraging healthy gums. Flossing is not recommended for children with their first teeth as it can be an unpleasant experience. However, once children have developed their permanent teeth, they should be encouraged to use dental floss. Again, the best way to encourage children to do things is to do them yourselves. Dental floss without the use of the wax covering is slightly preferable, as particles of wax can become dislodged and remain between the teeth.

Water Jets

Water jets are another effective method of removing particles from between the teeth, and often are enjoyed by children who don't like dental floss. Dental floss does a better job of cleaning if used correctly, however. Some children are frightened by the noise of the water jet, however; a period of time to adjust to the water jet should be given.

Fluoride

Fluoride is a natural element that is extremely effective in preventing tooth decay in children. Some have promoted fluoride as a miracle drug and others have attacked it because of its potential in extremely high doses of causing tooth damage. Fluoride will decrease, but not eliminate, tooth decay. Fluoride is found naturally in many water supplies and in many vegetables as well. In addition, a majority of cities in the United States have chosen to fluoridate their water supply. Because of these fluoridated water supplies, many packaged and canned foods in the supermarket also have measurable amounts of fluoride. Even if your community does not have a fluoridated water supply, you are undoubtedly receiving a fair amount of fluoride in the packaged foods that you buy.

The current recommendations are for supplementing infant feedings with fluoride drops in areas where the water supply is not fluoridated. Children between the ages of three and ten should receive about one milligram (usually one tablet) each day if the water supply is not fluoridated. Fluoride is required through age ten or so until the permanent teeth are in. Too much fluoride can discolor the teeth, so do not exceed these dosages. The recommended fluoride dose is slowly being decreased because of the increasing amount of fluoride in other sources of food. Fluoride is a prescription item and your physician should be aware of changing developments in the use of fluoride.

The First Trip to the Dentist
The time to first visit the dentist depends on the nature of your child's teeth. Examine your child's teeth yourself periodically. It is not difficult to see small holes in the child's teeth. Usually, teeth will not begin developing cavities before the age of three. If at the age of three you think you see holes in your child's teeth, by all means make a dental appointment. Although baby teeth are lost and replaced with permanent teeth beginning at about age six, severe damage to baby teeth can cause both dental pain and potential loss of adult teeth. Losing baby teeth prematurely may result in permanent teeth coming in crooked. If your children's teeth appear all right, a dental visit may be postponed until age four or so when the child will be less frightened by the dental examination. We recommend yearly visits to the dentist thereafter.

Permanent Teeth
Permanent teeth begin forming in the first few months of life, but do not erupt until the fifth or sixth year. The permanent teeth come in in approximately the same order as the baby teeth. In addition, the number of teeth will increase from 20 primary teeth to 32 permanent teeth. The eruption of permanent teeth generally does not end until an individual is in the twenties and the third molars (wisdom teeth) appear. There is no reason to have wisdom teeth removed routinely. If wisdom teeth become impacted or grow into other teeth, dental care may be necessary, but many people do have all 32 teeth.

Additional Reading
McGuire, Thomas, D.D.S., *The Tooth Trip*. New York: Random House-Bookwork, 1972.

PREVENTING ADULT DISEASES
The origins of the most serious medical problems of adults can usually be traced to habits and expectations developed in the early years. Tooth decay, accidents, and many infectious diseases can be effectively prevented, and the importance of doing so is obvious. Heart attack, stroke, high blood pressure, obesity, diabetes, cancer, emphysema, drug side effects, alcoholism, suicide, and homicide are the major national killers. There are effective ways of reducing the likelihood of developing every one of these problems; good health is a way of life. It is your responsibility to transmit the knowledge and attitudes that will serve your children over a lifetime.

Heart Attack and Arteriosclerosis
Once rare before middle life, heart attacks are now sometimes seen even in the twenties and thirties. A heart attack, sometimes called a *coronary thrombosis* or

myocardial infarction, results when a clot forms in one of the small blood vessels that supply blood and oxygen to the heart muscle. The clot forms on a narrowing in the blood vessel called an *arteriosclerotic plaque*. Thus, a heart attack is a form of arteriosclerosis, or "hardening of the arteries." Arteriosclerosis happens to all of us, and the process begins in the teens. In some people it happens faster; in others, slower. You can control the rate at which serious arteriosclerosis develops.

The risk factors for heart attacks are well established; they include obesity, cigarette smoking, high blood pressure, inactivity, diet, and stress. Each of these factors relates to the others, each is under the control of the individual, and each is susceptible to the influence of parents.

Both obesity and dietary fat intake are associated with the early onset of arteriosclerosis. The total body weight increases the load on the heart, and the dietary fats appear to cause the arteriosclerotic plaques to form more quickly. At any rate, for every pound greater than ten that an adult is over his or her ideal weight, life will be, on the average, one month shorter. Diabetes can be avoided in many individuals by maintaining a normal weight.

We describe in Problem 67 (Overweight) how fat children become fat adults; the number of fat cells is determined very early in life, usually in the first year. More important, however, is the fact that the attitudes that result in adult obesity begin at the dinner table, where tastes for foods develop. The cholesterol controversy continues, and we advise moderation with eggs and ice cream, use of unsaturated fat margarines rather than butter, and the use of low fat rather than whole milk. A well-balanced meal is still the best policy. Children don't buy groceries; if they are eating too much junk food, you are responsible. Rules do not have to be rigid; arteriosclerosis develops over a lifetime and good habits are not altered much by temporary indiscretions.

Controlling heart attacks requires more than dietary control. Adequate exercise also protects us from serious heart attacks. Exercise must be regular and lifelong. Stress also contributes to the high incidence of heart disease. Stress in our lives cannot be avoided but it can be dealt with if it is recognized. Many current techniques (from massage to meditation) are being developed to help individuals cope with stress. Parents can help their children cope and thereby teach them that they need not confront all problems alone and head-on.

High Blood Pressure and Stroke

A stroke is like a heart attack, except that the clot forms in a blood vessel that goes to the brain, and some of the brain tissue dies. Hardening of the arteries, arteriosclerosis, is almost always the cause. Prevention of stroke is like prevention of heart attacks, and dietary fat intake should be moderate. High blood pressure increases the chances of a heart attack, and increases the chances of a stroke even more.

Having high blood pressure is to the arteries what overinflation is to automobile tires; they don't last as long. High blood pressure is unusual in children, but is very common in adult life. And you can't tell if you have it, because the high pressure doesn't usually cause any symptoms. How can you prevent it if you don't know that you have it? Easy, but you have to do three things.

First, control your weight. Fat people need a stronger pumping action of the heart, and the blood is supplied at a higher pressure. Weight control will improve or prevent high blood pressure in a good percentage of people. Second, engage in regular exercise to build "reserves" into your circulatory system. This can reduce your blood pressure as well as make you feel better. Third, get a blood pressure check every year or so in adult life, starting at about age 21. But treatment of adult high blood pressure begins with development of the exercise habit and weight control in childhood.

Cancer

Unfortunately, many cancers can't be prevented. However, you do have control over preventing some cancers. Lung cancer is the best example; this is the most common fatal cancer and one of the hardest to treat; it results in about 20 percent of all cancer deaths. And almost all cases are caused by cigarette smoking. The cigarette tars and gases irritate the surface of the breathing tubes and after a period of time a cancer may begin to grow in the irritated area. Of extremely heavy smokers, one out of seven die of this cancer. To prevent it, don't smoke cigarettes. The examples and the attitude of the parents are critically important here; if you don't smoke, the chances are that your children won't either. If you must smoke, don't do it in front of your children. Children respect their parent's judgments and often imitate them. You improve their chances of not smoking by not smoking around them. More than one half of lung cancer and emphysema victims began as teenage smokers.

Nicotine also causes the blood vessels to constrict, and hardening of the arteries occurs at an earlier age in smokers. The tragic lung disease, emphysema, is almost always related to inhaled cigarette smoke. So there are three very important medical reasons why cigarette smoking is hazardous to your health: cancer, arteriosclerosis, and emphysema. Even moderate cigarette smokers lose two years of life expectancy. It is not only that cigarettes can kill you; it is the slow, lingering, painful way in which they do it.

Homicides

In the late teens and early twenties, only accidents cause more deaths than suicide and murder do. Murder is constantly dramatized as a purposeful crime, but it usually is not. Most frequently, it is spontaneous and results from temporary rage or miscalculation, often aggravated by alcohol. Fully 75 percent of all murder victims are known to their attackers, and a high percentage of best friends and family members are involved. The murderer often has not learned to assume responsibility for his or her acts, has grown up in a family where violent rage is common and sanctioned, and possesses a weapon capable of causing rapid death. Often there is a handgun in the home; many times there have been legal problems for the adolescent before the violent act. There is a pattern to senseless destructive behavior, and its origins are often early.

Suicide

Suicide is becoming a more common problem in our society. It is no longer unusual to find seven- and eight-year-olds attempting and committing suicide. Among adolescents, it is the third most common cause of death.

Most people think of committing suicide at some time. It is sometimes, but not always, a sign of mental illness. Because suicide is against the law and violates religious and moral codes, it is often a problem that families keep hidden. A suicide attempt, no matter how minor, is extremely serious and is a signal for a family to obtain professional help.

There are many reasons why a person attempts suicide. Often a major change or stress will occur in the person's life. The person must cope with this situation. A variety of coping strategies may be explored, including suicide. It is in this stage when people can be helped the most by offering your support.

Adolescents who attempt suicide are often isolated. They are loners, have few friends, and are often withdrawn. Frequently they will have only one close friend. Many have serious problems in school. A significant number are failing or experiencing discipline problems. Many live alone.

Following a seemingly minor altercation with a boyfriend, girlfriend, or parent, a suicide attempt will be made. At other times an attempt may follow an extremely angry exchange with a parent. The motivation behind such an act is complex. It may be an attention-seeking device, a manipulative act, an attempt at hurting a parent, or a reaction to a loss, anger, or guilt. It is always a cry for help. If an adolescent is crying for help, it does not mean that parents have failed; it means that help from a doctor, social worker, or other skilled counselor is needed at that moment.

Any child or adolescent who talks of suicide should be taken seriously. "You'll be sorry when I'm gone" should be listened to. While most suicide attempts are unsuccessful, 10 percent of these individuals will later kill themselves. Children and adolescents involved in frequent serious accidents should also receive professional counseling.

Alcohol

Alcohol is a useful sedative and has some social purposes. As a drug, it is even relatively safe when used as directed. If we were to prescribe it as a prescription drug, the label would read: "*Caution*: May cause drowsiness and altered judgment. Do not attempt productive work or driving after taking this drug. Do not exceed recommended dosage of 1½ ounces daily. May be habit-forming. Long-term or excessive use has been associated with ulcer, gastrointestinal hemorrhage, cirrhosis of the liver, inflammation of the pancreas, and atrophy (wasting) of the brain." Again, parents set the example, and again, we counsel moderation.

As the pattern of drug usage is shifting, more and more adolescents are turning to alcoholic beverages. Chronic alcoholism is now becoming common in adolescents. A chronic alcoholic needs help at any age.

Drugs

Nicotine, caffeine, and alcohol are the traditional American drugs. But there are others. And everyone likes to think that the other person's drug is terrible, while their own habit is not. We see teetotalling self-righteous zealots who are "drunk" their whole adult life on Valium. We see the alcoholic who finds his son's marijuana un-American. And the daughter who despises her parents' alcohol but uses "speed" to get up and "reds" (barbiturates) to get down. Medically, we find all drug habits psychologically equivalent. The long-term effects of marijuana and tranquilizers have not been studied as completely as those of alcohol and cigarettes, but may add up to the same devastating toll.

There is another side to the national drug problem that is of major medical importance. One out of six hospitalizations is for a drug side effect, and one out of seven hospitalized patients will have a drug reaction *while in the hospital.* We think that the history of this century will record its drug dependence as one of its worst features, and will remark upon the curious concept that there is a pill for everything. You will note from the discussions in Part II that, except for bacterial infections, there is a satisfactory pill for almost nothing. The average American goes too often to the doctor and too often to the medicine chest. We spend fortunes on overpromoted patent medicines and on prescription drugs of low value. We get taken. And, unless we are careful, our children will get taken also.

Consider two boys, each of whom scrapes his arm. The parents of one clean it and apply a bandage. The parents of the other take him to the emergency room of the hospital, where an intern, trying to be helpful, thinks it might be infected and gives an antibiotic. After five days, both scrapes are healed. Consider the psychological repercussions, because the family that used the emergency room has lost more than time and money. The antibiotic is credited with the cure! And the next time, the emergency room has changed from being a marginal decision to a necessity—to treat the infection that never was. The other boy has learned the real lesson: that a scrape will heal if cleaned and left alone, and that a certain measure of confidence in the natural healing properties of the body is warranted. Children learn drug dependence from their parents; you should never automatically encourage your child to use any drug, no matter how harmless.

Inactivity

We are a nation of television watchers and desk sitters, and it is bad for us. Our most serious diseases, such as arteriosclerosis and hypertension, are sometimes called "diseases of civilization." Our stomachs ulcer at the stress of it all, and our bowels won't work by themselves. Everything from hemorrhoids to stomach ulcers to middle-aged spread can be related to our lack of serious physical exercise.

Good physical exercise is a workout for the heart and blood vessels, not just the muscles. To work the heart, the exercise must be steady, moderately strenuous, and must last at least ten to twelve minutes. Bicycling , swimming, and jogging meet these requirements. Good exercise to fight the diseases of civilization must be regular, at least four or five times weekly, and must be a lifetime habit. Healthy exercise will reduce the resting pulse rate, a sign of greater efficiency of the heart, and will reduce the blood pressure. And at any particular exercise level the heart will not have to work as hard. Exercise, when regular and sustained, makes the heart more efficient. The best way to encourage your children to exercise is to exercise with them. It will benefit the whole family.

Chapter

9

The Home Pharmacy

As a society, we have relied far too long and far too often on drugs to solve our problems. Drugs have, of course, saved many lives. Medications for bacterial infections, epilepsy, cancer, heart failure, rheumatoid arthritis, diabetes, and other major illnesses have certainly changed the lives of many afflicted. However, there is almost unbelievable misuse of medications because of our social rituals, patients' demands, physicians' encouragement, and massive advertising.

The vast majority of all medical problems resolve themselves without the use of any medication. These illnesses include common colds, influenza, diarrhea, rashes, upset stomachs, headaches, and most of the other problems discussed in Part II. However, we are bombarded with advertisements implying that these problems can only be cured, or can be cured much quicker, by the use of some medication. One out of every eight television advertisements is for an over-the-counter medication. These claims are simply not true. For nearly every advertised drug, there is a cheaper alternative that is just as good or better; in many instances, the preferred alternative is nothing at all. You will find our recommendations under the "home treatment" section for every problem in Part II.

Finding a product on the shelf of a supermarket or pharmacy does not mean that it is either safe or effective. In 1966 the Food and Drug Administration commissioned a study to evaluate 400 common over-the-counter (nonprescription) drugs. More than 75 percent of these drugs were found to be less than effective for some or most of their claims. Products that have been on the market since before 1938 have never been subject to requirements for demonstrating safety or efficacy! Therefore, most of the estimated 250,000 to 500,000 (!)

products available on the shelves are less than effective and many are unsafe. Well-intentioned use of these products results in many deaths annually. The F.D.A. is currently taking steps to review available over-the-counter products. However, since their 1966 report, only one class of products, antacids, has been reviewed. Consequently, it will be many years before consumers can purchase medications with the knowledge that they are both safe and effective. The definition of safety can be only a relative one. All medications can cause serious side reactions. Aspirin, a potent and useful drug, causes more serious reactions and more deaths than any other medication. Be careful with *every* drug.

In this section, we discuss several medicines to use in treating common symptoms. Many of these are covered more extensively under discussion of the individual problem in Part II.

We believe that only two types of medication are essential for the home pharmacy when children are in the home. First are the fever and pain relievers aspirin and/or acetaminophen. Even these medications are potentially fatal and should be kept out of the reach of children. (Very few childproof caps are childproof. Often the best way to open a childproof cap that you are having trouble with is to ask your child to open it for you.)

Second, every home should have syrup of ipecac on hand. Syrup of ipecac can induce vomiting in children who have swallowed dangerous medications. It can be used immediately when a child has swallowed pills, liquid medication, or plants. For other poisonous substances, it may be dangerous to induce vomiting. Write the name of your poison control center on your telephone and in Problem 16 (Poisoning) now! Your poison control center can advise you if a household product that your child has taken can be safely removed by inducing vomiting.

In addition to these two medicines, have on hand Band-Aids, a vaporizer, elastic bandages, and hydrogen peroxide. Other common household drugs described below are included in our discussion to indicate their limitations. A drug on the shelf, whether intended for you or your child, is like keeping a loaded gun there. Dispose of leftover drugs now! By family discussion and by parental example, show that you understand what drugs do not do. Symptoms are not only nature's way of telling us that something is wrong, but also may be a part of the healing process. Often the cough, runny nose, or diarrhea is already helping the body get rid of the problem. Your child lives in a body brilliantly designed to restore health once it has been disturbed. Don't fool around with it.

ALLERGY

Antihistamine Compounds
These compounds are useful in children who have well-documented cases of allergic skin reactions to insect bites, allergic rhinitis, or hay fever, and are of dubious value for anything else. The discomfort of the hay fever should always be balanced against the risk of problems caused by the antihistamine compounds, which are usually dispensed in combination with a decongestant compound. The most common antihistamines are chlorpheniramine (Chlortrimeton), triprolidine (found in Actifed along with pseudoephedrine), diphenhydramine (Benadryl), and carbinoxamine (Rondec).

Side effects. Drowsiness is the most common side effect and can interfere with a child's schoolwork. While some parents feel that antihistamines are useful in helping children to get to sleep at bedtime, the children really never go into the sleep stage that is most restful while on antihistamines and, in fact, have an insufficient amount of the proper type of sleep. Antihistamines occasionally can cause hyperactivity in children. Follow package instructions for dosage.

COLD PREPARATIONS

With a cold or allergy, a runny nose is often the worst symptom. Although runny noses are a nuisance and not very aesthetic, they are seldom a serious problem and do help to carry the virus outside the body. One of the concerns with colds is that the swelling and secretions of a cold may block either the sinus outlets or the eustachian tube. Because sinuses are very poorly developed in very young children, there is not as much need to worry about sinusitis in children. However, if the eustachian tube, which drains the normal secretions from the middle ear into the child's nasal cavity, remains plugged for a day or so, a middle-ear infection may begin. It is easier for this tube to swell and close in younger children because it is shorter, narrower, and at a more horizontal angle than in older children. Whether this tube can be kept open sufficiently during a cold to prevent an ear infection is uncertain, but it is the basis for therapy with either nose drops or decongestants. Use of these agents is frequent, but controversial.

Nose Drops

Nose drops usually contain decongestants such as phenylephrine (Neosynephrine), ephredrine, or oxymetazoline (Afrin). These drugs work by causing the muscle in the walls of the blood vessels to constrict, decreasing blood flow. After many applications, these small muscles become fatigued and fail to respond. Finally, they are so fatigued that they relax entirely and the situation becomes worse than it was in the beginning. Generally, this fatigue process does not occur in the first three days, so most physicians recommend the use of nose drops only for a short temporary problem. The advantage of Afrin is that it is reputed to have a longer lasting effect than Neosynephrine, but it is far more costly. Neosynephrine comes in ⅛%, ¼%, ½%, and 1% solutions. Package instructions should be followed for dosage.

Perhaps the cheapest and safest nose drops can be made by mixing one half teaspoon of salt in a glass of water. Many physicians feel these to be as effective as medicated nose drops. But our favorite remedy for the runny nose is the handkerchief, used frequently and gently!

Oral Decongestants

Pseudo-ephedrine (Sudafed, Actifed) and ephedrine (Rondec) are commonly used decongestants. Again, their use in stuffy noses is to cause constriction of the blood vessels in the nose and therefore to decrease the stuffiness. Unfortunately, doses of these medications high enough to cause constriction of the blood vessels in the nose are also high enough to cause constriction of other blood vessels in the body, and can produce high blood pressure. Although these drugs are unlikely to produce high blood pressure at the recommended dosage levels, they are also unlikely to produce the necessary blood vessel constriction to give significant relief. At this time there is no convincing evidence that the use of these decongestants prevents the complications of sinusitis or middle-ear infection. Because of their relative safety in appropriate doses and because of the theoretical possibility that they do assist once a person has developed sinusitis or an earache (otitis media), they are commonly used for this purpose. Children who have recurrent bouts of ear infections may be placed on decongestants at the first sign of a cold with the hope that perhaps another ear infection may be avoided. We consider middle-ear infections serious enough to justify the use of these relatively safe medications in some such circumstances, although their effectiveness is unproved. We do not recommend the routine use of decongestants for all colds or stuffy noses.

Cough Syrups

The cough is a natural reflex that helps clear the child's lung of mucous secretions that are accumulating because of an infection. The cough then is one of the body's defenses. There are two types of commonly available cough medications.

The first type of cough medication is commonly known as an expectorant. An example is glycerol guaiacolate (Robitussin, 2-G). Its purpose is to help liquefy the secretions in the lungs and help the cough reflex to remove these secretions from the lungs. The principle of liquefaction of secretions is extremely important, especially in such illnesses as croup. However, there is little evidence to indicate that any cough syrup is very effective in producing this liquefaction. Vaporizers are far more useful for liquefying secretions. Many antihistamine drugs are combined with other drugs in "cough preparations," without any definite evidence of their effectiveness. Examples are Benylin expectorant (diphenhydramine and alcohol) and Conar (noscapine).

The second type of cough medication suppresses the cough. The cough reflex is a natural defense that usually should be encouraged. There are, however, certain times when coughing may interfere with the child's getting better. The most common example is when coughing interferes with the child getting to sleep. If a child is unable to sleep, a cough suppressant, such as dextromethorphan (Romilar) may be used. Many other preparations have dextromethorphan but usually in combination with other drugs not shown to be effective (Dorcal, Novahistine, DMX, phenergan expectorant with dextromethorphan, Rondec-DM). Codeine also suppresses cough in children. Although codeine is a relatively safe narcotic, dextromethorphan is just as good and causes less sleepiness and depression of breathing. Occasionally during the daytime, children may have coughing that is so prolonged and so severe that it begins to cause chest pain; this may be another indication for suppressing the cough.

CONSTIPATION

There is hardly ever a time when you should treat constipation in children with drugs. Prune juice, every grandmother's favorite remedy, is still effective in relieving constipation. And constipation (Problem 66) is very seldom a real problem. Prune juice acts by drawing a large amount of water into the intestines, thereby helping to soften hard stools. Food high in fiber or bran content is also extremely effective. While laxatives (such as Maltsupex, Milk of Magnesia, Ex-lax, Colace, mineral oil, and Metamucil) are used commonly in children they are only very rarely required. Mineral oil is perhaps the cheapest and most effective but is dangerous in infants and toddlers because of the potential problems it can cause if vomited and inhaled into the lungs.

There is virtually no indication for giving a child an enema. An enema for a child can be extremely frightening, and rare serious complications have occurred.

DIARRHEA

The proper management of diarrhea is discussed elsewhere (see Problem 83). Medication is of little use in the treatment of ordinary diarrhea. Compounds such as kaolin and pectin (frequently found in preparations such as Kaopectate) will help change a liquid stool into a more gelatinous stool. However, during periods of diarrhea, the total amount of water lost and the total number of stools produced will be about the same. We do not see the necessity of using these types of preparations merely to change the form of the stool. They do not decrease the diarrhea nor the water lost. Some parents, however, find that leakage out of diapers is less of a problem with a more formed bowel movement.

Paregoric-containing preparations (such as Parapectolin and Parelixir) are also not recommended for use in children. Paregoric is a narcotic that decreases the activity of the digestive tract. This increased activity of the digestive tract is a defense mechanism that usually should not be suppressed. In addition, narcotic overdose with paregoric can occur, and drowsiness and nausea can be caused. And, like most other narcotics, paregoric can produce constipation. Lomotil contains a narcoticlike compound that is also not recommended for children.

EYE IRRITATIONS

Eye irritations in children seldom require the use of over-the-counter preparations (Visine, Murine). "Pink eye" and its treatment is discussed in Problem 78 (Eye Burning, Itching, and Discharge).

PAIN AND FEVER

Pain and fever in childhood are generally signs of an infection. For specific problems of pain and fever, refer to the appropriate problem in Part II. Aspirin or acetaminophen may assist in providing relief of these symptoms.

Aspirin

Aspirin is one of the oldest, safest, and most useful medications available. Certain individuals are particularly sensitive to aspirin. These individuals may experience gastrointestinal disturbances, including bleeding, following the use of aspirin. Very rarely, patients may actually have wheezing induced by aspirin; this is an allergy. On the other hand, there are side effects that all individuals will experience if aspirin is taken in too high a dosage. The most common complaint of aspirin overdosage in older children is ringing of the ears, although this is an unreliable sign in younger children. In younger children, aspirin overdosage initially causes very rapid breathing, followed after a period of time by slowed breathing, lethargy, and unresponsiveness. This is seen only when large amounts of aspirin have been taken. Giving an infant twice the recommended dosage for one dose only is an accident that should not cause alarm. However, if adult aspirin is mistakenly administered rather than baby aspirin, four times the dosage has been given and your physician or the poison control center should be contacted immediately.

There is no indication for the use of aspirin combinations such as aspirin, phenacetin and caffeine, or aspirin and caffeine in children (APC tablets, Anacin).

It is a common mistake to believe that there is liquid aspirin. Aspirin is not available in liquid preparations; it is only available in tablets or in Aspergum.

Acetaminophen (Tylenol, Tempra, Liquiprin, Datril, Valadol)

Acetaminophen is a very effective medication for fever reduction in children. It is not quite as effective as aspirin for reducing pain. Acetaminophen is used frequently in children because it is safer than aspirin and because it is easier to administer as a liquid. However, in extremely high doses, even acetaminophen can be fatal by causing massive liver damage.

Dosage. The dosages of acetaminophen and aspirin are identical. Each can be given in a dosage of 60 mg (one grain) per year of age of the child. Thus, a two-year-old child can receive 120 mg (two grains) of either aspirin or acetaminophen every four hours. After age 10, the adult dose has been reached. *Caution*: Acetaminophen is available in many concentrations. A teaspoon of one preparation (drops) can contain four times as much drug as a teaspoon of another preparation (elixir). Read the label carefully!

POISONING

To induce vomiting, use syrup of ipecac. Any time your child swallows a large number of pills or liquid medication, ipecac can be given. Give the child a glass of water or milk immediately after giving a tablespoon of syrup of ipecac in young children (or two tablespoons in older children) to induce vomiting. If there has been no vomiting in 20 minutes, repeat with another tablespoon of ipecac in young children or two tablespoons in older children. If after 40 minutes there is no vomiting, it will be necessary for the child to be seen by a physician in order to have his or her stomach emptied. Ipecac in and of itself can produce problems if it is not vomited up.

There are other methods of inducing vomiting in children such as mixing mustard with warm water and forcing them to drink it, or by touching the back of the child's throat; these are less aesthetic but sometimes as good. For any item other than medication, a call to the poison control center or your physician should be made *before* attempting to induce vomiting (see Problem 16, Oral Poisoning); with medicines, call right after inducing the vomiting.

STERILIZING AGENTS AND ANTISEPTICS (HYDROGEN PEROXIDE AND IODINE)

The best way to clean a dirty wound is to scrub it with soap and water. Hydrogen peroxide, which foams and cleanses as you work it into the wound, is also a good cleansing agent. It should not be used in strengths greater than 3%, so watch out for bottles sold at higher strengths for bleaching hair.

Although iodine is a good agent and kills germs, it is irritating to the skin and sometimes winds up in little children's mouths; it is a dangerous poison. In addition, some people are allergic to iodine. Betadine is a nonstinging iodine preparation, but reasonably expensive. Soap, water, and hydrogen peroxide will take you a long way in dealing with the common scrapes and sores that all children get. Mercurochrome has a pretty color but is not effective. In only rare instances are antibiotic ointments more effective than soap and water.

Band-Aids are for children what medals are for adults. They are worn proudly as symbols of surviving major confrontations with the ground. As such, they may be awarded when the child feels they are necessary. Here is another example where you can encourage your child to make a decision about the application of a treatment. For wounds in areas likely to have heavy exposure to dirt, Band-Aids (and occasionally gauze dressings) may be necessary in order to prevent further contamination and the possibility of infection.

VAPORIZERS

A vaporizer is one of the best investments you can make. It efficiently provides the steam necessary for the relief of croup and is soothing for many other coughs. A cold-steam vaporizer is preferable since there is no possibility of a child being burned by hot steam. It is not necessary to add any medication to the vaporizer. These preparations make the room smell nice but do not add to the therapy offered by the steam alone.

VITAMINS

We mention these only to emphasize that vitamin supplementation is *not* required for most children. An ordinary diet, balanced with foods from each of the major groups, contains far more vitamins than the growing body requires. Vitamin-D supplementation is recommended for infants during the period of breast feeding, but that is all. Minerals are also abundantly present in common foods. (See Problem 70, Weakness and Tiredness, for a list of iron-containing foods.) Fluoride needs to be provided if the water supply is deficient, as outlined in Chapter 8. The American child taking vitamin and mineral supplements secretes the most expensive urine in the world, since that is where excess materials end up.

GIVING MEDICINE

The medical encounter frequently results in instructions to give the child some medication. There are a number of factors to keep in mind whenever you give your child medicine; here are some of the more important ones.

- Do you understand the instructions? Check before leaving the office. If the instructions on the medication bottle differ from what the physician or pharmacist said, call your physician immediately. If you are confused, call the physician or the pharmacist.

- Be sure of the strength of the medication. Some common medications appear in many different concentrations, and the wrong strength may be dangerous.

- Be sure your child is not allergic to the medication. Even the most careful physician occasionally forgets that a child may be allergic to penicillin and may prescribe it. Do not give your child anything that you know he or she is allergic to.

- Be as precise as possible in your measurements. Teaspoons vary greatly in size. When most physicians prescribe a teaspoon, they mean to prescribe five cubic centimeters (cc) of medication. Kitchen measuring spoons are more accurate. Many pharmacies sell small plastic measuring devices or give them away.

- Never give a child medication intended for another person.

- Never give a child medication if the expiration date has passed.

- Never tell a child that medication is candy. As soon as your back is turned, children will sometimes try to get as many of these candies into their mouths as possible.

- Do not tell a child a medication tastes good when you know it doesn't. This will help get the first dose into the child, but you will have an impossible time with the second.

Some of your most interesting moments with your children will be spent trying to give them medications. An average child can spit an average medication a seeming distance of 15 feet. While this may be good practice for the annual North Carolina Watermelon Pit Spitting Contest, medication on the walls has seldom been known to do the child any good. Getting medication into your children will be a great test of your ingenuity. Remember, you are older, wiser, more clever, and ultimately bigger. But here are some hints so that you don't have to use force. For younger infants, you can mix some medications in with applesauce or ice cream. Medications usually do not give a pleasant flavor to milk and we discourage this practice; most children are familiar with how their milk tastes and are suspicious of funny-tasting milk. Cranberry juice is a good place to hide medication. Finally, older children should be required to take medication as a matter of course. They should not need to be threatened or bribed any more than they need to be bribed or threatened when it is their bedtime. Children over the year of three and one half can begin to be treated as adults with regard to taking medications. Development of proper respect for medication is important at this age. So, start talking to them about the importance of medication to help them through their illness; do not talk of medication as either magic or rewards. And emphasize the importance of taking medication as directed, not more or less.

TINCTURE OF TIME

Used prudently, this is the most important medicine. It is the only known cure for the common cold, as well as most of the other problems of everyday life. With time, things get better. In the remainder of this book we try to tell you how to use time, and how long it should take.

Why do we, as a society, use drugs rather than time, even though time usually works and the drugs usually don't? Sure, we are impatient, confused by the complexities of science, and hustled by the advertisers. But let's not ignore the biggest reason. We use drugs, and sometimes the doctor, to prove that we care for our child. The statements "I'll run down and get something from the drugstore" or "You're going to the doctor first thing in the morning" are part of our everyday life. We must have something to do, if we care, for a sick child; in our society we have equated caring with the giving of drugs.

Consider the consequences of such actions. The child receives a pill rather than a parent. He or she learns that a symptom requires a drug. Colds, scrapes, headaches, and constipation are associated with the need to imbibe a pill or some odious fluid. Later, the parent is disturbed when the child wants pills, shots, or fluids to cure boredom, unhappiness, or agitation, or just to interact socially with friends. And, although time will take the symptom away, the drug will take the credit. The child fails to learn that the body is strong, and thinks instead that health is frail and only precariously maintained by an intake of chemicals.

If you care for your child, your instruction in health maintenance must express these truths. With a sick child, you can care by spending time instead of money. Nondrug treatments, such as encouraging fluids, running the vaporizer, and cleaning and soaking the wound will give you plenty to do. Most medical problems are learning experiences. If you and your child react and interact appropriately, the lessons can be very positive, and can lead to emotional growth and physical confidence. The choice is yours, and the consequences are immense. It is drug dependence or personal independence. We hope that the guidelines of the remainder of this book will help your family toward the goal of personal self-reliance and independent living.

Part

II

The Child and the Common Complaint

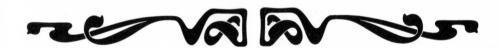

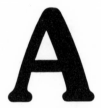

A

Interpretation of Childhood Complaints

HOW TO USE THIS PART

In Part II, you will find general information and decision charts for most of the common medical problems of children. The general information of the left-hand page will give you background on the specific medical problem; also it will provide instructions for home treatment, as well as information on what to expect at the doctor's office, if you go. The charts on the right-hand page will help you decide whether to use home treatment or to consult a physician. To gain the most benefit from this part of the book, use these simple guidelines.

Emergencies. Before dealing with any medical problem at home, the first question to ask is whether or not emergency action is necessary. Often the answer is obvious. The great majority of complaints are quickly recognized as minor; the true emergency is hard to ignore. The information in Section B, Emergencies, presents a common-sense approach to several problems that require immediate action. Decision charts assume that emergency symptoms have been considered first.

Finding the right chart for your medical problem. Determine the "chief complaint" or major symptom—for instance, a cough, an earache, or chest pains—and look it up in the table of contents, the index, or inside the front cover. Then turn to the appropriate page.

Multiple problems. If you have more than one problem you may have to use more than one decision chart. For example, if you have a bad sore throat, a slight cough, and a runny nose, look up your most serious complaint first, then the next most serious, etc. You may notice some duplication of questions in the decision charts, especially when the symptoms are closely related. If you use more than one chart, take the most "conservative" advice; if one chart recommends home treatment and another advises a visit to the physician, then go to the doctor.

Using the charts. First read all of the general information on your particular problem; then go to the decision chart. Start at the top and follow the arrows. Skipping around may result in errors. Each question assumes that all questions before have been answered. The general information under the medical problem will help you understand the questions in the chart. If this general material is ignored, a question may be misinterpreted and the wrong course of action selected.

If the chart indicates home treatment. Don't assume that an instruction to use home treatment guarantees that the problem is trivial and may be ignored. Home therapy must be approached conscientiously if it is to work. If over-the-counter medicines are suggested, look them up in the index and read about dosage and side effects in Chapter 9 before you use them.

There are times when home treatment is not effective despite conscientious application; in these cases, a physician should be consulted. The length of time that you should wait before consulting a doctor is indicated in the general information for each problem. Do not hesitate to call the physician earlier if in your judgment your child's illness appears troublesome. The home treatment that we include in these pages is what most physicians recommend as a first approach to these problems. If it doesn't work, think the problem through again. If you are seriously worried about your child's condition, call the doctor.

If the chart indicates that you should consult a physician. This does not necessarily mean that the illness is serious or dangerous. Often you are directed to the doctor because a physical examination should be performed or because certain facilities of the physician's office are needed. The chart will refer you to a physician with different levels of urgency. "See physician now" means right away. "See physician today" indicates that the visit should be on the same day. "Make appointment with physician" indicates a less urgent situation; the visit should be scheduled, but may take place any time during the next few days. Sometimes a phone consultation with the physician can help. Sometimes we will give you the medical terminology related to a specific problem. With this information, you will be able to "translate" the terms your doctor may use during your visit or telephone call.

With these guidelines, you will be able to use the decision charts to quickly locate the information you need. Look over the charts for several complaints; you will quickly get the knack of finding the answers you need.

Trust your own judgment. Remember that you know your child best. If your child appears quite sick, be sure to get the necessary help; common sense is your best guide in such matters.

THE SICK CHILD

Sudden illness in a child can be very frightening. Children who are playing and well one moment may appear completely devoid of energy the next. It is a testimony to the strength of children that they have the resiliency to recover as quickly as they have become ill. As a general rule, all ill children under the age of four months should be immediately brought to the physician. Illness in this age group is far more serious and may progress far more rapidly than in older children.

All experienced parents quickly learn to recognize what the early signs of illness are in their children. For some, it is a dazed or glassy-eyed look; for others, it is lethargy or bags under the eyes; for others, it is a pale or "pre-vomit white" color. In general, observation and common sense will tell you how sick your child is. An extremely active child who begins to slow down may be showing early signs of an illness, whereas a quiet child who becomes fussy or irritable should be suspected of having an illness. The following areas should be assessed whenever considering illness in your child.

- *Activity.* What is the child's activity like now compared to what it usually is at this time of the day? Is your child's sleep pattern disturbed? Is your child playing the way he or she usually plays?

- *Is your child eating normally?* All children have some food finickiness, but severely ill children will refuse almost all food.

- *If there is vomiting or diarrhea present, what is its nature?* If a child loses an excessive amount of fluid from vomiting or diarrhea, dehydration can result. The larger the amount of fluid lost in the vomitus or diarrhea, the greater is the likelihood of dehydration. Not only the frequency but the amount is important to consider in your evaluation. If there is blood in either the vomiting or diarrhea this is cause to contact your physician. If the vomiting is extremely violent, this is another indication for contacting your physician.

- *Has the child urinated?* Infrequent urination or dark yellow urine are signs that the child is becoming dehydrated.

- *What is the child's skin turgor like?* Gather the skin on your child's stomach together using your five fingers. When you release it, it should immediately spring back. Dehydrated skin does not have the elasticity of normal skin. If there is a question in your mind, compare the sick child's skin with another child's or your own. The skin of a dangerously dehydrated child is like the skin of a very old person.

- *Are your child's eyes and mouth moist?* A dry mouth or eyes that appear sunken are signs of dehydration that require immediate attention by your physician.

- *What is your child's temperature?* Fever is discussed extensively in Section E. A high fever can make your child feel quite uncomfortable and increase fluid requirements. Except in instances of physical exertion, a fever is a sign of illness in a child.

- *What is your child's heart rate?* Children have a higher heart rate than adults, and the heart rate increases further with fever. It may decrease after severe head injury. In general, pulse rates over 130 or under 60 when a child is resting warrant an immediate physician visit.

- *How fast is your child breathing?* The rate at which your child breathes decreases as the child becomes older. Breathing rates are far higher after activity; when evaluating your child's breathing rate, the child should be resting. While many newborns have breathing rates of 50 to 60, by the age of a year resting rates are usually between 25 and 35. A rate over 40 at rest is of concern except in children under a year old. By age six resting respiratory rates should be below 30 and by age 10, below 25. Fever is a common cause of an elevated breathing rate, so assess your child's breathing rate at rest after you have attempted to reduce the fever.

As you become more experienced with illnesses in your children, these observations, and many of your own that are far more subtle, will become intuitive. You will soon learn that you are the best judge of illness in your child. Physicians can only help in diagnosing the specific causes of the illness. The purpose of Part II of this book is to assist you in managing many of the more commonly recognized illnesses on your own.

B

Emergencies

Emergencies require prompt action, not panic. What action you should take depends on the nature of the problem and the facilities available. If there are massive injuries or if your child is unconscious, you must get help immediately. Go to the emergency room if it is close by. If it isn't, you can often obtain help over the phone by calling an emergency room or the rescue squad. If you think that a child has swallowed poison, the emergency room is the first place to call if you do not have the phone number of a poison control center.

The most important thing is to be prepared to go or to phone. Record the phone numbers of the nearest emergency facility, poison control center, and rescue squad in the front of this book. Know the best way to reach the emergency room by car. Develop these procedures *before* an actual emergency arises.

When to call an ambulance. Usually, the slowest way to reach a medical facility is by ambulance. It must go both ways and is not twice as fast as a private car. If your child can readily move or be moved and a private car is available, use the car and have someone call ahead.

The ambulance brings with it a trained crew, who know how to lift a patient to minimize the chance of further injury. Oxygen is usually available, splints and bandages are carried, and, in some instances, lifesaving resuscitation may be used en route to the hospital. Thus, the child who is gravely ill, who has a back or head injury, or who is severely short of breath may benefit from the care afforded by the ambulance attendants.

In our experience, ambulances are often used as expensive taxis. The type of accident or illness, the facilities available, and the distance involved are all important factors in deciding whether an ambulance should be used.

The decision charts in the rest of this book assume that no emergency signs are present. Emergency signs "overrule" the charts and dictate that medical help should be sought immediately. Be familiar with the following emergency signs.

Major injury. Common sense tells us that the child with an obviously broken leg or a large chest wound deserves immediate attention. Emergency facilities exist to take care of major injuries. They should be used, and promptly.

Unconsciousness and coma. Obviously, any child in a state of coma or semiconsciousness should be brought immediately to the nearest medical facility. Coma is most often due to a medication or other toxic product taken by mouth, a seizure, drowning, severe head trauma, or a severe allergic reaction. Any medication or other suspected material that might have been taken should be brought to the medical facility with you. Children breathing with difficulty should have their mouths cleared. Artificial respiration can be given at the rate of ten breaths per minute either through the mouth or the nose.

Choking. If an object has become lodged in your child's windpipe, choking may ensue. Violent coughing will often dislodge the object. Various procedures which may dislodge the object include a sharp slap on the back, holding the child upside down while slapping, or a rapidly applied bear hug to the lower chest. Attempting to dislodge an object that is partially obstructing breathing by using your finger may lead to complete obstruction. So long as the child is able to breathe it is best to proceed to the emergency room.

Active bleeding. Most cuts will stop bleeding if pressure is applied to the wound. Unless the bleeding is obviously minor, a wound that continues to bleed despite the application of pressure requires attention in order to prevent unnecessary loss of blood. The average adult can tolerate the loss of several cups of blood with little ill effect, but children can tolerate only smaller amounts, proportional to their body size. Remember that active and vigorous bleeding can almost always be controlled by the application of pressure directly to the wound and that this is the most important part of first aid for such wounds.

Stupor or drowsiness. A decreased level of mental activity, short of unconsciousness, is termed *stupor*. A practical way of telling whether the severity of stupor or drowsiness warrants urgent treatment is to note the child's ability to answer questions. If he or she is not sufficiently awake to answer questions concerning what has happened, then urgent action is necessary. Children are difficult to judge, but the child who cannot be aroused needs immediate attention.

Disorientation. Within medicine, disorientation is described in terms of time, place, and person. This simply means that the child cannot tell the date, the location, or who he or she is. The child who does not know his or her own identity is in a more difficult state than one who cannot give the correct date. Disorientation may be part of a variety of illnesses and is especially common when a high fever is present. The child who becomes disoriented and confused deserves immediate medical attention.

Shortness of breath. Shortness of breath is described more extensively in Problem 76. As a general rule, a child deserves immediate attention if there is shortness of breath while resting. However, in young adults the most frequent cause of shortness of breath at rest is the hyperventilation syndrome, which is not a serious concern. Nevertheless, if it cannot be confidently determined that shortness of breath is due to the hyperventilation syndrome then the only reasonable course of action is to seek immediate aid.

Severe pain. Surprisingly enough, severe pain is rarely the symptom that determines that a problem is serious and urgent. Most often it is associated with other symptoms that indicate the nature of the condition; the most obvious example is pain associated with a major injury, such as a broken leg, which itself clearly requires urgent care. The severity of pain is subjective and depends on the particular child; often the magnitude of the pain has been altered by emotional and psychological factors. Nevertheless, severe pain demands urgent medical attention, if for no other reason than to relieve the pain.

Much of the art and science of medicine is directed at the relief of pain, and the use of emergency procedures to secure this relief is justified even if the cause of the pain eventually proves to be inconsequential. However, the person who frequently complains of severe pain from minor causes is in much the same situation as the boy who cried "wolf"; calls for help will inevitably be taken less and less seriously by the doctor. This situation is a dangerous one, for there may be more difficulty in obtaining help when it is most needed.

Work out a procedure for medical emergencies. Develop and test it before an actual emergency arises. If you plan your actions ahead of time, you will decrease the likelihood of panic and increase the probability of receiving the proper care quickly.

Poisoning. Poisoning is described in Problem 16. Seldom does the delay of a few moments make any difference in the eventual outcome. However, making a hasty wrong decision can be dangerous. Many poisons do their damage while being swallowed (acids, strong alkalis, drain and oven cleaners) and vomiting should *not* be induced. Other poisons (turpentine, gasoline, furniture polish) cause damage from their vapors and again vomiting should *not* be induced. Medication can be safely vomited. Always bring the poison with you to the doctor or emergency room.

Seizures (convulsions). Seizures are discussed in Problem 72. During the seizure it is most important to protect the child from injury. Except for children known to have recurrent seizures, a prompt medical visit is required.

C

Common Injuries

1. **Cuts (Lacerations)**   148
   A stitch in time.

2. **Puncture Wounds**   150
   The rusty nail and other hazards.

3. **Animal Bites**   152
   Rabies is rare.

4. **Scrapes and Abrasions**   154
   Soap, water, air, and time.

5. **Tetanus Shots**   156
   How often is often?

6. **Is a Bone Broken?**   158
   When an X-ray?

7. **Ankle Injuries**   160
   Few are serious.

8. **Knee Injuries**   162
   Does it wobble?

9. **Wrist, Elbow, and Shoulder Injuries**   164
   Can you use it?

10. **Head Injuries**   166
    Observation is the name of the game.

11. **Burns**   168
    Pain, ice, and healing.

12. **Infected Wounds and Blood Poisoning**   170
    Normal recovery can concern you.

13. **Insect Bites or Stings**   172
    Breathing can be a problem.

14. **Fishhooks**   174
    Push it through or pull it out?

15. **Smashed Fingers**   176
    Car doors and paper clips.

1
Cuts
(Lacerations)

Most cuts affect only the skin and the fatty tissue beneath it. Usually they heal without permanent damage. However, injury to internal structures such as muscles, tendons, blood vessels, ligaments, or nerves presents the possibility of permanent damage. Your physician can decrease this likelihood.

A cut on the face, chest, abdomen, or back is potentially more serious than one on the legs or arms (extremities). Luckily, most lacerations do occur on the extremities. Cuts on the trunk or face should be examined by a physician unless the injury is very small or extremely shallow. If you see fat protruding from the wound, see the doctor.

You may find it difficult to determine whether major blood vessels, nerves, or arteries have been damaged. Numbness, blood pumping vigorously from the wound, or a tingling or weakness in the affected limb all call for examination by a physician.

Signs of infections—such as pus oozing from the wound, fever, extensive redness and swelling—will not appear for at least 24 hours. Bacteria need time to grow and multiply. If these signs do appear, a physician must be consulted.

Stitching (suturing) a laceration is a ritual in our society. The only purpose in suturing a wound is to pull the edges together to hasten healing and minimize scarring. If the wound can be held closed without the use of stitches, they are not recommended, since they themselves injure tissue to some extent.

Home Treatment

Cleanse the wound. Soap and water will do, but be vigorous. Hydrogen peroxide (3%) may also be used. Make sure that no dirt, glass, or other foreign material remains in the wound. This is very important. Antiseptics such as Mercurochrome and merthiolate are unlikely to help, and some are painful. Iodine will kill germs, but is not really needed and is also painful. (Betadine is a modified iodine preparation that is painless, but costly.)

The edges of a clean, minor cut can usually be held together by "butterfly" bandages or "steristrips" (preferred)—strips of sterile paper tape. Apply either of these bandages so that the edges of the wound join without "rolling under."

In a young child who drools, facial wounds are often too wet to treat with bandages, so the doctor's help is usually needed. Because of potential disfigurement, all but minor facial wounds should be treated professionally. Often stitching is required in young children who are apt to pull off bandages or in areas that are subject to a great deal of motion, such as the fingers or joints. Cuts in the palm are also prone to infection so do not attempt home treatment unless the cut is shallow.

Stitching must take place within eight hours of the injury, because germs begin to grow in the wound and can be trapped under the skin to fester. Thus the chart says "See physician now." Decide immediately whether to see a physician or treat at home. Also refer to Problem 5 (Tetanus Shots).

Removing Stitches

Your doctor will tell you when the stitches are to be removed. Unless there is some other reason to return to the doctor, you can perform this simple procedure. First, gently lift the stitch away from the skin by grasping a loose end of the knot; tweezers help. Sometimes in order to accomplish this, a scab must be removed by soaking. Next, cut the stitch at the end as close to the skin as possible and pull it out. A pair of small, sharp scissors or a fingernail clipper work well. It is important to get as close as possible to the skin so that as little as possible of the stitch that was outside the skin is pulled through the skin. This reduces the chance of contamination and infection.

What to Expect at the Doctor's Office

The wound will be thoroughly cleansed and explored to be sure that no foreign particles are left in the wound and that blood vessels,

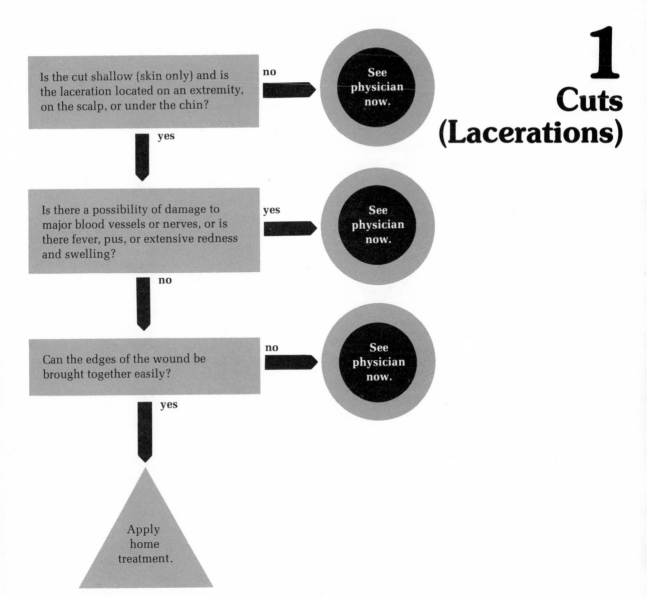

Is the cut shallow (skin only) and is the laceration located on an extremity, on the scalp, or under the chin?

no → See physician now.

yes ↓

Is there a possibility of damage to major blood vessels or nerves, or is there fever, pus, or extensive redness and swelling?

yes → See physician now.

no ↓

Can the edges of the wound be brought together easily?

no → See physician now.

yes ↓

Apply home treatment.

nerves, or tendons are undamaged. The physician may use an anesthetic to deaden the area. Be aware of any allergy to lidocaine (Xylocaine) or other local anesthetics; report any possible allergy to the physician. The physician will determine need, if any, for a tetanus shot and decide whether antibiotics are needed (usually not). Lacerations that may require a surgical specialist include those with injury to tendons or major vessels, especially when this damage has occurred in the hand. Facial cuts may also require a surgical specialist if a good cosmetic result appears difficult to obtain.

2
Puncture Wounds

Puncture wounds are those caused by nails, pins, tacks, and other sharp objects. The most important question is whether a tetanus shot is needed. Consult Tetanus Shots (Problem 5) to determine this. Occasionally puncture wounds do occur in which further medical attention is required.

Most minor puncture wounds are located in the extremities, particularly in the feet. If the puncture wound is located on the head, abdomen, or chest, a hidden internal injury may have occurred. Unless a wound in these areas is obviously minor, see a physician.

Injury to a nerve or to a major blood vessel is rare but can be serious. Injury to an artery may be indicated by blood pumping vigorously from the wound; injury to a nerve usually causes numbness or tingling in the wounded limb, beyond the site of the wound. Major injuries such as these occur rarely with a narrow implement such as a needle; they are more likely with a nail, ice pick, or larger instrument.

To avoid infection, be absolutely sure that nothing has been left in the wound. Sometimes, for example, part of a needle will break off and remain in the foot. If there is any question of a foreign body remaining, the wound should be examined by the physician.

Signs of infection do not occur immediately at the time of injury; they usually take at least 24 hours to develop. The formation of pus, a fever, or severe swelling and redness are indications that the wound should be seen by a physician.

Many physicians feel that puncture wounds of the hand, if not very minor, should be treated with antibiotics. Once started, infections deep in the hand are difficult to treat and many lead to loss of function. Call the physician for advice if a puncture wound of the hand (not the fingers) has occurred.

Home Treatment

Clean the wound to prevent infection. Let it bleed as much as possible to carry foreign material to the outside, since you cannot scrub the inside of a puncture wound. Do not apply pressure to stop the bleeding unless there is a large amount of blood loss and a "pumping," squirting bleeding. The wound should be washed thoroughly with soap and warm water and checked as thoroughly as possible for remaining foreign objects. Hydrogen peroxide (3%) can also be used to cleanse the wound.

Soak the wound in warm water several times a day for four to five days. The object of the soaking is to keep the skin puncture open as long as possible, so that any germs or foreign debris can drain from the open wound. If the wound is allowed to close, an infection may form beneath the skin but not become apparent for several days. Consult Tetanus Shots (Problem 5).

What to Expect at the Doctor's Office

The physician will answer the questions on the opposite chart by history and examination. The wound will be surgically explored if necessary. More frequently, it will be observed for a reaction to a foreign body over the next few days. If a metallic foreign body is suspected, X-rays may be taken. Be prepared to tell the physician the date of the last tetanus shot. Most physicians will recommend home treatment. Antibiotics will only rarely be suggested. In puncture wounds caused by buckshot, the shot may be left in the skin. Occasionally glass or wood may be left in for a period of time to give the body time to push it to the surface.

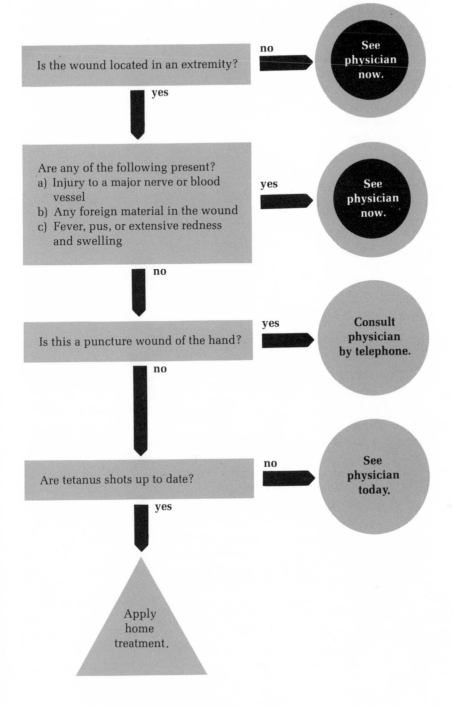

Is the wound located in an extremity?

no → See physician now.

yes ↓

Are any of the following present?
a) Injury to a major nerve or blood vessel
b) Any foreign material in the wound
c) Fever, pus, or extensive redness and swelling

yes → See physician now.

no ↓

Is this a puncture wound of the hand?

yes → Consult physician by telephone.

no ↓

Are tetanus shots up to date?

no → See physician today.

yes ↓

Apply home treatment.

2
Puncture Wounds

3
Animal Bites

The question of rabies is uppermost following an animal bite. The main carriers of rabies are wild animals, especially skunks, foxes, bats, raccoons, and possums. Rabies is also carried, though rarely, by cattle, dogs, and cats, but it is extremely rare in squirrels, chipmunks, rats, and mice. Although 3000–4000 animals are found each year with rabies, only one or two humans annually contract the disease in the United States. Rabid animals act strangely, attack without provocation, and may foam at the mouth. Be concerned if the attacking animal has any of these characteristics.

Any bite by an animal other than a pet dog or cat requires consultation with the physician as to whether or not the use of antirabies vaccine will be required. If the bite is by a dog or a cat, if the animal is being reliably observed for sickness by its owner, and if its immunizations are up to date, then consultation with the physician is not required. If the bite has left a wound that might require stitching or other treatment, consult Cuts (Problem 1) or Puncture Wounds (Problem 2). You should also check Tetanus Shots (Problem 5). Facial wounds should be checked by a physician because of potential cosmetic disfigurement.

Home Treatment

An animal whose immunizations are up to date is, of course, unlikely to have rabies. However, arrange for the animal to be observed for the next 15 days to make sure that it does not develop rabies. Most often, the owners of the animal can be relied on to observe it. If the owners cannot be trusted, then the animal must be kept for observation by the local public agency charged with that responsibility. Many localities require that animal bites be reported to the health department. If the animal should develop rabies during this time, a serious situation exists and treatment by a physician must be started immediately.

For the wound itself, use soap and water. Treat bites as cuts (see Problem 1) or puncture wounds (Problem 2), depending on its appearance. The best approach to animal bites is to avoid getting them. We have suggested some ways in which parents can teach their children to get along with dogs and avoid bites on pp. 108–109.

What to Expect at the Doctor's Office

The physician must balance the usually remote possibility of exposure to rabies against the hazards of rabies vaccine or antirabies serum. An unprovoked attack by a wild animal or a bite from an animal that appears to have rabies may require both the rabies vaccine and the antirabies serum. The extent and location of the wounds also play a part in this decision; severe wounds of the head are the most dangerous.

A bite caused by an animal that has then escaped will often require the use of at least the rabies vaccine. This is one of the most difficult decisions in medicine. Rabies vaccine is administered in 14 to 21 daily injections, which are followed by booster injections 10 to 20 days after the initial series. The vaccine will often cause local skin reactions as well as fever, chills, aches, and pain. Severe reactions to the vaccine are rare. The antirabies serum, unfortunately, has a high risk of serious reactions. The serum is given both directly into the wound and by intramuscular injections.

Many physicians give a tetanus shot if the child is not "up to date" because tetanus bacteria can (rarely) be introduced by an animal bite. Be sure you know when your child's last tetanus shot was received.

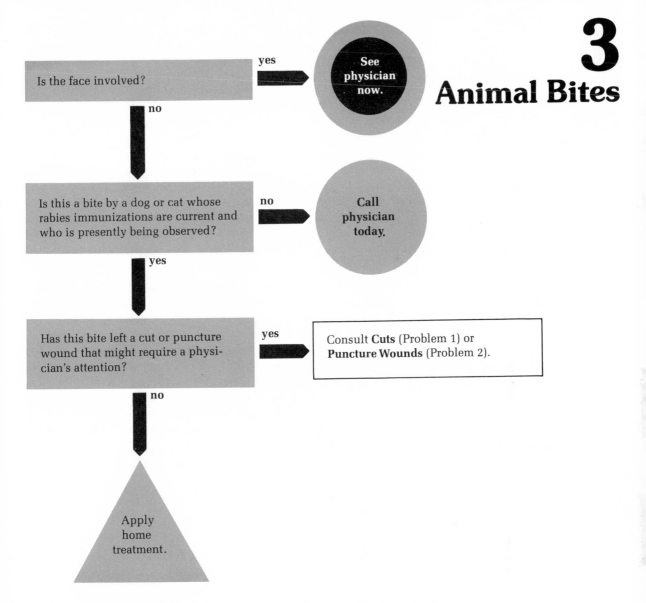

Is the face involved? — yes → **See physician now.**

no ↓

Is this a bite by a dog or cat whose rabies immunizations are current and who is presently being observed? — no → **Call physician today.**

yes ↓

Has this bite left a cut or puncture wound that might require a physician's attention? — yes → Consult **Cuts** (Problem 1) or **Puncture Wounds** (Problem 2).

no ↓

Apply home treatment.

3
Animal Bites

4

Scrapes and Abrasions

Scrapes and abrasions are shallow. Several layers of the skin may be torn or even totally scraped off, but the wound does not go far beneath the skin. Abrasions are usually caused by falls onto the hands, elbows, or knees, but skateboard and bicycle riders frequently find ways to get abrasions on just about any part of their bodies. Since abrasions expose millions of nerve endings, all of which send pain impulses to the brain, they are usually much more painful than cuts.

Home Treatment

Remove all dirt and foreign matter. Washing the wound with soap and warm water is the most important step in treatment. Hydrogen peroxide (3%) may also be used to cleanse the wound. Most scrapes will "scab" rather quickly; this is nature's way of "dressing" the wound. The use of Mercurochrome, iodine, and other antiseptics does little good and is usually painful. The use of adhesive bandages may be necessary for a wound that continues to ooze blood, but should be discontinued as soon as possible to allow the air and sun to the wound.

Loose skin flaps, if they are not dirty, may be left to help form a natural dressing. If the skin flap is dirty, cut it off carefully with nail scissors. (If it hurts, stop! You're cutting the wrong tissue.) Watch the wound for signs of infection—pus, a fever, or severe swelling or redness—but don't be worried by redness around the edges; this indicates normal healing. Infection will not be obvious in the first 24 hours; serious infection without fever is rare. Pain can be treated for the first few minutes with an ice pack in a plastic bag or towel applied over the wounds as needed. The worst pain subsides fairly quickly, and aspirin or acetaminophen can then be used if necessary.

What to Expect at the Doctor's Office

The physician will make sure that the wound is free of dirt and foreign matter. Soap and water and hydrogen peroxide (3%) will often be used. Sometimes a local anesthetic is required to reduce the pain of the cleansing process. An antibacterial ointment such as Neosporin or Bacitracin is sometimes applied after cleansing the wound. Betadine is a painless iodine preparation that is also occasionally used. Tetanus shots are not required for simple scrapes, but if your child is overdue, it is a good chance to get caught up.

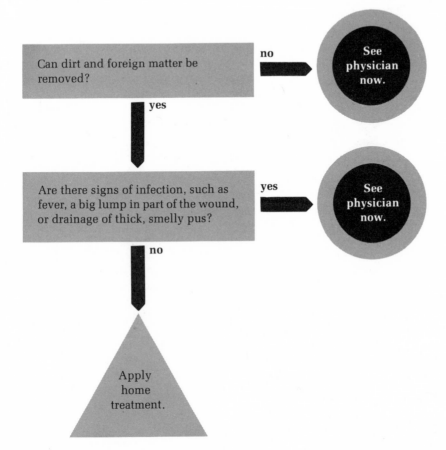

5
Tetanus Shots

Parents often bring their children to the doctor's office or emergency room simply to get a tetanus shot. Often the wound is minor and needs only some soap and water. If the shot is not needed, you don't need a doctor. The chart on the facing page illustrates the essentials of the current United States Public Health Service recommendations. It can save you and your children several visits to the doctor.

The question of whether or not a wound is minor may be troublesome. Wounds caused by sharp, clean objects such as knives or razor blades have less chance of becoming infected than those in which dirt or foreign bodies have penetrated and lodged beneath the skin. Abrasions and minor burns will not result in tetanus. The tetanus germ cannot grow in the presence of air; the skin must be cut or punctured for the germ to reach an airless location.

If your child has never had a basic series of three tetanus shots, then you should see the doctor. Sometimes a different kind of tetanus shot is required if you have not been adequately immunized. This shot is called *tetanus immune globulin*, and is used when immunization is not complete and there is a significant risk of tetanus. This shot is more expensive, more painful, and more likely to cause an allergic reaction than is the tetanus booster. So keep a record of your family's immunizations in the back of this book and know the dates.

During the first tetanus shots (usually a series of three injections given in early childhood), immunity to tetanus develops over a three-week period. This immunity then slowly declines over many months. After each booster, immunity develops more rapidly and lasts longer. If your child has had an initial series of five tetanus injections, immunity will usually last at least ten years after every booster injection. Nevertheless, if a wound has left contaminated material beneath the skin and not exposed to the air, and if your child has not had a tetanus shot within the past five years, a booster shot is advised to keep the level of immunity as high as possible.

In the United States, tetanus immunization remains very important, since the tetanus germ is quite common and the disease (lockjaw) is so severe. Be absolutely sure that each of your children has had the basic series of three injections and appropriate boosters. Since the immunity lasts so long, adults usually get away with a long period between boosters, but with children it should be "by the book." (See p. 112.)

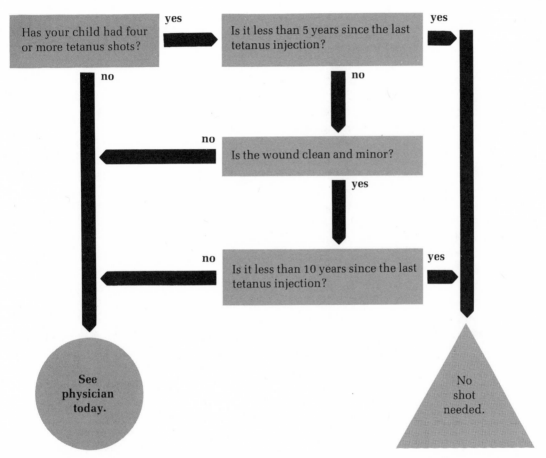

Has your child had four or more tetanus shots?

yes → Is it less than 5 years since the last tetanus injection?

yes →

no ↓

Is the wound clean and minor?

no ←

yes ↓

Is it less than 10 years since the last tetanus injection?

no ←

yes →

no (from first question) ↓

See physician today.

No shot needed.

6

Is a Bone Broken?

Neither parent nor doctor can always tell by eye whether or not a bone is broken. We have found fractures when we were not expecting them and not found them when we were sure a bone was broken. So you need an X-ray any time that there is a reasonable suspicion of a fracture. The chart on the facing page is a guide to "reasonable suspicion." In the majority of fractures, the bone fragments are already aligned for good healing. Thus prompt manipulation of the fragments is not necessary. If the injured part is protected and resting, a delay of several days before casting does no harm. Remember that the cast does not have healing properties; it just keeps the fragments from getting joggled too much during the healing period. Possible fractures are discussed further in Ankle Injuries (Problem 7), Knee Injuries (Problem 8), and Wrist, Elbow, and Shoulder Injuries (Problem 9).

A fracture can injure nearby nerves and arteries. If the limb is cold, blue, or numb, see the doctor now! Fractures of the pelvis or thigh are particularly serious. Check out all injuries to these areas with the doctor. Fortunately, these fractures are relatively rare except when great force is involved, as in automobile accidents. In these situations the need for immediate help is obvious. For head injuries, see Problem 10.

Paleness, sweating, dizziness, and thirst can indicate shock, and immediate attention is needed.

A crooked limb is an obvious reason to check for fracture. The arm bent halfway between elbow and wrist or the leg bent at mid-calf clearly indicates a fracture. Pain that prevents use of the injured limb suggests the need for an X-ray. Soft-tissue injuries usually allow some use of the limb, although there are exceptions to this rule.

Although large bruises under the skin may be caused by soft-tissue injuries alone, marked bruising in a limb that may have a fracture means that you should see the doctor.

Common sense tells us that when great force is involved the possibility of a broken bone is increased. The most common example is the automobile accident, which often gives us the unwanted opportunity to witness the results of great forces applied to the human body. The child who has fallen twenty feet out of a tree is much more likely to have a broken limb than the child who has stumbled and fallen. The severity of the accident is helpful information to have, but some bones break with very little provocation.

Children's bones are younger and hence more flexible and resilient than those of adults. Instead of outright breaks, young bones often bend or splinter like young tree limbs and hence are called "greenstick" fractures. Young bones are also still growing. The growth plates of all bones are at the ends. Consequently, an injury to a bone near the end must be treated more cautiously since growth plate damage may stop limb growth.

Home Treatment

Apply ice packs. The immediate application of cold will help to decrease swelling and inflammation. If a broken bone is suspected, the involved limb should be protected and rested for at least 48 hours. To rest a bone effectively, the joint above and below the bone should be immobilized. If you suspect a fracture of the lower arm, the splint should prevent the wrist and elbow from moving. Magazines, cardboard, and rolled newspaper will all serve. Do not wrap tightly or circulation will be cut off. During this time the limb should be cautiously tested to determine persistence of pain on movement and the return of function. A limb that cannot be used at all is more likely to be broken.

Any injury that is still painful after 48 hours should be examined by a physician. Minutes and hours are *not* crucial unless there is misalignment or injury to arteries or nerves. A limb that is adequately protected and rested is likely to have a good outcome even if a fracture is present and casting or splinting is delayed. Give your child aspirin or acetaminophen for pain.

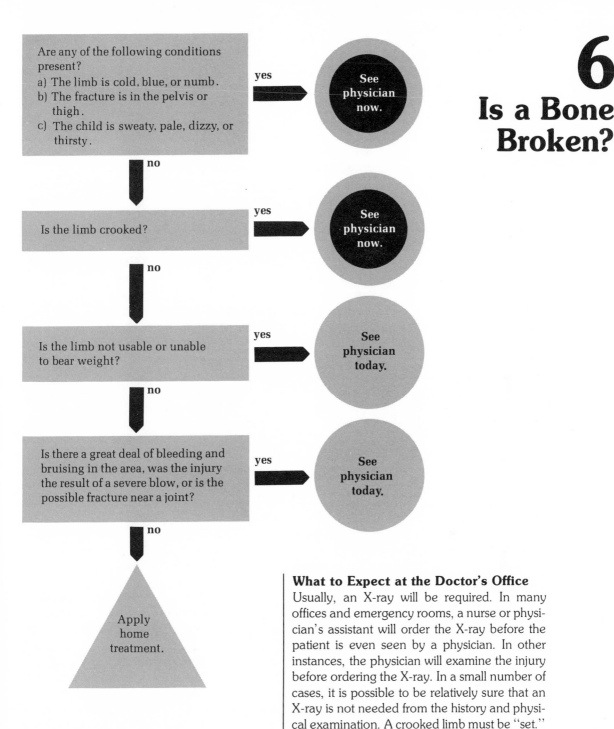

6
Is a Bone Broken?

Are any of the following conditions present?
a) The limb is cold, blue, or numb.
b) The fracture is in the pelvis or thigh.
c) The child is sweaty, pale, dizzy, or thirsty.

yes → **See physician now.**

no

Is the limb crooked?

yes → **See physician now.**

no

Is the limb not usable or unable to bear weight?

yes → **See physician today.**

no

Is there a great deal of bleeding and bruising in the area, was the injury the result of a severe blow, or is the possible fracture near a joint?

yes → **See physician today.**

no

Apply home treatment.

What to Expect at the Doctor's Office

Usually, an X-ray will be required. In many offices and emergency rooms, a nurse or physician's assistant will order the X-ray before the patient is even seen by a physician. In other instances, the physician will examine the injury before ordering the X-ray. In a small number of cases, it is possible to be relatively sure that an X-ray is not needed from the history and physical examination. A crooked limb must be "set." Sometimes this requires general anesthesia. Pinning the fragments together surgically so that they will heal well is required for certain fractures, like elbow fractures.

7
Ankle Injuries

Ligaments are tissues that connect the bones of a joint to provide stability during the joint's action. When the ankle is twisted severely, either the ligament or the bone must give way. If the ligaments give, they may be stretched (strained), partially torn (sprained), or completely torn (torn ligaments). If the ligaments do not give, then one of the bones around the ankle must break (fracture).

Strains, sprains, and even some minor fractures of the ankle will heal well with home treatment. Even some torn ligaments may do well without a great deal of medical care; operations to repair them are rare. For practical purposes, the immediate attention of the doctor is only necessary when the injury has been severe enough to cause obvious fracture to the bones around the ankle or to cause a completely torn ligament. This is indicated by a deformed joint with abnormal motion. Fractures are more likely in a fall from a considerable height or in automobile or in bicycle accidents. They are *not* likely to happen when the ankle is twisted while walking or running.

The typical ankle sprain swells either around the bony bump at the outside of the ankle or about two inches in front of and below it. The usual sprain does not need prolonged rest, casting, or X-rays. Except for obvious deformities of the ankle suggesting a severe fracture, home treatment should be started promptly. Detection of any damage to the ligaments is difficult immediately after the injury because of the amount of swelling that may be present. Since it is easier to do an adequate examination of the foot after the swelling has gone down, and since no damage is done by resting a mild fracture or torn ligament, there is no need to rush to the doctor.

Pain "tells" you what to do with ankle injuries. If what the child is doing hurts, don't do it. If pain prevents any standing on the ankle for more than 24 hours, see the doctor. If little progress is being made so that pain makes weight bearing difficult at 72 hours, see the doctor. Swelling is not a good guide as to what to do with an ankle injury. Sprains and torn ligaments usually swell quickly because there is bleeding into the tissue around the ankle. The skin will turn blue-black in the area as the blood is broken down by the body. The amount of swelling will not differentiate between sprains, tears, and fractures. The common chip fractures around the ankle are variable and often the swelling is considerably less than with a sprain. Remember these basic facts: Home treatment is adequate for all ankle injuries except for some fractures and complete ligament tears. Even if a fracture is present, if the ankle is rested and protected, no harm will be done by waiting and watching it.

Home Treatment

RIP is your key word: rest, ice, and protection. Elevate the ankle and keep it elevated. Do *not* let the child return to play as soon as the pain becomes bearable. Apply ice in a towel to the injured area and leave it there for at least 30 minutes. If there is any evidence of swelling after the first 30 minutes, then ice should be applied for 30 minutes on and 15 minutes off through the next few hours. If pain subsides completely in the elevated position, then weight bearing may be attempted cautiously. If pain is present when bearing weight, then weight bearing should be avoided for the first 24 hours. Heat may be applied, but only after 24 hours.

If crutches are used, adjust the crutches so that the shoulder support is two finger-breadths short of the armpit. The weight should be taken on the hand, not the armpit, where the crutch could damage blood vessels and nerves. If at the end of the first 24 hours the pain prevents any weight bearing, then see the doctor. If pain is present but not severe, then continue using the crutches until walking can be accomplished with little discomfort, usually two or three days. During this time, an elastic bandage may be used, but this will not prevent reinjury if full

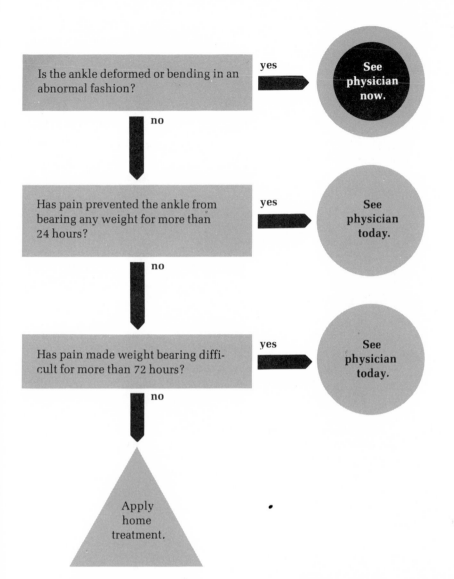

Is the ankle deformed or bending in an abnormal fashion?

yes → **See physician now.**

no

Has pain prevented the ankle from bearing any weight for more than 24 hours?

yes → **See physician today.**

no

Has pain made weight bearing difficult for more than 72 hours?

yes → **See physician today.**

no

Apply home treatment.

activity is resumed. Do not stretch the bandage so that it is very tight and interferes with blood circulation. Taping generally should not be attempted in children; if it is done incorrectly, it may cut off circulation to the foot. The ankle should feel relatively normal by about 10 days. Be warned, however, that full healing will not take place for from four to six weeks. (The same is true of a fracture.) If strenuous activity, such as organized athletics, is to be pursued during this time, then the ankle should be taped by someone experienced in this technique.

What to Expect at the Doctor's Office

The doctor will examine the motions of the ankle to see if they are abnormal and may take an X-ray. If there is no fracture, it is likely that a continuation of home treatment will be recommended. Home treatment may also be recommended if a minor chip fracture is noted. For other fractures, a cast will be necessary or, rarely, an operation to put the bones back together. Depending on the nature and extent of a ligament injury, an operation may be required to repair a completely torn ligament.

8
Knee Injuries

The ligaments of the knee may be stretched (strained), partially torn (sprained), or completely torn (torn ligament). Unlike the ankle, torn ligaments in the knee need to be repaired surgically as soon as possible after the injury occurs. If surgery is delayed, the operation is more difficult and less likely to be successful. For this reason, the approach to knee injuries is more cautious than for ankle injuries. If there is any possibility of a torn ligament, go to the doctor. Fractures in the area of the knee are less common than around the ankle and all need to be cared for by a doctor.

Significant knee injuries usually occur during a sports activity, when the knee is more likely to experience twisting and side contact; these are responsible for most ligament injuries. (Deep knee bends stretch knee ligaments and may contribute to knee injuries; they should be practiced cautiously.) Serious knee injuries occur when the leg is planted on the ground and a blow is received to the knee from the side. If the foot cannot give, the knee will. There is no way to totally avoid this possibility in athletics. The use of shorter spikes and cleats help, but elastic knee supports and wraps give virtually no protection.

When ligaments are completely torn, the lower leg can be wiggled from side to side when the leg is straight. Compare the injured knee to the opposite knee to get some idea of what amount of side-to-side motion is normal. Your examination will not be as skilled as that of the doctor, but if you think that the motion may be abnormally loose, see the doctor. If the cartilage within the knee has been torn, then the normal motion of the knee may be blocked, preventing it from being straightened out. Although a torn cartilage does not need immediate surgery, it deserves prompt medical attention. The amount of pain and swelling does not indicate the severity of the injury. The ability to bear weight, to move the knee through the normal range of motion, and to keep the knee stable when wiggled is more important. Typically, strains and sprains hurt immediately and continue to hurt for hours and even days after the injury. Swelling in strains and sprains tends to come on rather slowly over a period of hours, but may reach rather large proportions. When a ligament is completely torn, there is intense pain immediately, which subsides until the knee may hurt little or not at all for a while. Usually, there is significant bleeding into the tissues around the joint when a ligament is torn so that swelling tends to come on quickly and be impressive in its quantity. The best policy when there is a potential injury to the ligament is to have the child avoid any major activity until it is clear that this is a minor strain or sprain. Home treatment is intended only for minor strains and sprains.

Home Treatment
RIP again is the key word—rest, ice, and protection. Get the child off the knee and elevate it. Apply ice in a towel for at least 30 minutes to minimize swelling. If there is more than slight swelling or pain, despite the fact that the knee was put immediately to rest and ice was applied, see the doctor. If this is not the case, then ice should be on the knee for 30 minutes and then off for 15 minutes for the next several hours. Limited weight bearing may be attempted during this time with a close watch for increased swelling and pain. Heat may be applied after 24 hours. By 24 hours, the knee should look and feel relatively normal, and after 72 hours this should clearly be the case. Remember, however, that a strain or sprain is not completely healed for four to six weeks and that it requires protection during this healing period. Elastic bandages will not give adequate support but will ease symptoms a bit and remind the child to be careful with the knee.

What to Expect at the Doctor's Office
The knee will be examined for range of motion and the lateral stability will be tested by stressing the knee from side to side. A massively swollen knee may have blood removed from the joint with a needle. Torn ligaments need

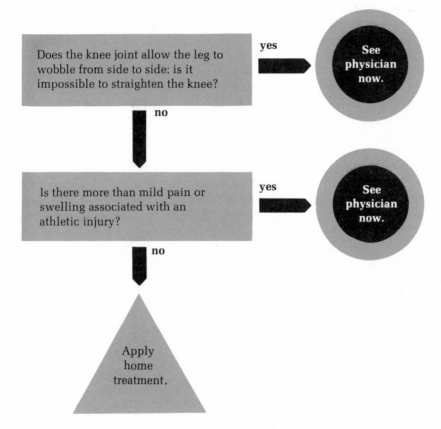

Does the knee joint allow the leg to wobble from side to side; is it impossible to straighten the knee?

yes → See physician now.

no ↓

Is there more than mild pain or swelling associated with an athletic injury?

yes → See physician now.

no ↓

Apply home treatment.

surgical repair. X-rays may be taken, but are not always helpful. For injuries that appear minor, home treatment will be advised. Pain medications are sometimes, but not often, required.

9

Wrist, Elbow, and Shoulder Injuries

The ligaments of these joints may be stretched (strained) or partially torn (sprained), but complete tears are rare in children. This is because the weakest points of long bones in children are the soft cartilage growth plates at the bone ends. Trauma will often result in injury to these growth plates; injuries to bone ends must be treated cautiously. Fractures may occur at the wrist, are less frequent around the elbow, and are uncommon around the shoulder. Injuries to wrist and elbow occur most often during a fall, when the weight of the body is caught on the outstretched arm. Injuries to the shoulder usually result from direct blows.

The wrist is the most frequently injured of these joints. Strains and sprains are common and the small bones in the wrist may be fractured. Fractures of these small bones may be difficult to see on an X-ray. The most frequent fracture of the wrist involves the ends of the long bones of the forearm and is easily recognized because it causes an unnatural bend near the wrist. Physicians refer to this as the "silver fork deformity."

The most frequent elbow injury is the "pulled elbow," which is often not even suspected. A young child (usually less than five years old) is noted cradling one arm in the other and holding the elbow. Parents often think that the arm is paralyzed, since the child cannot lift the affected arm. The fact that the toddler may have been pulled along by the arm an hour before is often not remembered, although this is what caused the injury. In the case of a pulled elbow, the palm of the hand is facing down toward the floor or inward toward the belly; if the palm is turned upward, it is unlikely that a pulled elbow is the problem, since the cure for a pulled elbow is to turn the palm upward. The cure is frequently performed unknowingly by the child, parent, nurse, or X-ray technician before the child is seen by the doctor. A pulled elbow does not show up on an X-ray.

The collarbone (clavicle) is a frequently fractured bone in children; fortunately, it has remarkable healing powers. Parents will often notice the fracture because of the child's inability to raise the arm on the affected side. The shoulders may also appear uneven. This fracture occurs in newborns as well as in older children. Bandaging is all the treatment required.

The shoulder separation often seen in high school athletes is perhaps the most common injury of the shoulder. It is a stretching or tearing of the ligament that attaches the collarbone to one of the bones that forms the shoulder joint. It causes a slight deformity and extreme tenderness at the end of the collarbone. Sprains and strains of other ligaments occur, but complete tearing is rare as are fractures. Dislocations of the shoulder are rare outside of high school athletics, but are best treated early when they do occur.

In summary, severe fractures and dislocations are best treated early. These usually cause deformity, severe pain, and limitation of movement. Other fractures will not be harmed if the injured limb is rested and protected. Complete tears of ligaments are rare; strains and sprains will heal with home treatment.

Home Treatment

Partial dislocation of elbow (pulled elbow). Bend the elbow so that the forearm and upper arm form a right angle. With one hand, hold the elbow and steady it so it cannot move. With the other hand, grasp the child's hand and wrist and turn the palm upward, while gently pulling away from the body at the elbow. Some doctors prefer a quick, forceful twist, but we think a gentle turn does as well. Initially, this turning will cause discomfort. A click is then felt or even heard. If treatment occurs soon after the injury, then immediate relief of pain is usual. If treatment is delayed, then some soreness usually remains for a short period. Great force is not required for this treatment. If success does not come easily, see your doctor.

164

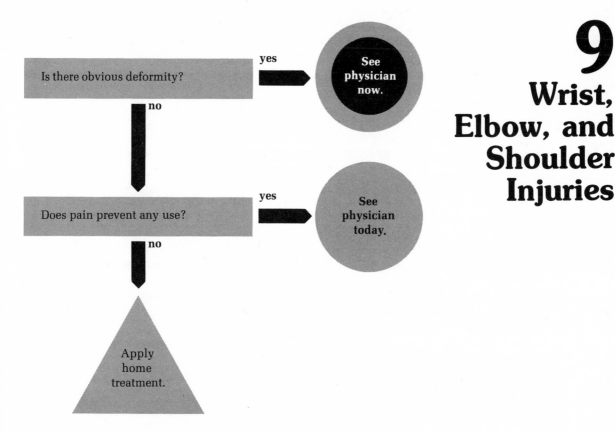

Is there obvious deformity? — **yes** → **See physician now.**

no ↓

Does pain prevent any use? — **yes** → **See physician today.**

no ↓

Apply home treatment.

Wrist, Elbow, and Shoulder Injuries

Sprains and strains. RIP is the key word— rest, ice, and protection. Rest the arm and apply ice for at least 30 minutes. If the pain is gone and there is no swelling at the end of this time, the ice may be discontinued. A sling for shoulder and elbow injuries and a partial splint for wrist injuries will give protection and rest to the injury while allowing the child to move around. Ice wrapped in a towel applied for 30 minutes on and 15 minutes off may be continued through the first eight hours if swelling appears. Heat may be applied *after* 24 hours. The injured joint should be usable with little pain within 24 hours and should be almost normal by 72 hours. If not, see the doctor. Complete healing takes from four to six weeks and activities with a likelihood of reinjury should be avoided by the child if possible during this time.

What to Expect at the Doctor's Office

An examination and sometimes X-rays will be performed. A broken bone may require a cast. The pulled elbow will be fixed if you didn't fix it already. A sling may be devised. Pain medication is sometimes given, but aspirin or acetaminophen are about as good and are less hazardous.

10
Head
Injuries

Every child will experience a bang on the head sometime in life and many children seem to bump their heads every few days. Many of these injuries will be minor, such as those from walking into a table or falling from the couch. Other head injuries will occur in bicycle, baseball, and automobile accidents. All head injuries are potentially serious, but few ever lead to problems. The major concern in a head injury in which the skull is not clearly and obviously damaged is the occurrence of bleeding inside the skull. The accumulation of blood inside of the skull will eventually compress the brain and cause damage. Fortunately, nature has carefully cushioned the valuable contents of the skull. In infants, the fontanel or soft spot serves as a safety valve to help diminish the severity of head injuries. Careful observation is the most valuable tool for diagnosing serious head injury. This can be done as well at home as at the hospital; there is some risk either way and it is your choice.

Home Treatment
Ice applied to a bruised area may minimize swelling. Children often develop "goose eggs" anyway. The size of the bump does not indicate the severity of the injury.

The initial observation period is crucial. Bleeding into the head can be very rapid within the first 24 hours and may continue for as long as 72 hours or more. Some bleeding may occur very slowly; this is called a *subdural hematoma* and may produce chronic headache, persistent vomiting, or personality changes months after the injury.

Observation of your child begins with the accident. If your child was knocked unconscious or cannot remember the events immediately before or after the accident, it is evidence of a concussion and the child should be brought to the doctor.

How does your child act? Increased lethargy, alternating alert and drowsy periods during the day, persistent vomiting, and unresponsiveness are all signs of possible bleeding within the skull. Vomiting usually occurs at least once after any significant head injury. If repeated vomiting occurs, see the physician. The seriously affected child also cannot be easily roused.

How does your child look? Children who appear persistently pale, sweaty, or weak should be brought to the doctor. Look also for unequal pupil size, which can be caused by pressure on the brain created by blood within the skull. Some children have pupils that are unequal all the time; this is normal for them. If the pupils become unequal after an injury, however, it is a serious sign. A slow (less than 60) or irregular pulse is a sign of internal bleeding.

In the case of a typical minor head injury, a child falls off a table and bangs his or her head. A bump may immediately develop. The child remains conscious and cries immediately. For a few minutes, the child is unconsolable and may vomit once or twice over the first few hours. Some sleepiness from the excitement may be noted; the child may nap but is easily aroused. Neither pupil is enlarged and the vomiting ceases shortly. The child does not appear pale and the pulse is strong and regular. Within eight hours the child is back to normal except for the tender and often prominent "goose egg."

A serious head injury is more likely to occur with more severe trauma, such as falling from a roof, being hit by a baseball, bicycle, skateboard, or automobile accidents. The child may or may not have lost consciousness. The child often becomes lethargic but may seem to recover only to become lethargic again. A pupil may or may not enlarge. Vomiting is often repeated. The child may appear pale and the pulse may be irregular or slow (below 70).

In serious accidents, injury to the chest, abdomen, or extremities must not be overlooked.

You should reassess your child's condition frequently. If there are any suspicious signs in your child, consult the physician by phone at once. Since most accidents occur in the evening hours, children will be asleep several hours after most accidents; you can look in on them periodically to check their pulse, pupils,

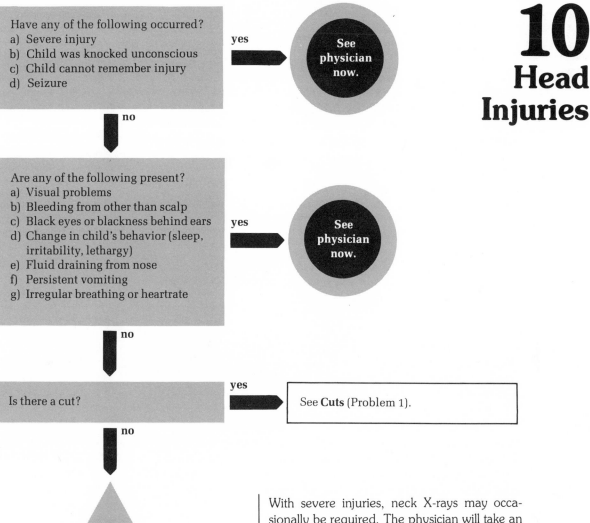

Have any of the following occurred?
a) Severe injury
b) Child was knocked unconscious
c) Child cannot remember injury
d) Seizure

yes → See physician now.

no

Are any of the following present?
a) Visual problems
b) Bleeding from other than scalp
c) Black eyes or blackness behind ears
d) Change in child's behavior (sleep, irritability, lethargy)
e) Fluid draining from nose
f) Persistent vomiting
g) Irregular breathing or heartrate

yes → See physician now.

no

Is there a cut?

yes → See **Cuts** (Problem 1).

no

Apply home treatment.

and arousability if you are concerned. With minor head bumps, nighttime checking is usually not necessary.

What to Expect at the Doctor's Office

The diagnosis of bleeding within the skull cannot be made with great accuracy. Skull X-rays are seldom helpful except in detecting whether a fragment of bone from the skull has been pushed into the brain, but this situation is rare.

With severe injuries, neck X-rays may occasionally be required. The physician will take an extensive history on the nature of the accident, and in addition assess the child's general appearance and take repeated blood pressures and pulse rates. In addition, the head, eyes, ears, nose, throat, neck, and nervous system will be examined. The physician will also check for other possible sites of injury such as the chest, abdomen, and arms and legs. Where internal bleeding is likely but not certain, the child may be hospitalized for observation. During this observation period, the child's pulse, pupils, and blood pressure will be checked periodically. In short, the doctor will observe and wait, much as would be done at home. Use of medications, which may obscure the situation, will be avoided.

11
Burns

How bad is a burn? Burns are classified as first, second, or third degree, according to the depth of the burn. First-degree burns are superficial and cause the skin to turn red. A sunburn is usually a first-degree burn. Second-degree burns are deeper and result in splitting of the skin layers or blistering. Scalding with hot water or a very severe sunburn with blisters are common instances of second-degree burns. Third-degree burns destroy all layers of the skin and extend into the deeper tissues. They are painless because nerve endings have been destroyed. Charring of the burned tissue is usually present.

First-degree burns may cause a lot of pain but are not a major medical problem. Even when they are extensive, they seldom give rise to lasting problems and seldom need a doctor's attention.

Second-degree burns are also painful, and extensive second-degree burns may cause significant fluid loss. Scarring, however, is usually minimal, and infection usually is not a problem. Second-degree burns can be treated at home if they are not extensive. Any second-degree burn that involves an area larger than the child's hand should be seen by a doctor. In addition, a second-degree burn that involves the face or hands should be seen by a physician; these might result in cosmetic problems or loss of function.

Third-degree burns result in scarring and present frequent problems with infection and fluid loss. The more extensive the burn, the more difficult these problems. All third-degree burns should be seen by a physician, since not only do they possibly lead to scarring and infection, but skin grafts are often needed.

Home Treatment

Apply cold water or ice immediately. This reduces the amount of skin damage caused by the burn and also eases pain. The cold should be applied for at least five minutes and continued until pain is relieved or for one hour, whichever comes first. Be careful not to apply cold so long that the burned area turns numb, since frostbite can occur! It may be reapplied if pain returns. Aspirin or acetaminophen may be used to reduce pain. Blisters should not be broken. If they burst by themselves, as they often do, the overlying skin should be allowed to remain as a wet dressing. The use of local anesthetic creams or sprays is not recommended, since they may slow healing. Also, some patients develop an irritation or allergy to these drugs. Any burn that continues to be painful for more than 48 hours should be seen by a physician.

What to Expect at the Doctor's Office

The physician will establish the extent and degree of the burn and will determine the need for antibiotics, hospitalization, and skin grafting. An antibacterial ointment and dressing, with frequent changes and checks for infections, will often be recommended. Extensive burns may require hospitalization and third-degree burns may eventually require skin grafts.

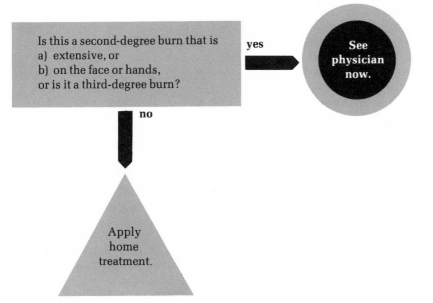

Is this a second-degree burn that is
a) extensive, or
b) on the face or hands,
or is it a third-degree burn?

yes

See physician now.

no

Apply home treatment.

12
Infected Wounds and Blood Poisoning

"Blood poisoning" is not a current medical term. There is a folk saying that red streaks running up the arm or leg from a wound are blood poisoning and that the patient will die when the streaks reach the heart. In fact, such streaks are only an inflammation of the lymph channels carrying away the debris from the wound. They will stop when they reach local lymph nodes in the armpit or groin and do not, by themselves, indicate blood poisoning. However, they usually are worth checking with your doctor.

Blood poisoning, to a physician, means bacterial infection in the bloodstream, and is termed *septicemia*. Fever is a better guide to this rare occurrence. A local wound should only give a very minor temperature elevation unless infected. If there is a fever, see the doctor.

An infected wound usually festers beneath the surface of the skin, resulting in pain and swelling. Bacterial infection requires at least a day, and usually two or three days, to develop. Therefore, a late increase in pain or swelling is a legitimate cause for concern. If the festering wound bursts open, pus will drain out. This is good, and the wound will usually heal well. Still, this demonstrates that an infection was present, and the doctor should evaluate the situation unless it is clearly minor.

An explanation of normal wound healing will be helpful. First, the body pours out serum into a wound area. Serum is yellowish and clear, and later turns into a scab. Serum is frequently mistaken for pus, which is thick, cheesy, smelly, and never seen in the first day or so. Second, inflammation around a wound is normal. In order to heal an area, the body must remove the debris and bring in new materials. Thus, the edges of a wound will be pink or red, and the wound area may be warm, without an infection. Third, the lymphatic system is actively involved in debris clearance, and pain along lymph channels or in the lymph nodes themselves may be present without infection.

Home Treatment

Keep a wound clean. If it is unsightly or in a location where it gets dirty easily, bandage it, changing bandages daily; if not, leave it open to the air. Soak and clean it gently with warm water for short periods—three or four times daily to remove debris and keep the scab soft. Children like to pick at scabs and often will fall on a scab. In these instances, Band-Aids are useful. The simplest wound of the face requires three to five days for healing. The healing period is five to seven days for the chest and arms and seven to nine days for the legs. Larger wounds, or those that have gaped open and must heal across a space, take correspondingly longer to heal. Children heal more rapidly than adults do.

What to Expect at the Doctor's Office

An examination of the wound and regional lymph nodes will be done, and the child's temperature will be taken. Sometimes cultures of the blood or of the wound are performed, and sometimes antibiotics are prescribed. If there is a suspicion of bacterial infection, then cultures may be taken before the antibiotics are given. If a wound is festering it may be drained either with a needle or a scalpel. This procedure is not very painful and actually relieves discomfort. For severe wound infections, hospitalization may be needed.

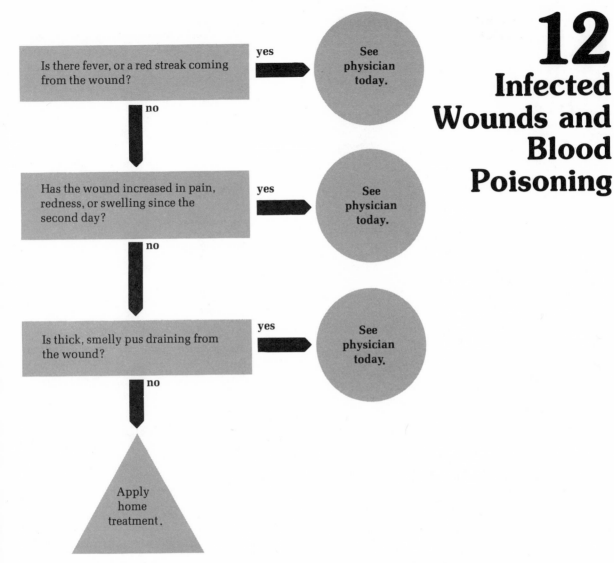

12
Infected Wounds and Blood Poisoning

Is there fever, or a red streak coming from the wound?

yes → See physician today.

no

Has the wound increased in pain, redness, or swelling since the second day?

yes → See physician today.

no

Is thick, smelly pus draining from the wound?

yes → See physician today.

no

Apply home treatment.

13
Insect Bites or Stings

Most insect bites are trivial, but some insect bites or stings may cause reactions either locally or in the basic body systems. Local reactions may be uncomfortable, but do not pose a serious hazard. In contrast, systemic reactions occasionally may be serious and may require emergency treatment.

There are three types of systemic reactions. All are rare. The most common is an asthma attack, causing difficulty breathing and perhaps audible wheezing. Hives or extensive skin rashes following insect bites are less serious but indicate that a reaction has occurred and a more severe reaction might occur if the child is bitten or stung again. Very rarely, fainting or loss of consciousness may occur. If a child has lost consciousness, you must assume that the collapse is due to an allergic reaction. This is an emergency. If a child has had any of these reactions in the past, he or she should be taken immediately to a medical facility if stung or bitten.

Bites from poisonous spiders are rare. The female black widow spider accounts for many of them. This spider is glossy black with a body of approximately one half inch in diameter, a leg span of about two inches, and a characteristic red hourglass mark on the abdomen. The black widow spider is found in wood piles, sheds, basements, or outdoor privies. The bite is often painless and the first sign may be cramping abdominal pain. The abdomen becomes hard and boardlike as the waves of pain become severe. Breathing is difficult and accompanied by grunting. There may be nausea, vomiting, headaches, sweating, twitching, shaking, and tingling sensations of the hand. The bite itself may not be prominent and may be overshadowed by the systemic reaction. Brown recluse spiders cause painful bites and serious local reaction, but are not nearly as dangerous as black widows. Brown recluse spiders are slightly smaller than black widows; they have a white "violin" pattern on their backs.

If the local reaction to a bite or sting is severe or a deep sore is developing, then a physician should be consulted by telephone. Children frequently have more severe local reactions than do adults.

Tick bites are common. The tick lives in tall grass or low shrubs and hops on and off of passing mammals, such as deer or dogs. In some localities, ticks may carry Rocky Mountain spotted fever, but most tick bites are not complicated by subsequent illness. Ticks will commonly be found in the scalp. Refer to Problem 48, Ticks and Chiggers.

Home Treatment
Apply something cold promptly. Ice or cold packs may be used. Delay in application of cold results in a more severe local reaction. Aspirin or other pain relievers may be used. Antihistamines, such as Chlor-Trimeton or Benadryl, can be helpful by relieving the itch somewhat. If the reaction is severe, the physician may be consulted by telephone.

What to Expect at the Doctor's Office
The physician will inquire what sort of insect or spider has inflicted the wound and will search for signs of systemic reaction. If a systemic reaction is present, adrenalin by injection is usually necessary. Rarely, measures to support breathing or blood pressure will be needed; these measures require the facilities of an emergency room or hospital.

If the problem is a local reaction, the physician will examine the wound for signs of death of tissue or infection. Occasionally, surgical drainage of the wound will be needed. In other cases, pain relievers or antihistamines may make the patient more comfortable. Adrenalin injections are occasionally used for very severe local reactions.

If there has been a severe allergic reaction, desensitization shots may be initiated. In addition, emergency kits can be purchased to help the person with a serious allergy.

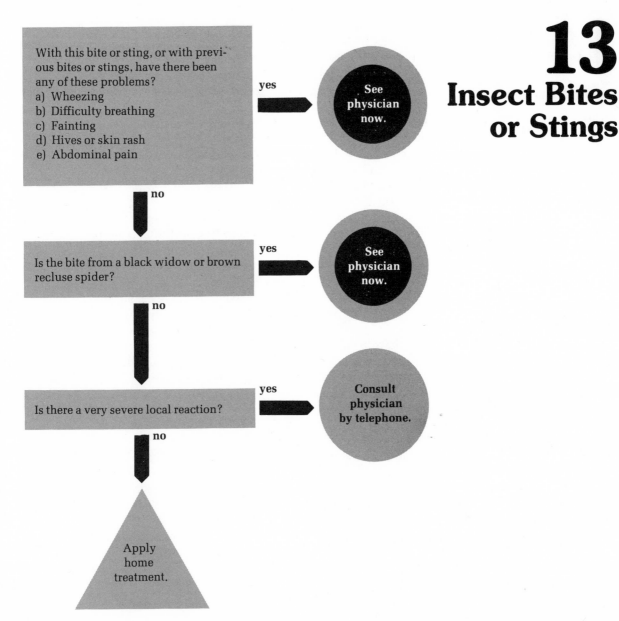

With this bite or sting, or with previous bites or stings, have there been any of these problems?
a) Wheezing
b) Difficulty breathing
c) Fainting
d) Hives or skin rash
e) Abdominal pain

yes → **See physician now.**

no ↓

Is the bite from a black widow or brown recluse spider?

yes → **See physician now.**

no ↓

Is there a very severe local reaction?

yes → **Consult physician by telephone.**

no ↓

Apply home treatment.

13
Insect Bites or Stings

14
Fishhooks

The problem, of course, is the barb. While the fish seem to get loose easily enough, children usually stay hooked. If you and the child can keep calm, you can remove the fishhook unless it is in the eye. (No attempt should be made to remove hooks that have actually penetrated the eyeball; this is a job for the doctor.) You will need the child's confidence and cooperation in order to avoid a visit to the doctor. The advantage of the doctor's office is a local anesthetic and extra hands to help hold the child. Remember that the injection of the anesthetic will hurt some, so this is not a choice between pain and no pain.

Home Treatment

Occasionally the hook will have come all the way around so that it lies just beneath the surface of the skin. If this is the case, often the best technique is simply to push the hook on through the skin, cut it off just behind the barb with wirecutters, and remove it by pulling it back through the way it entered.

On other occasions, the hook will be embedded only slightly and can be removed by simply grasping the shank of the hook (pliers help), pushing slightly forward and away from the barb, and then pulling it out. Sometimes, neither of these maneuvers will do the trick. In these cases, the method illustrated on the opposite page usually removes the hook quickly and very nearly painlessly. First a loop of fish line is put through the bend of the fishhook so that at the appropriate time a quick jerk can be applied and the hook can be pulled out directly in line with the shaft of the hook. (A) Holding onto the shaft, push the hook slightly in and away from the barb so as to disengage the barb. (B and C) Holding this pressure constant to keep the barb disengaged, give a quick jerk on the fish line and the hook pops out. If you are successful, then be sure that the child's tetanus shots are up to date (see Problem 5, Tetanus Shots). Treat the wound as in the home treatment section for Problem 2 (Puncture Wounds). If you are not successful, then the hook can be pushed all the way through and out so that the barb can be cut off with wirecutters as described above. However, this may be a bit more painful than the average child can tolerate with equanimity. If all else fails, a visit to the doctor should solve the problem. Note that a pair of needlenose pliers with a wire-cutting blade should be part of your fishing equipment.

What to Expect at the Doctor's Office

The doctor will use one of the three methods above to remove the hook. If necessary, the area around the hook can be infiltrated with a local anesthetic before the hook is removed. Often the giving of a local anesthetic is more painful than just removing the hook without the anesthetic.

If the hook is in the eye, it is likely that the help of an ophthalmologist (eye specialist) will be needed and it may be necessary to remove the hook in the operating room.

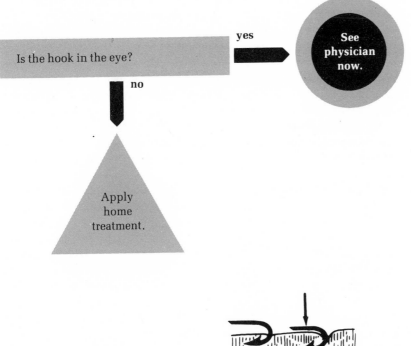

Is the hook in the eye?

yes — See physician now.

no

Apply home treatment.

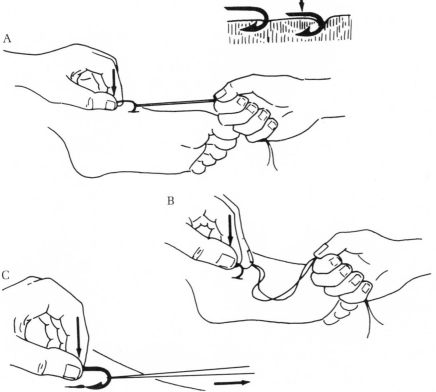

A

B

C

Drawing adapted from George Hill, *Outpatient Surgery.* Philadelphia: W. B. Saunders, 1973.

15
Smashed Fingers

Children always seem to be smashing their fingers in car doors or desk drawers or with hammers or baseballs. If the injury involves only the end segment of the finger (called the terminal phalanx) and does not involve a significant cut (see Problem 1, Cuts), then these injuries seldom need the help of a doctor. A painful problem that you can easily fix is blood under the fingernail (subungual hematoma). The method is described in the home treatment section below.

Fractures of the bone in this end segment are not treated unless they involve the joint. Many physicians feel that it is unwise to splint the finger even if there is a fracture of the joint. While the splint will decrease pain, it may also increase the stiffness of the joint after healing. However, if the fracture is not splinted, then pain may persist longer and your child may end up with a stiff joint anyway. You should discuss these advantages and disadvantages of splinting with your doctor.

If the injury involves other parts of the finger and if the child can move the finger easily, then apply home treatment of an ice pack for the swelling and aspirin or acetaminophen for the pain.

Fingernails are often dislocated in these injuries. It is not necessary to have the entire fingernail removed. The nail that is detached should be clipped off to avoid catching it painfully on other objects. Nail regrowth will take from four to six weeks.

Home Treatment

If there is a large amount of blood under the fingernail causing pain, this problem can often be relieved simply. Bend open an ordinary paper clip. (Hold the paper clip with a pair of pliers.) Heat one end using a candle or a cigarette lighter. When the tip is quite hot, touch it to the nail and it will melt its way right through the fingernail, leaving a small, clean hole. Steady the hand holding the pliers with the opposite hand so that the paper clip goes only through the nail and not into the flesh below. The blood trapped beneath the nail can now escape through the small hole and the pain will be relieved as the pressure is released. If the hole closes and the blood reaccumulates, then the procedure can be repeated using the same hole once again.

What to Expect at the Doctor's Office

The finger will be examined; an X-ray is likely if it appears that more than the end segment is involved. If there is a fracture involving the last joint on the finger, you should expect a discussion of the advantages and disadvantages of splinting the finger. Often splinting of one finger is accomplished by bandaging it together with the adjacent finger. If the finger is splinted, then periods of exercise should be included to preserve mobility. Severe injuries of fingers may occasionally require surgery in order to preserve function.

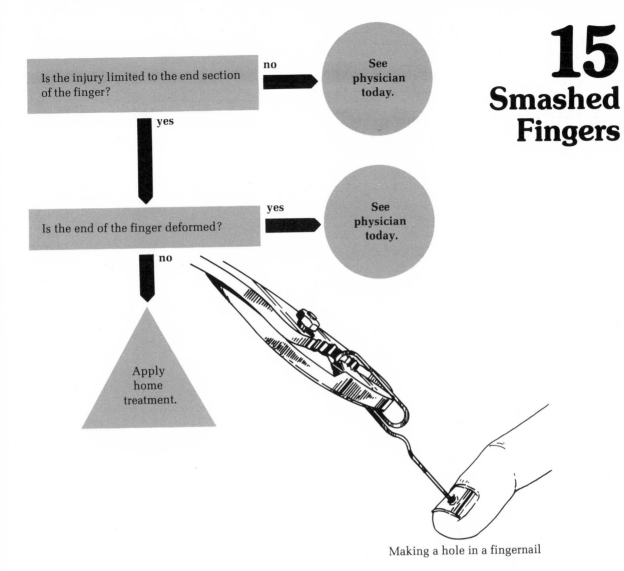

| Is the injury limited to the end section of the finger? | —no→ | See physician today. |

yes ↓

| Is the end of the finger deformed? | —yes→ | See physician today. |

no ↓

Apply home treatment.

Making a hole in a fingernail

D
Poisons

16. Oral Poisoning   **180**

What to do on the way to the doctor.

16
Oral
Poisoning

Although poisons may be inhaled or absorbed through the skin, for the most part they are swallowed. The term *ingestion* refers to oral poisoning.

Most poisoning can be prevented. Children almost always swallow poison accidentally. Keep harmful substances, such as medications, insecticides, caustic cleansers, and organic solvents like kerosene, gasoline, or furniture polish, out of the reach of little hands. The most damaging are strong alkali solutions used as drain cleaners (Drano), which will destroy any tissue with which they come in contact.

Treatment must be prompt to be effective, but while speed is important, accurate identification of the substance is equally so. *Don't panic.* Call the doctor or poison control center immediately and get advice on what to do. Attempt to identify the substance without causing undue delay. Always bring the container with you to the emergency room. Life-support measures take precedence in the case of the unconscious child, but the ingested substance must be identified before proper therapy can be instituted.

Suicide attempts cause many significant medication overdoses in teemagers. Any suicide attempt is an indication that help is needed. Such help is not optional, *even if the patient has "recovered"* and is in no immediate danger. Most successful suicides are preceded by unsuccessful attempts.

Home Treatment

All cases of poisoning require professional help. Someone should call immediately. If the child is conscious and alert and the ingredients swallowed are known, there are two types of treatment: those in which vomiting should be induced, and those in which it should not. Vomiting can be very dangerous if the poison contained strong acids, alkalis, or petroleum products. These substances can destroy the esophagus or damage the lungs as they are vomited. Neutralize them with milk while contacting the physician. If you don't have milk, give the child some water or milk of magnesia.

Vomiting is a safe way to remove medications and suspicious plants. It is more effective and safer than using a stomach pump and can be induced by a parent. Vomiting can sometimes be achieved immediately by stimulating the back of the throat with a finger (don't be squeamish!), or by giving two to four teaspoonfuls of *syrup* (*not* extract) of ipecac, followed by as much liquid as the child can drink. Vomiting follows usually within twenty minutes but, since time is important, using your finger is sometimes quicker. Or you can try both. Mustard mixed with warm water also works. If there is no vomiting in 25 minutes, repeat the dose of syrup of ipecac. Collect the vomitus so that it may be examined by the physician.

Before, after, or during first aid, contact a physician. Many communities have established poison control centers to identify poisons and give advice. These are often located in emergency rooms. Find out if such a center exists in your community and, if so, record the telephone number both on the chart and in the front of this book. Quick first aid and fast professional advice are your best chance to avoid a tragedy.

If an accidental poisoning has occurred, make sure that it doesn't happen again. Refer to Chapter 8 for information on "childproofing" your house.

What to Expect at the Doctor's Office

Significant poisoning is best managed at the emergency room. Treatment of the conscious child depends on the particular poison and whether vomiting has been achieved successfully. If indicated, the stomach will be evacuated by vomiting or by the use of a stomach pump. Children who are unconscious or have swallowed a strong acid or alkali will require admission to the hospital. With those who are not admitted to the hospital, observation at home is important.

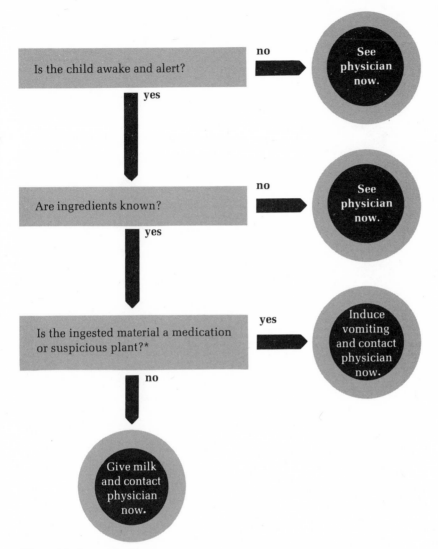

Is the child awake and alert? — no → See physician now.

yes ↓

Are ingredients known? — no → See physician now.

yes ↓

Is the ingested material a medication or suspicious plant?* — yes → Induce vomiting and contact physician now.

no ↓

Give milk and contact physician now.

*Do *not* induce vomiting
if the child has swallowed any
of the following:

Acids: battery acid, sulphuric acid,
hydrochloric acid, bleach, hair
straightener, etc.

Alkalis: Drano, drain cleaners, oven
cleaners, etc.

Poison control center telephone number _____
Emergency room telephone number _____

E
Fever

17. Fever   189
    What goes up will come down.

Many people, including physicians, speak of fever and illness as if they were one and the same. Surprisingly, an elevated temperature is not necessarily a sign of illness. Normal body temperature varies from individual to individual. If we measured a large number of healthy childrens' body temperatures while they were all resting, we would find a difference between the lowest and highest child of about 1.5°F. This is another reminder that children are individuals, and there is nothing either magical or accurate about the figure 98.6°F (37°C).

Normal body temperature varies greatly during the day. Temperature is generally lowest in the morning upon awakening. Many things will elevate body temperature including food, excess clothing, excitement, and anxiety. Vigorous exercise can raise body temperature to as much as 103°F. Severe exercise, without water or salt, can result in a condition known as heat stroke, with temperatures above 106°F. Other mechanisms also influence body temperature. Hormones, for example, account for a monthly variation of body temperature in ovulating women. The normal temperature is 1° to 1.5°F higher in the second half of the menstrual cycle. In general, children have higher body temperatures than adults do and seem to have greater daily variation because of their greater amounts of excitement and activity.

The most common causes for persistent fevers in children are viral and bacterial infections such as colds, sore throats, earaches, diarrhea, urinary infections, roseola, chickenpox, mumps, measles, and occasionally pneumonia, appendicitis, and meningitis.

A viral infection can result in a normal temperature or a temperature of 105°F. The height of the temperature is *not* a reliable indicator of the seriousness of the underlying infection.

Taking Your Child's Temperature

Either Fahrenheit or centigrade thermometers are acceptable. Rectal temperatures are usually more accurate and are about 0.5°F higher than oral temperatures. Oral temperature can be affected by hot or cold foods, routine breathing, and smoking. Generally, oral thermometers can be recognized by the longer bulb at the business end of the thermometer. The length of the bulb is to provide for a greater surface area and a faster, more accurate reading. Rectal thermometers have a shorter, rounder bulb to facilitate entry into the rectum.

Rectal thermometers can be used to take oral temperatures, but require a longer period in the mouth to achieve the same degree of accuracy as the oral thermometer. While oral thermometers can be used to take rectal temperatures, their shape is not ideal for younger children and we do not recommend their use in children.

Lubricants can facilitate placement of rectal thermometers. You need not bury the thermometer. Only an inch or so need be inside the child's rectum. The mercury will rise within seconds on a rectal thermometer since the rectum closely contacts the thermometer. Remove the thermometer when the mercury is no longer rising after a minute or two is up. Children should be placed on their stomachs when rectal temperatures are being taken. You should place a hand on their bottom to prevent them from moving.

Parents frequently ask us what temperature should be considered dangerous, or at what temperature a child should be brought to the doctor if no other symptoms are present. Consult a doctor immediately for the following:

- Fever in a child less than four months.

- Fever of more than 105°F if the home treatment measures described below fail to reduce the temperature at least partly. This is not because this temperature signifies a serious underlying condition, but because temperatures more than 105°F may be potentially damaging if they persist. Any temperature of 106°F should be evaluated by a physician promptly.

- Fever persisting for more than five days.

Febrile Seizures (Fever Fits)

The danger of an extremely high temperature is the possibility that the fever will cause a seizure (convulsion). All of us are capable of "seizing" if our body temperatures become too high. Febrile seizures are relatively common in normal, healthy children; about 3–5 percent will experience a febrile seizure. However, although common, they should not be minimized and must be treated with respect.

Febrile seizures occur most often in children between the ages of six months and four years. Illnesses that cause rapid elevations to high temperatures, such as roseola, have been frequently associated with febrile seizure. Rarely, a seizure is the first sign of a serious underlying problem such as meningitis.

During a seizure the brain, which is normally transmitting electrical impulses at a fairly regular rhythm, begins misfiring because of the overheating and causes involuntary muscular responses termed a seizure, convulsion, fit, or "falling out spell." The first sign may be a stiffening of the entire body. Children may have rhythmic beating of a single hand or foot, or any combination of the hands and feet. The eyes may roll back and the head may jerk. Urine and feces may pass involuntarily.

Most seizures last only from one to five minutes. There is very little evidence that such a short seizure is of any long-term consequence. On the other hand, prolonged seizures of more than 30 minutes are often a sign of a more serious underlying problem. Less than half of all children who have a short febrile seizure will ever experience a second, and less than half who experience a second will ever have a third.

Although a "seizing" child is a terrifying sight to a parent, the dangers to the child during a seizure are small. The following common-sense rules should be followed during a seizure.

- Protect your child's head from hitting anything hard. Place the child on a bed.

- Considerable damage can be done by forcing objects into the child's mouth to prevent biting of the tongue. Surprisingly, cut tongues are both uncommon and heal quickly.

- Make sure the child's breathing passage is open. Forcing a stick in your child's mouth does not ensure an open airway. In order to facilitate breathing, (1) clear the nose and mouth of vomitus or other material, and (2) pull the head backward slightly to "hyperextend" the neck. Artificial respiration is almost never necessary. These techniques are best learned in demonstrations. In a true emergency, hyperextend the neck and breathe ten times each minute through the child's nose while keeping the mouth covered (or through the child's mouth while keeping the nose pinched with your finger). Only blow air in; the child will blow the air out naturally.

- Begin fever reduction (discussed below) and seek medical attention immediately. Fortunately, once the seizure has stopped the child is usually temporarily resistant to a second seizure. However, since there are exceptions to this rule, medical attention is critical.

After the seizure has subsided, the child may be very groggy and have no recollection of what has occurred. Others may show signs of extreme weakness and even paralysis of an arm or leg. This paralysis is almost always temporary, but must be carefully evaluated.

A good physician will do a careful study to determine the cause of a febrile seizure. For the first febrile seizure, this will usually include a spinal tap (lumbar puncture) and fluid analysis to make certain that the seizure was not caused by meningitis. Following the termination of the fever, the physician will stress the importance of fever control for the next few days and will often place the child on anticonvulsant medications. For further discussion, see Problem 72 (Seizures).

The Meaning of the Chill
A chill is another symptom of a fever. The feeling of being hot or cold is maintained by a complex system of nerve receptors in our skin and in a part of our brain known as the hypothalamus. This system is sensitive to the difference between the body temperature and the temperature outside. Cold can be sensed in two different ways, either by lowering the environmental temperature or by raising the body temperature. The body responds in a similar manner to a fever as it would if the outside temperature dropped. All of the normal systems that increase heat production, such as shivering, become active.

Eating has already been mentioned as a means of increasing heat production, and hunger may be experienced. The body tries to conserve heat by causing constriction of the blood vessels near the skin. Children will sometimes curl up in a ball to conserve heat. Goose bumps are intended to raise the hairs on our body to form a layer of insulation. Don't bundle up your child in blankets if he or she shivers or becomes chilled; this will only cause the fever to go higher. Use home treatment as described below.

Home Treatment
There are two ways in which to reduce a fever: sponging and medication.

Sponging. Evaporation has a cooling effect on the skin and hence on the body temperature. Evaporation can be enhanced by sponging the skin with water. Although alcohol evaporates more rapidly, it is somewhat uncomfortable for the child and the vapors can be dangerous. Generally, sponging with tepid water (water that is comfortable to the touch) will be sufficient. Heat is also lost by conduction if a child is sponged or sitting in a tub. Conduction is the process in which heat is lost to a cooler environment (the bathwater or air) from the warmer environment of the body. A comfortable tub of water (70°) is sufficiently lower than the body temperature to encourage conduction. Although cold water will work somewhat faster, the discomfort of the procedure makes this less desirable. The child will tolerate cold bathing and sponging for a much shorter period.

Medication. Medication should not be given by mouth to a seizing or unconscious child. A child who has just had a seizure can be given an aspirin suppository. Most aspirin suppositories come in five-grain sizes, and approximately 1¼ to 1½ grains per year of age can be given—somewhat higher than the recommended dose for oral aspirin. The suppository can be cut lengthwise using a warm knife, to give the proper dose.

Temperature can be controlled in the conscious, alert child with either aspirin or acetaminophen (Tylenol, Tempra, Liquiprin, Valadol, Datril, Tenlap, etc.). Remember that fever is the body's way of naturally responding to a variety of conditions including infection. A fever may signify the response of a body's immune system to an infection and thus be the visible manifestation of a beneficial effect. Nonetheless, fevers do make children uncomfortable. Controlling a fever that is sufficiently high to interfere with a child's eating, drinking, sleeping, or other important activities will make the child feel better. In short, if your child seems to be suffering from the fever, treat it. If the fever is mild and the child shows no effects, it may be unnecessary to treat.

Aspirin is universally familiar, effective, and reliable. It does *not* come in a liquid preparation. A few individuals are allergic to aspirin and may experience severe skin rashes or gastrointestinal bleeding. All people will suffer if they take too much aspirin. Early signs of excess aspirin include rapid breathing and ringing in the ears. All aspirin kept at home should be in child-proof bottles. Since there really are no totally child-proof bottles, aspirin should be kept out of the child's reach. An excessive dose of aspirin can be fatal and has in fact been responsible for more childhood deaths than any other medication.

"Baby aspirin" contains 1¼ grains or 75 mg per tablet. Children can take approximately 1 grain or 60 mg per year of life, up to ten years, and 10 grains every four to six hours after age 10. By the time a child is five, an adult aspirin or four baby aspirin (5 grains) can be given. Toxic effects will begin to develop at less than twice the recommended dosage so you must handle this medication with respect.

Acetaminophen unfortunately carries the nickname of "liquid aspirin," but it is a completely different medication. The advantage of acetaminophen is that it can be given in either liquid or tablet form. Acetaminophen is as effective as aspirin in fever reduction. It is not as effective as aspirin for other purposes, such as reducing inflammation, and hence is not recommended for conditions like arthritis. Fewer people are allergic to acetaminophen, and not as many gastrointestinal disturbances are caused. However, if your child has never had nausea, abdominal pain, or other gastrointestinal problems with aspirin this is probably not an important consideration. Although acetaminophen carries the reputation of being safer than aspirin, overdoses can be fatal. There are no "safe" drugs. Acetaminophen causes liver damage at high doses and consequently can cause death.

Acetaminophen is available in drops, suspension, and tablets. The concentration of the drops is much higher than the suspension and therefore must be administered cautiously. An unsuspecting person used to a different preparation of acetaminophen can create a problem by using the wrong dosage on your child. The recommended dosage is 60 mg per year of life every four to six hours, the same as aspirin. But tablets contain 325 mg and should not be confused with baby aspirin tablets, which contain only 75 mg.

Since aspirin and acetaminophen are different medications that exert their effects in slightly different manners, they can be used together when one is not effective in maintaining proper temperature control. The dosages are the same but the aspirin and acetaminophen are given together every six hours or staggered so that one or the other is given every three hours.

Feed a Cold, Starve a Fever?

This folk remedy probably came from individuals clever enough to notice the relationship between food and temperature elevation. However, there are many reasons why children should be fed during a fever. The increased heat increases caloric requirements since calories are being consumed rapidly at the higher body temperature. More important, there is an increased demand for fluid. Liquids should never be withheld from a feverish child. If a child will not eat because of the discomfort caused by fever, it is still essential to continue to encourage that he or she drink fluids.

Fevers get easier to control as your child gets older. The child's temperature regulatory center matures and, in addition, the child loses a layer of brown fat, located between the backbones, that is responsible for a great deal of heat insulation in the infant.

What to Expect at the Doctor's Office

This will depend on how long your child has had a fever and how sick your child appears. An examination to determine whether an infection is present will evaluate skin, eyes, ears, nose, throat, neck, chest, and belly. If no other symptoms are present and the exam does not reveal an infection, watchful waiting may be advised. If the fever has been prolonged or the child appears ill, tests of the blood and urine may be done. A chest X-ray or spinal tap may be needed. Specific infections will be treated appropriately; fever will be treated as discussed in Home Treatment.

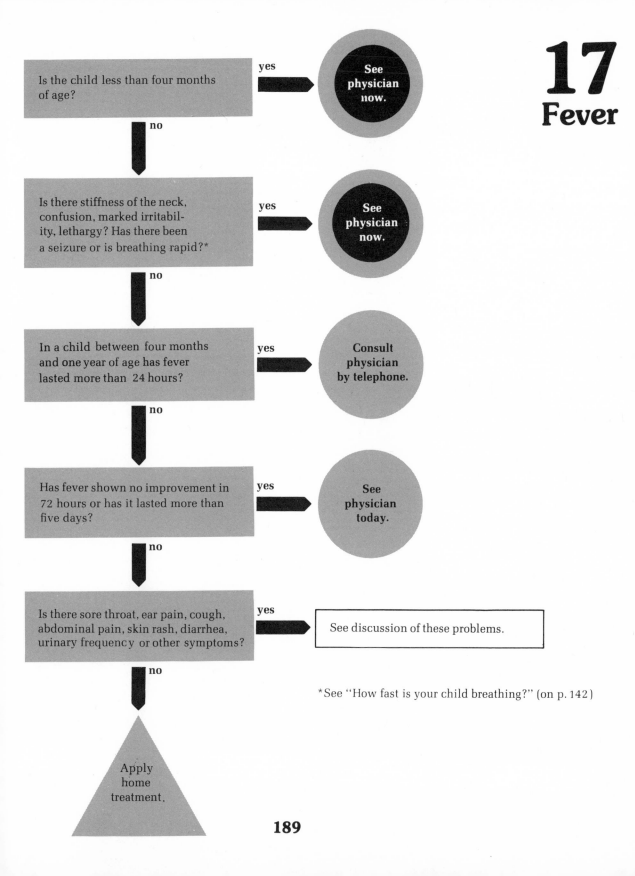

Is the child less than four months of age?

yes → See physician now.

no

Is there stiffness of the neck, confusion, marked irritability, lethargy? Has there been a seizure or is breathing rapid?*

yes → See physician now.

no

In a child between four months and one year of age has fever lasted more than 24 hours?

yes → Consult physician by telephone.

no

Has fever shown no improvement in 72 hours or has it lasted more than five days?

yes → See physician today.

no

Is there sore throat, ear pain, cough, abdominal pain, skin rash, diarrhea, urinary frequency or other symptoms?

yes → See discussion of these problems.

no

Apply home treatment.

*See "How fast is your child breathing?" (on p. 142)

17
Fever

F

Allergies

Allergy was first described at the turn of the century by a pediatrician named Clemens von Pirquet. The term *allergy* meant "changed activity" and described changes that occurred after contacting a foreign substance. Two types of change were noticed, one of which was beneficial. The benefit occurred from the development of protection against a foreign substance after having been once exposed to it. This response prevents us from developing many infectious diseases for a second time and provides the scientific basis for most immunizations. The other type of response was known as a hypersensitivity response, is generally not beneficial, and is the response for which the term allergy is generally used.

Allergy is now known to be possible even without previous exposure to the substance. All persons are capable of allergic responses; for example, anyone given a transfusion with the wrong type of blood will have an allergic reaction.

However, the term allergy is overused. When your eyes smart in Los Angeles, they are not allergic to the air, but are experiencing a direct chemical irritation from the pollutants. Similarly, skin coming in contact with some plants or chemicals experiences direct damage and not an allergic response. Physicians often blame milk or food allergy for vomiting, diarrhea, colic, crying, irritability, fretfulness, or sneezing in infants. While allergy can cause these symptoms, so can countless other things.

Over the next few pages we will discuss common allergies (such as those to food, insects, drugs, pets, pollen, and dust), the common allergic problems (such as asthma, hay fever, hives, and other skin problems) and the medical treatments available.

FOOD ALLERGY

Almost any food can produce an allergic response; only breast milk appears to be incapable of causing an allergy. Even in this case, as one scrutinizes the medical literature very carefully, a 1928 report can be found which incriminates beans in a mother's diet, detected in the breast milk, as a cause of allergy in an infant. Food allergy is not the only cause of digestive upsets, and gets blamed for much that it does not cause. For example, some children are born without an important digestive enzyme, known as lactase, which is necessary to digest the sugars present in milk. Other children lose the ability to make lactase after the age of three or four. The absence of lactase can produce diarrhea, abdominal pain, and vomiting after the drinking of milk. This is only one example of a digestive problem that can be confused with food allergy; there are many others.

Symptoms of Food Allergy

Food allergy may produce swelling of the mouth and lips, hives, skin rashes, vomiting, diarrhea, blood loss from the intestinal tract, asthma, allergic rhinitis (runny nose), and shock (extremely rarely). Of course, many other allergens besides food can cause these problems, making it difficult to prove that a particular food is the culprit. The best approach for detecting food allergy is for the parent to think like Sherlock Holmes. If your child's lips swell only after eating strawberries, you have your suspect!

Foods Responsible for Allergy

Cow's milk is frequently blamed for food allergy by parents, pediatricians, and allergists. Since almost any symptom can be blamed on allergy, and since infants consume so much cow's milk, it is easy to see why milk is so quickly blamed. Infant intestines are capable of absorbing proteins that older children's digestive tracts would not absorb. These proteins may set up altered reactions or allergies.

Controversy exists over the relationship of early exposure to cow's milk and the later development of asthma. Some physicians have maintained that avoidance of cow's milk will delay or eliminate the development of asthma. Others have found the opposite. The only agreement is that the children most likely to develop allergies, including asthma, come from families with other allergic members. Cow's milk may have some effects on children likely to develop allergies but probably should not be of particular concern in children with no family history of allergy.

Cow's milk can cause allergic responses in infants, with diarrhea and even blood loss through the intestines, but very rarely. This situation is a clear indication for removal of cow's milk, if the severe diarrhea is documented by a physician. The necessary tests are simple and require analysis of the stools (feces). Stool analysis should be repeated after the child has been taken off cow's milk.

Other foods that have been associated with allergic reactions in children include wheat, eggs, citrus fruits, beef and veal, fish, and nuts. Severe reactions are very rare in children; parents need not be anxious about giving their children new foods. Families with a strong history of allergy can introduce new foods to an infant one every few days so that if an allergy develops, the cause is obvious.

Soybean Substitutes for Milk

The amount of soybean formula produced in this country exceeds the amount necessary to provide for children with a cow's milk allergy! Milk allergy consists of an altered response to the cow's milk protein, producing vomiting and/or diarrhea, and is extremely rare. Intolerance to cow's milk because of lack of the enzyme lactase to digest the sugar lactose will produce bloating, abdominal pain, vomiting, and/or diarrhea. This intolerance is also rare.

There are two possible explanations for the purchase of soybean preparations. First, parents may buy them because they like them. They are nutritious and children tolerate them well. However, they tend to be more expensive than cow's milk. The other reason for the high consumption of soybean formula is that parents have been instructed to substitute for cow's milk formulae at the slightest suspicion of an allergy. Every childhood symptom known has been attributed to cow's milk allergy—but the condition is rare.

Before you go out and spend more money on a soybean formula, make sure that your physician has determined that the child really needs it. Many stories of children getting better on a soybean preparation result from the child spontaneously recovering from whatever was formerly producing the troublesome symptom.

ASTHMA

Asthma is a severe allergic disorder, and is discussed further under its most prominent symptom—wheezing (see Problem 26). The wheezing in asthma is caused by spasm of the muscles in the walls of the smaller air passages in the lungs. An excess amount of mucus production further narrows the air passages and can aggravate the difficulty in getting the air out. Infections and foreign bodies in the air passages can mimic asthma. All wheezing in children is potentially serious and should be evaluated by a medical professional, at least for the first few occurrences. Asthma tends to occur in families where other members have either asthma, hay fever, or eczema.

An attack can be triggered by an infection, by an emotionally upsetting event, or by exposure to an *allergen*. Common allergens include house dust, pollen, mold, food, and shed animal materials or "animal danders." It is sometimes easy to identify airborne allergens to which a person is susceptible. Some children will wheeze only around cats, others only during a particular pollen season. (Pollens most often cause seasonal hay fever or allergic rhinitis, rather than asthma.) Most often, there is no clear reason for a particular asthmatic attack. If asthma is severe, it is desirable to identify the offending allergens if possible.

Treatment of Asthma

The treatment of asthma varies according to the severity of the problem. Some children have only one or two episodes of asthma and are never troubled again. We wonder if we should even call these asthma attacks. Other children will have daily attacks, which severely compromise their growth and development.

While some doctors maintain that children never truly outgrow asthma, the evidence is otherwise. More than half of the children diagnosed as having asthma will never have an asthmatic attack as an adult. Another ten percent will have only occasional attacks during adult life.

Therapy provides relief of symptoms, often dramatically so, but must also work to remove the cause, be it allergic, infectious, or emotional. Symptomatic relief of asthma is provided through a variety of prescription medications, including epinephrine, isoproterenol, ephedrine, aminophylline, prednisone, and others.

Several different prescription drugs are often combined, but we see no reason to begin treatment with such combination drugs. Many of these compounds have phenobarbital added to counteract some of the stimulating effects of the other medicines included; we could keep on adding new medications to counteract the side effects of the previous medication forever. All of these drugs are powerful, and all cause side effects. Minimal side effects may be acceptable to relieve major symptoms. If side effects are intolerable, then a new treatment plan can be made. Try to avoid combination drugs.

Corticosteroid drugs (steroids, prednisone) are effective in severe asthmatics. They block the smooth muscle contractions that narrow the airway passages. They have many and severe side effects, including growth retardation, and should be used only after full discussion with your physician.

Antihistamines are not useful in the treatment of asthma. In fact, the drying of secretions by antihistamines may actually cause airway plugging.

Nebulizers (spray medicines) can be potentially abused and can even have fatal reactions. They should be used sparingly in children, and only in those not responding to medication by mouth. Freon-containing nebulizers should not be used.

Cromolyn is a relatively new drug that is taken by inhalation. Unlike other inhaled drugs it is not useful during an attack but can prevent future attacks. Cromolyn should be used only in children with severe asthma who are requiring high dosages of oral medications. Many children on corticosteroid drugs have been able to reduce steroid dosage by using Cromolyn. Cromolyn seems to work particularly well in children sensitive to inhaled allergens and in children who develop asthma after exercise.

Asthma is a complicated subject. If you have an asthmatic child, your physician will need to spend a great deal of time discussing management of the illness with you.

Allergen Avoidance

A relatively clean and dust-free house is healthy for all, but essential for the allergic. Rugs, furniture, drapes, bedspreads, and other items that are particular dust-catchers should be vacuumed regularly. An asthmatic child's room should be particularly allergen-free, since sleeping requires eight to ten hours in the room. Except in very severe cases we do not recommend changing the entire household furnishings to reduce potential allergen exposure. Even then, removal of items should progress on a rational basis after suspected allergens have been identified. Children and pets may do fine together, although it is best not to allow pets to sleep in an allergic child's room. Toy animals should be kept clean;

washable ones are the best. A home without stuffed animals seems to some like a morning without sunshine and orange juice, but please avoid products that may be stuffed with animal hair. Finally, don't forget to change heating filters and air-conditioner filters regularly.

Infection Control
Since infections can trigger asthma, a physical examination is important during any first or frequently recurring attacks. Antibiotics should not be given unless a definite infection is present.

Hydration Therapy
Water and other fluids taken by mouth are very important. Water can help loosen the mucus in the lungs and make breathing easier. Mist is not too helpful during asthmatic attacks because the affected airway passages are beyond the reach of the mist. Vaporizers are most useful for problems of the upper air passages of ears, nose, sinuses, mouth, and throat.

Supportive Therapy
Severe asthma is strenuous for parents and family, as well as for the affected child. Assistance is often required to manage the emotional consequences of asthma for the whole family. Do not hesitate to seek this assistance; social workers and other counselors can be invaluable here.

Exercise and Asthma
Asthmatics can participate in athletics; five athletes with asthma recently have won gold medals in Olympic swimming. Swimming appears to be far and away the best exercise and best sport for the asthmatic child. Exercise programs with long and steady energy requirements seem to work the best, and swimmers come into contact with allergens rather less often than in most other sports.

ALLERGIC RHINITIS (HAY FEVER)
Allergic rhinitis is the most common allergic problem. A stuffy runny nose, watering itchy eyes, headache, and sneezing are all common. The cause in infants is often dust or food, and in adults, dust or pollens. Most individuals are troubled only in pollen season; ragweed is particularly troublesome. The problem seems to run in families.

Treatment is directed toward both symptomatic relief and avoidance of the offending allergen. The first line in symptomatic relief is the use of tissues or handkerchiefs; often this is not enough. Drugs that will reduce symptoms may be prescribed or purchased over the counter; all have some side effects.

Antihistamines block the action of histamine, a substance released during allergic reactions. They also have a drying effect and improve nasal stuffiness. They also may be useful in reducing itching, helping motion sickness, or decreasing vomiting. The antihistamines used most often in allergic rhinitis are diphenhydramine (Benadryl), chlorpheniramine maleate (Chlor-Trimeton), tripelennamine (Pyribenzamine) and brompheniramine (Dimetane). These four drugs are from three different classes of antihistamine compounds. Individuals respond differently to different drugs and a trial of the different types of antihistamines may be necessary to determine the most effective type.

The most common side effect of antihistamines is drowsiness, and this may interfere with a child's schoolwork. Antihistamines should not be used as sleeping pills because the drowsiness they produce *decreases* the amount of deep sleep necessary for normal rest.

ATOPIC DERMATITIS (ECZEMA)

Atopic dermatitis, known commonly as eczema, is an allergic skin condition characterized by dry, itching skin. This itching often leads to scratching. The scratching then produces weeping, infected skin. Dried weepings lead to crusting. This weeping and crusting condition is medically referred to as eczema. Sufficient scratching will produce a thickened, rough skin, which is characteristic of longstanding atopic dermatitis.

Atopic dermatitis runs in families with asthma and allergic rhinitis. Like asthma, a variety of conditions can aggravate it. These conditions include infection, emotional stress, food allergy, and sweating.

Infants seldom exhibit any signs of this problem at birth. The first signs may be red, chapped cheeks. Often infants can rub these itchy areas and cause secondary infections.

As the child grows older, the atopic dermatitis can spread. It may be found on the back of the legs and front of the arms. Adults often have problems with their hands; this is especially true of people whose hands are in frequent contact with water. Water tends to have a drying effect on the skin and tends to aggravate the dry skin-itch-scratch-weep-crust cycle.

Therapy is based upon avoidance of allergens and maintenance of good skin care.

- Avoid wool, which tends to aggravate itching.

- Avoid excessively warm clothing, which will cause sweat retention and aggravate itching.

- Keep the child's fingernails clipped short.

- Avoid bathing with soap and water in moderate to severe cases, since these tend to dry the skin. Instead use non-lipid containing cleansers. Some cleansers with cetyl alcohol aid in preventing drying of the skin (Cetaphil lotion).

- Avoid all oil or grease preparations. They occlude the skin and increase sweat retention and itching.

- Avoiding cow's milk is often suggested; make sure this really works for your child before permanently changing to more expensive feedings. When trying your child on any milk avoidance diet, make *no* other changes in food or other care for a full two weeks unless absolutely necessary.

- Itching is often worse at bedtime. Aspirin is an effective and inexpensive medication for reducing itching. Antihistamines also reduce itching but should be used only if necessary.

- Steroid creams are useful in severe cases. When possible, steroids should be used only for a short period of time. Prolonged use of steroids on the skin can produce numerous side effects, including growth retardation and skin discoloration.

- Antibiotics are sometimes necessary to clear up badly infected skin.

- Emotional factors may need attention; they may be the key to successful therapy.

- There has been no benefit demonstrated from either skin testing or hyposensitization.

ALLERGY TESTING AND HYPOSENSITIZATION

The purpose of allergy testing is to help decide what is causing the allergy; it is not a treatment, and as a test it is not always accurate. Once an allergy test is positive, there are two treatment approaches: avoidance and hyposensitization (desensitization).

Avoidance is sometimes, though not usually, possible. Seldom is a child allergic to cats and nothing else, and usually such an isolated allergy is noted by alert parents and children. Avoiding dusts, pollens, trees, and flowers is next to impossible, so hyposensitization is sometimes reasonable if the problem is severe. Hyposensitization involves injecting a tiny amount of the offending allergen. Gradually larger and larger amounts are injected until the child is able to tolerate exposure to the allergen with only mild symptoms.

Hyposensitization works in many cases, but there are many problems. Local reactions at the site of the injection are common, but can be minimized by injecting through a different needle from the one used to withdraw the material from the bottle. Hyposensitization requires weekly injections for months or years. It may be considered for children with moderate or severe asthma or severe hay fever, but appears unwarranted, as does the preliminary skin testing, for children with mild asthma or with mild allergic rhinitis.

G

The Ears, Nose, and Throat

Is It a Virus, Bacteria, or an Allergy?   200

18. Colds and Flu   202
Sorry, there are no miracle drugs.

19. Sore Throat   204
It takes a culture to tell the cause.

20. Earaches   206
Crying in the night.

21. Ear Discharges   208
Wax and swimming.

22. Hearing Loss   210
Check it out.

23. Runny Nose   212
Allergic or viral?

24. Cough   214
An important reflex.

25. Croup   216
A bark like a seal.

26. Wheezing   218
Asthma and allergies.

27. Hoarseness   220
Frog in the throat.

28. Swollen Glands   222
A result and not a cause.

29. Nosebleeds   224
How to press and for how long.

30. Bad Breath   226
Not a problem for mouthwash.

31. Mouth Lesions   228
They'll usually go away.

32. Toothaches   230
A preventable pain.

IS IT A VIRUS, BACTERIA, OR AN ALLERGY?

The following sections discuss upper respiratory problems, including colds and flu, sore throats, ear pain or stuffiness, runny nose, cough, hoarseness, swollen glands, nosebleeds. A central question is important to each of these complaints: Is it caused by a virus, or bacteria, or an allergic reaction? In general, only for bacterial infection does the doctor have more effective treatment than is available at home. The fact to remember is that viral infections and allergies do *not* improve with treatment by penicillin or other antibiotics. To demand a "penicillin shot" for a cold or allergy is to ask for a drug reaction, risk a more serious "super-infection," and waste time and money. Among common problems well treated at home are:

- The common cold—often termed "viral URI (Upper Respiratory Infection)" by doctors.
- The flu when uncomplicated.
- Hay fever.
- Mononucleosis—infectious mononucleosis or "mono."

Medical treatment *is* commonly required for:

- Strep throat.
- Ear infection.

How can you tell these conditions apart? The table below and the charts for the following problems will usually suffice. Here are some brief descriptions.

Viral syndromes. Viruses usually involve several portions of the body and cause many different symptoms. Three basic patterns (or syndromes) are common in viral illnesses.

Viral URI: This is the "common cold." It includes some combination of the following: sore throat, runny nose, stuffy or congested ears, hoarseness, swollen glands, and fever. One symptom usually precedes the others and another (usually hoarseness or cough) may remain after the others have disappeared.

The flu: Fever may be quite high. Headache can be severe; muscle aches and pain (especially low back and eye muscles) are equally troublesome.

Viral gastroenteritis: This is the "stomach flu" with nausea, vomiting, diarrhea, and crampy abdominal pain. It may be incapacitating and can mimic a variety of other more serious conditions including appendicitis.

Overlap between these three syndromes is not unusual. Your child's illness may sometimes have features of each.

Hay fever. The seasonal runny nose, sneezing, and itchy eyes are well known. As with viruses, this disorder is treated simply to relieve symptoms; given enough time the condition runs its course without doing any permanent harm. Allergies tend to recur whenever the pollen or other allergic substance is encountered. (See Section F on Hay fever.)

Strep throat. Most strep throats will be accompanied by soreness of the throat. However, symptoms outside the respiratory tract can occur, most commonly fever and swollen lymph glands in the neck (from draining the infected material). The rash of scarlet fever sometimes may help to distinguish a streptococcal (strep) from a viral infection. Abdominal pain or headaches may be associated with a strep throat. This disorder must be diagnosed and treated, since serious heart and kidney complications can follow if adequate antibiotic therapy is not given. (See Sore Throat, Problem 19.)

IS IT A VIRUS, BACTERIA, OR AN ALLERGY?

	Virus	Bacteria	Allergy
Runny nose?	Often	Rare	Often
Aching muscles?	Usually	Rare	No
Headache?	Often	Often	Rare
Fever?	Often	Often	No
Cough?	Often	Sometimes	Rare
Croup?	Usually	Rare	No
Recurs at a particular season?	No	No	Often
Do antibiotics help?	No	Yes	No
Can the doctor help?	Seldom	Yes	Sometimes

Remember, viral infections and allergies do not improve with treatment by penicillin or other antibiotics.

18
Colds and Flu

All children have "colds" and most parents become experts in the treatment of their children's common viral upper respiratory infections rather quickly. Colds are almost invariably caused by viruses and do not require or respond to antibiotic treatment. An uncomplicated cold can hardly be considered an illness. In fact, a great many viral infections in children are so mild that no symptoms at all are noticed. Viruses can cause headaches (Problem 63), runny noses (Problem 23), sore throats (Problem 19), muscle aches (Problem 59), cough (Problem 24), vomiting (Problem 82), and diarrhea (Problem 83), among other symptoms. These individual problems may be consulted for further discussion.

Most parents are worried about "complications." These do, of course, occur, but are fortunately much less common than the uncomplicated illness. The most frequent is a blockage in the tube that drains the middle ear and, consequently, an ear infection. Other parents worry about colds progressing to a pneumonia. The observant parent will be able to tell when a child is developing a complication of a cold. Children with a developing complication are often more fussy and may be taking their food poorly. Younger children may tug at their ears or cry frequently if an ear infection is starting. Older children may complain of pain in their ears. A breathing rate greater than 40 per minute is also an indication that a cold may be becoming complicated.

Parents are also frequently concerned that their children may have too many colds. Most healthy, average children have between six and nine viral infections each year. Some of these colds will be very short and mild, while others may last a week or longer. Children with frequent colds seldom have anything seriously wrong with them. These children do *not* need gamma globulin shots. Children who have real problems with their immune defense system most often have extremely serious illnesses rather than frequent mild illnesses. The child's immune system is being made stronger with each cold, so even the sniffles have their positive side.

Home Treatment

Rest is needed by a tired child, but most children will restrict themselves adequately. We see no reason for a child to be kept in bed if the child feels well enough to be up and about. If a child feels well enough to go to school, he or she should be allowed to do so. Of course, if the child is coughing or having other problems that will interfere with schoolwork, it may be better to keep the child at home rather than to have the child sent home in the middle of the day. Colds are usually the most contagious a day or two *before* symptoms appear, so that keeping a child home until all symptoms are gone is pointless; the other children have already been exposed.

The child should receive plenty of fluids during the time of the cold. Don't worry about solid food if the child is not hungry. Fever should be treated appropriately (see Section E, pp. 183–189). For treatment of other symptoms, please refer to the discussion of those specific problems.

What to Expect at the Doctor's Office

Simple colds do not require a visit to the doctor. If you are suspicious that your child may be developing a complication such as an earache or pneumonia, a thorough examination will be performed at the physician's office. Children prone to frequent ear infections should be treated differently at the start of a cold. Discuss strategy with your physician; decongestants or nose drops will often be suggested.

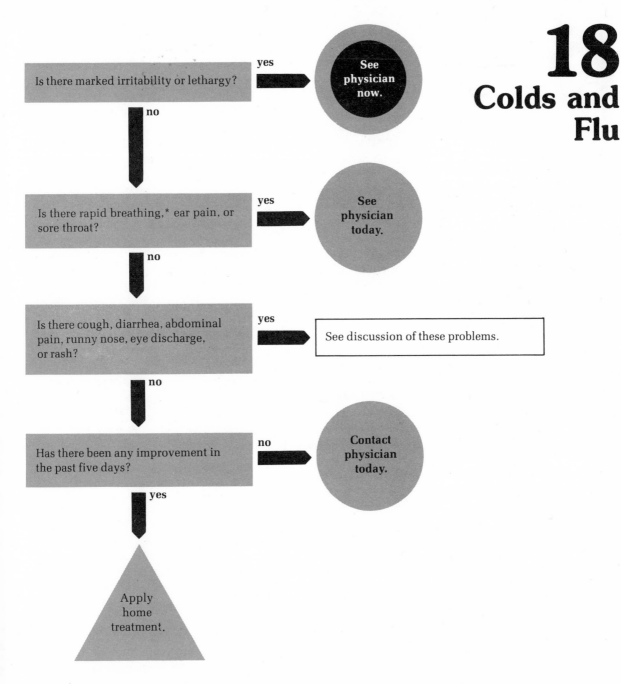

Is there marked irritability or lethargy?

yes → **See physician now.**

no ↓

Is there rapid breathing,* ear pain, or sore throat?

yes → **See physician today.**

no ↓

Is there cough, diarrhea, abdominal pain, runny nose, eye discharge, or rash?

yes → See discussion of these problems.

no ↓

Has there been any improvement in the past five days?

no → **Contact physician today.**

yes ↓

Apply home treatment.

*See "How fast is your child breathing?" (on p. 142)

19
Sore Throat

Sore throat is one of the most common complaints of childhood. Very often a sore throat is accompanied by a fever, a headache, or even abdominal pain. Infants seldom have a sore throat, but as children approach school age sore throats become more frequent.

Sore throats can be caused by either viruses or bacteria. Often, especially in the winter, sleeping with an open mouth or mouth breathing can cause drying and irritation of the throat. This type of irritation always subsides quickly after the pharynx becomes moist again.

Viral sore throats, like other viral infections, cannot be treated with antibiotics and must run their course. Cold liquids for pain and aspirin or acetaminophen for pain and fever are often helpful. Older children and adolescents frequently develop a viral sore throat known as *infectious mononucleosis* or "mono." Despite the formidable sounding name of this illness, complications seldom occur. The sore throat is often more severe and is often prolonged beyond a week, and the child may feel particularly weak. Occasionally, the spleen, one of the internal organs in the abdomen, may enlarge during mononucleosis and resting will be important. A viral sore throat that does not resolve within a week might be caused by the virus responsible for mononucleosis.

Virtually all sore throats caused by bacteria are due to the streptococcal bacteria. These sore throats are commonly referred to as *strep throat*. A strep throat should be treated with an antibiotic because of two types of complications. First, an abscess may form in the throat. This is an extremely rare complication but should be suspected if the child has extreme difficulty in swallowing, has an excess of salivation, or has difficulty opening his or her mouth. The second and most significant complications of strep throat occur from one to four weeks after the pain in the throat has disappeared. It is these complications that are of concern to parents and physicians. One of these complications causes an inflammation of the kidney. It is

not certain that antibiotics will prevent this complication but the antibiotics will prevent the strep from spreading to other family members or friends. Of greatest concern is the complication of rheumatic fever, less common today than in the past but still a significant problem in many parts of the country. Rheumatic fever is a complicated disease that causes painful swollen joints, unusual skin rashes, and heart damage in half of its victims. Rheumatic fever can be prevented by antibiotic treatment of a strep throat.

Unfortunately, it is not possible to definitely distinguish a viral sore throat from a strep throat on the basis of symptoms. Neither the height of the fever, the appearance of the throat, nor the amount of pain present will prove whether a sore throat is due to a virus or strep. The only method of distinguishing viral from strep throat is through a throat culture. In many parts of the country, a throat culture can be obtained without a physician's office visit fee. If you have no other concerns about your child and merely need to know whether the child has a strep throat, you should inquire about obtaining a throat culture without a full office visit.

Frequent and recurrent sore throats are common, especially in children between the ages of five and ten. There is no evidence that removing the tonsils decreases this frequency!

Home Treatment
Cold liquids, aspirin, and acetaminophen are effective for the pain and fever. Many home remedies include saltwater gargles and honey or lemon in tea. Time is the most important healer for pain; a vaporizer makes the waiting more comfortable for some.

What to Expect at the Doctor's Office
A throat culture will be taken. Most physicians will delay treating a sore throat until the culture results are known; delaying treatment by one or two days does not increase the risk of developing rheumatic fever. Furthermore, antibiotic treatment has not been shown to be effective in reducing the discomfort of a sore throat, but only the complications. Since the majority of sore throats are due to viruses, treat-

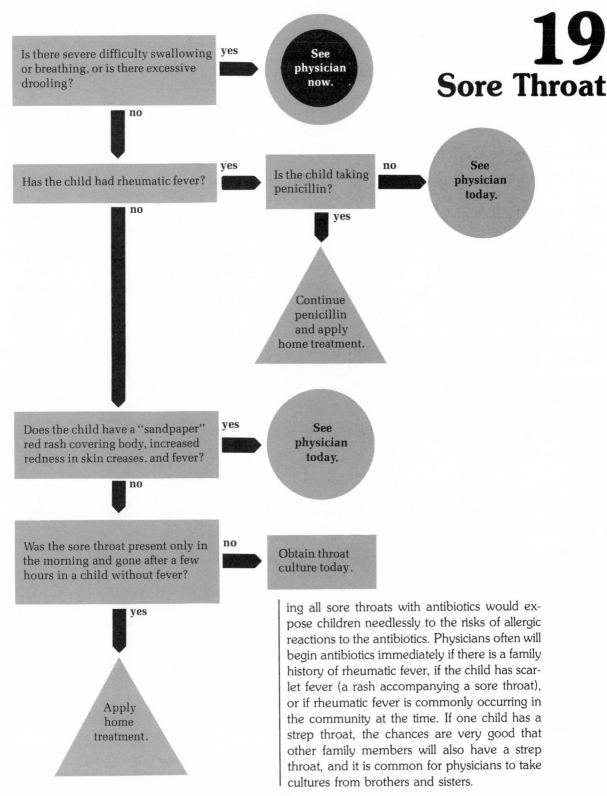

Is there severe difficulty swallowing or breathing, or is there excessive drooling?

yes → **See physician now.**

no ↓

Has the child had rheumatic fever?

yes → Is the child taking penicillin?

no → **See physician today.**

yes ↓ Continue penicillin and apply home treatment.

no ↓

Does the child have a "sandpaper" red rash covering body, increased redness in skin creases, and fever?

yes → **See physician today.**

no ↓

Was the sore throat present only in the morning and gone after a few hours in a child without fever?

no → Obtain throat culture today.

yes ↓ Apply home treatment.

ing all sore throats with antibiotics would expose children needlessly to the risks of allergic reactions to the antibiotics. Physicians often will begin antibiotics immediately if there is a family history of rheumatic fever, if the child has scarlet fever (a rash accompanying a sore throat), or if rheumatic fever is commonly occurring in the community at the time. If one child has a strep throat, the chances are very good that other family members will also have a strep throat, and it is common for physicians to take cultures from brothers and sisters.

20
Earaches

Most children will have at least one earache while growing up, and many will have frequent earaches. Ear pain is caused by a buildup of fluid and pressure in the child's middle ear. Under normal circumstances, the middle ear is drained by a short narrow tube (the eustachian tube) into the nasal passages. Often during a cold the eustachian tube will become swollen shut; this occurs most easily in small children in whom the tube is smaller. Many infants are given bottles of milk while lying flat in bed; drinking milk while lying down may also cause an irritation of the eustachian tube and may cause it to close. When the tube closes, the normal flow of fluid from the middle ear is prevented and the fluid begins to accumulate. Bacteria grow rapidly in this stagnant fluid and hence a bacterial infection often results.

The symptoms of an ear infection may include fever, ear pain, fussiness, increased crying, irritability, or pulling at the ears. Since infants cannot tell you that their ears hurt, increased irritability or ear pulling should make a parent suspicious of ear infection.

Ear pain and ear stuffiness can also result from high altitudes, as when descending in an airplane. Here again, the mechanism for the stuffiness or pain is obstruction of the eustachian tube. Swallowing will frequently relieve this pressure. Closing the mouth and holding the nose closed while pretending to blow one's nose is another method of opening the eustachian tube.

Parents are often concerned about hearing impairment after ear infections. While most children will have a temporary and minor hearing loss during and immediately following an ear infection, there is seldom any permanent hearing loss with adequate medical management.

Home Treatment

Ear infections require antibiotic treatment and hence a physician visit. However, parents can begin pain and fever treatment with aspirin or acetaminophen immediately upon suspecting an ear infection.

What to Expect at the Doctor's Office

An examination of the ear, nose, and throat as well as the bony portion of the skull behind the ears, known as the mastoid, will be performed. Pain, tenderness, or redness of the mastoid signifies a serious infection.

Therapy will generally consist of an antibiotic as well as an attempt to open the eustachian tube by medication. Nose drops can help clear the tube by decreasing the swelling. Decongestants may also be of value, although this has not definitely been proven. Antihistamine preparations are seldom useful except in a child known to be allergic. Antibiotic therapy generally will be prescribed for at least a week, while other treatments will usually be given for a shorter period. Be sure to give all of the antibiotic prescribed, and on schedule.

Occasionally fluid in the middle ear will persist for a long period without infection. In this event, there may be a slight decrease in hearing. This condition is known as *serous otitis media* and is usually not treated with antibiotics, but with attempts to open the eustachian tube and allow drainage. If this condition persists, the physician may resort to placement of ear tubes in order to establish proper functioning of the middle ear once again. Placing ear tubes sounds frightening, but this is actually a simple and very effective procedure.

Most physicians will wish to reexamine your child's ears to make sure the infection has completely cleared and to make sure that the child's hearing has returned to normal.

20
Earaches

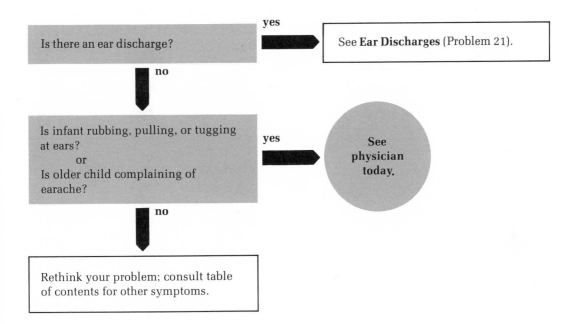

Is there an ear discharge? — **yes** → See **Ear Discharges** (Problem 21).

no ↓

Is infant rubbing, pulling, or tugging at ears?
or
Is older child complaining of earache? — **yes** → See physician today.

no ↓

Rethink your problem; consult table of contents for other symptoms.

21
Ear Discharges

In a young child or in an older child who has been complaining of ear pain, a white or yellow discharge is often the sign of a ruptured eardrum. Sometimes the parents will find that there is dry crusted material on the child's pillow. Here again, a ruptured ear drum should be suspected. These children should be brought to a physician for antibiotic therapy. Do not be unduly alarmed; the ruptured eardrum is actually the first stage of a natural healing process, which the antibiotics will help. Children have remarkable healing powers and most eardrums will heal completely within a matter of weeks.

In the summertime, ear discharges are commonly caused by "swimmer's ear," an irritation of the ear canal and not a problem of the middle ear or eardrum. Children will often complain that their ears are itchy. In addition, tugging on the ear will often cause pain; this can be a helpful clue to an inflammation of the outer ear and canal, such as swimmer's ear. The urge to scratch inside the ear is very tempting but must be resisted. We especially caution against the use of hairpins or other such instruments to accomplish the scratching, since injury to the eardrum can result.

Ear wax is almost never a problem unless attempts are made to "clean" the child's ear canals. Ear wax functions as a protective lining for the ear canal. Taking warm showers or washing the external ears with washcloths dipped in warm water provides enough vapor to prevent the buildup of wax that is thick and caked. Children often like to push things in their ear canal and they may pack the wax tightly enough to prevent vibration of the eardrum and hence interfere with hearing. Well-meaning parents armed with a cotton swab on a stick often accomplish the same awkward result.

Home Treatment

Packed-down ear wax can be removed by using warm water flushed in gently with a syringe, available at the drugstore. A water jet set at the very lowest setting can also be useful, but can be frightening to young children and is dangerous at higher settings. We do not advise that parents attempt to remove impacted ear wax unless they are dealing with an older child and can see the impacted, blackened ear wax. Wax softeners such as Cerumenex or ordinary olive oil are useful; all of the commercial products can be irritating if not used properly. Cerumenex, for example, must be flushed out of the ear within 30 minutes. Washing should never be attempted if there is any question about the condition of the eardrum.

Although swimmer's ear (or other causes of similar "otitis externa") is often caused by a bacterial infection, this infection does not often require antibiotic treatment, since the infection is very shallow. Effective treatment is to place a cotton wick soaked in Burrow's solution in the ear canal overnight, followed by a brief irrigation with 3% hydrogen peroxide followed by warm water. Success has also been reported with merthiolate mixed with mineral oil (enough to make it pink), followed by the hydrogen peroxide and warm water rinse. For particularly severe or itching cases or persistence beyond five days, a doctor's visit is advisable.

What to Expect at the Doctor's Office

A thorough examination of the ear will be performed. In severe cases a culture for bacteria may be taken. Corticosteroid and antibiotic preparations to be placed in the ear canal may be prescribed, or one of the regimens described above under Home Treatment may be advised. Oral antibiotics will usually be given if a perforated eardrum is causing the discharge.

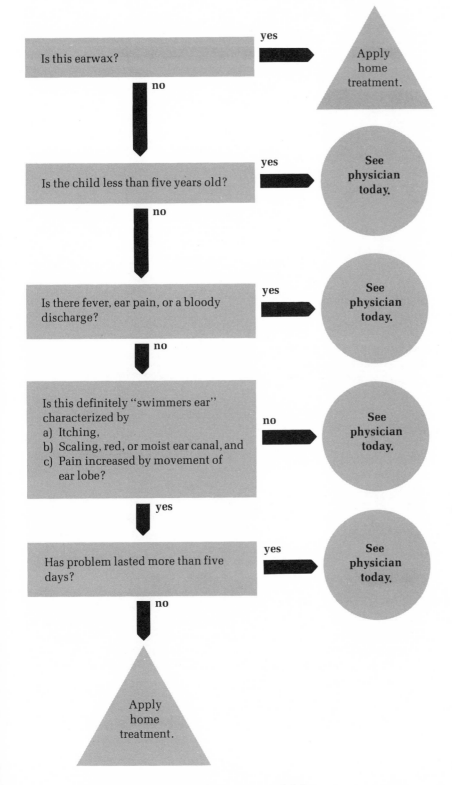

Is this earwax?

yes → Apply home treatment.

no

Is the child less than five years old?

yes → See physician today.

no

Is there fever, ear pain, or a bloody discharge?

yes → See physician today.

no

Is this definitely "swimmers ear" characterized by
a) Itching,
b) Scaling, red, or moist ear canal, and
c) Pain increased by movement of ear lobe?

no → See physician today.

yes

Has problem lasted more than five days?

yes → See physician today.

no

Apply home treatment.

22
Hearing Loss

Problems with hearing may be divided into two broad categories: sudden and slow. When a child of five or older complains of difficulty in hearing developing over a short period of time, then the problem is usually a blockage in the ear of one type or another. On the outside of the eardrum, such blockage may be due to the accumulation of wax, a foreign object that the child has put in the ear canal, or an infection of the ear canal. On the inside of the eardrum, fluid may accumulate and cause blockage because of an ear infection caused by a virus or bacteria.

In the other category are hearing problems that are slow in developing or are present from birth and become evident over a long period of time. Many parents become concerned that their infant or small child is not hearing normally. Hearing can now be tested in a child of any age through the use of computers to analyze changes in brain waves in response to sounds. More simply, a child with normal hearing will react in a characteristic manner to a noise. A hand clap, horn, or whistle may be used to produce the sound. From birth up to three months, the infant will blink or open the eyes, move arms or legs, turn the head, or begin sucking in response to sound. If a child is moving or vocalizing before the sound is made, these activities may stop. At three months, children begin to attempt to find a sound by moving the head and looking for it. The ability to find the sound no matter where it is (below, behind, or above the child) may not be fully developed until the age of two.

Normal speech development relies upon hearing. A child whose speech is developing slowly or not at all may, in fact, have difficulty in hearing. Children who babble continually beyond a year without forming words should also be suspected of hearing difficulties.

Home Treatment

The need for an accurate ear examination usually necessitates a trip to the doctor. However, if the problem is known with certainty to be due to wax accumulation, this may be effectively treated at home. The ear is simply flushed gently with tepid or warm water and the wax washed out. Ear syringes or other devices for squirting water into the ear canal are available in drugstores. A water jet set *at the very lowest setting* can be used with considerable success, but we do not recommend it for young children because of the frightening noise. Wax softeners, such as Cerumenex, may be needed when the wax is hard and impacted; follow the instructions on the label. (Debrox has gained a reputation for irritating ear canals, perhaps unjustly.) A few words of warning: First, the water must be as close to body temperature as possible; the use of cold water may result in dizziness and vomiting. Second, you are assuming that the eardrum is intact and undamaged. Washing should never be attempted if there is any question about the condition of the eardrum.

Caution must be advised with respect to removing foreign bodies. Unless the object is easily accessible and removing it clearly poses no threat of damage to ear structures, do not try to remove. Sharp instruments should never be used in an attempt to remove foreign bodies. Many times efforts to remove objects at home lead to pushing the object further into the ear or to damage of the eardrum itself.

What to Expect at the Doctor's Office

A thorough examination of both ears often reveals the cause of the hearing loss. If it does not, then the physician may test the hearing in the manner described above or, if the child is older, recommend audiometry (an electronic hearing test).

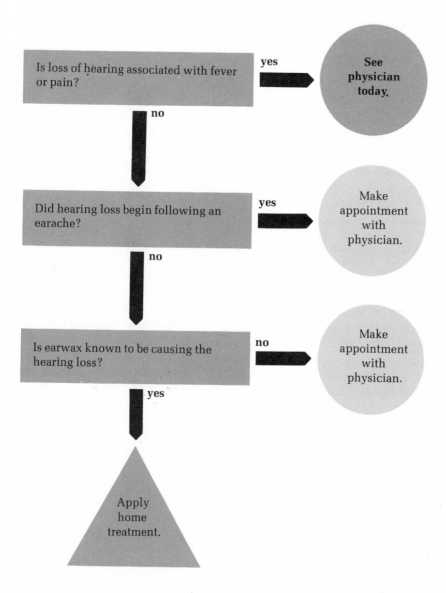

Is loss of hearing associated with fever or pain?

yes → **See physician today.**

no

Did hearing loss begin following an earache?

yes → Make appointment with physician.

no

Is earwax known to be causing the hearing loss?

no → Make appointment with physician.

yes

Apply home treatment.

23
Runny Nose

A runny nose is one of the most frequent occurrences of childhood. Many infants will have a runny nose and sneezing during the first two weeks of life. The cause of this is unknown but it is certainly a natural phenomenon.

Children will also have runny noses during episodes of crying and sometimes after exercising. Runny noses in these instances are temporary and of no concern.

The hallmark of the common cold is the runny nose. It is intended by nature to help the body fight the virus infection. Nasal secretions contain antibodies, which act against the viruses. The profuse outpouring of fluid carries the virus outside the body.

Allergy is another common cause of runny noses. Children whose runny noses are due to an allergic basis are deemed to have *allergic rhinitis*, better known as hay fever. The nasal secretions in this instance are often clear and very thin. Children with allergic rhinitis will often have other symptoms simultaneously, including sneezing, and itching, watery eyes. They will rub their noses so often that a crease in the nose may appear. This problem lasts longer than a viral infection, often for weeks or months, and occurs most commonly during the season when pollen particles or other allergens are in the air. A great many other substances may aggravate allergic rhinitis including house dusts, molds, and animal danders.

The runny nose may also be due to a small object that a young child has pushed into the nose. Usually, but not always, this will produce a discharge from only one nostril. Often the discharge will be foul smelling and yellow or green.

Another common cause of runny noses as well as stuffy noses is prolonged use of nose drops. This problem of *excess medication* is known as *rhinitis medicamentosum*. Nose drops containing substances like ephedrine should never be used for longer than three days. This problem can be avoided by switching the child to saline nose drops (made by placing a teaspoon of salt in a pint of water) over the next few days.

Complications from the runny nose are due to the excess mucus. The mucus may cause a postnasal drip and a cough that is most prominent at night. The mucus drip may plug the eustachian tube between the nasal passages and the ear, resulting in ear infection and pain. It may plug the sinus passages, resulting in secondary sinus infection and sinus pain.

Home Treatment

Two major types of drugs are used to control a runny nose. Decongestants such as pseudoephedrine and ephedrine act to shrink the mucus membranes and to open the nasal passages. Antihistamines act to block allergic reactions and decrease the amount of secretion. Decongestants make some children overly active and antihistamines may cause drowsiness as well as interfere with sleep. Because of the complications of the medications, runny noses should be treated only when they are severely impairing the child's comfort. Often a tissue is the best approach; it has no side effects, costs less, and helps get the virus outside the body!

Should you choose to treat a runny nose, topical decongestants (nose drops) are suitable. Saline nose drops are fine for young infants. As children get older they can graduate from 1/4% to 1/2% Neo-Synephrine nose drops, or may take Afrin nose drops. These nose drops should never be used for longer than three consecutive days. An oral decongestant that can be purchased over the counter is Sudafed; it should not be used longer than a week without consulting your physician.

Complications such as ear and sinus infection may be prevented by ensuring that the mucus is thin rather than thick and sticky. This helps to prevent plugging of the nasal passages. Increased humidity in the air with a vaporizer or humidifier helps to liquefy the mucus. Inside a house heated air is often very dry; cooler air contains more moisture and is preferable. Drinking a great deal of liquid will also help liquefy the secretions.

If symptoms persist beyond three weeks, your physician should be contacted.

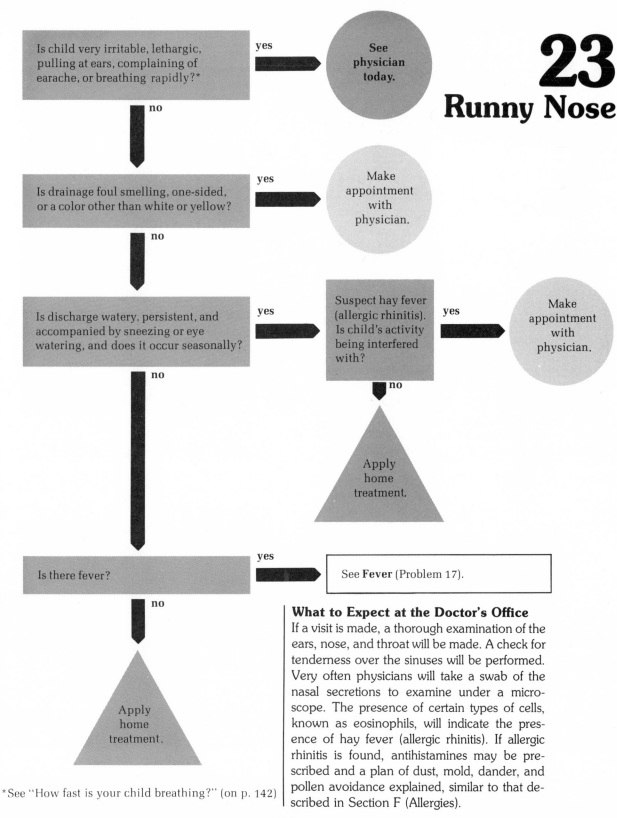

Is child very irritable, lethargic, pulling at ears, complaining of earache, or breathing rapidly?*

yes → See physician today.

no ↓

Is drainage foul smelling, one-sided, or a color other than white or yellow?

yes → Make appointment with physician.

no ↓

Is discharge watery, persistent, and accompanied by sneezing or eye watering, and does it occur seasonally?

yes → Suspect hay fever (allergic rhinitis). Is child's activity being interfered with?

yes → Make appointment with physician.

no ↓

Apply home treatment.

no ↓

Is there fever?

yes → See **Fever** (Problem 17).

no ↓

Apply home treatment.

*See "How fast is your child breathing?" (on p. 142)

23
Runny Nose

What to Expect at the Doctor's Office

If a visit is made, a thorough examination of the ears, nose, and throat will be made. A check for tenderness over the sinuses will be performed. Very often physicians will take a swab of the nasal secretions to examine under a microscope. The presence of certain types of cells, known as eosinophils, will indicate the presence of hay fever (allergic rhinitis). If allergic rhinitis is found, antihistamines may be prescribed and a plan of dust, mold, dander, and pollen avoidance explained, similar to that described in Section F (Allergies).

213

24.
Cough

Coughing, of course, has several causes. In very young infants, coughing is unusual and may indicate a serious lung problem. In older infants who are prone to swallowing foreign objects, an object may become lodged in the windpipe and cause coughing. Young children also tend to inhale bits of peanut and popcorn, which can produce coughing and serious problems in the lung. However, most coughs are produced by infections, usually viral.

Is it pneumonia? This question worries parents more than any other. Pneumonia is a serious infection of the lung that often requires antibiotics and hence needs the doctor. Fortunately, it is rare when the only symptom is a cough. A rapid breathing rate is often the best indicator of a pneumonia, and this problem may follow an ordinary upper respiratory infection (such as a cold) by a few days. So, if the fever from a simple cold doesn't go down after a few days, see the doctor.

The cough reflex is one of the body's best defense mechanisms. An irritation of the breathing tubes will trigger this reflex, and a violent rush of air helps clear material from the breathing tubes. Hence, material in the lungs that should not be present is removed by the coughing. Consequently, much of the treatment directed at coughing is directed at increasing the ability of the lungs to clear out unnecessary material.

Often, a minor irritation in the breathing tubes will trigger a cough reflex even when there is no material to be expelled. At other times, mucus from the nasal passages will drip into the breathing tubes at night (postnasal drip) and will start the cough reflex. Coughing that is interfering with a child's sleep can be counterproductive and this is the only type of cough that should be stopped.

Home Treatment
The reason for home treatment is to liquefy the secretions in the breathing tubes in order to enhance clearing unwanted materials from the lungs. The mucus in the breathing tubes may be made thinner by several means. Increased humidity in the air may help, and a cool mist vaporizer can often provide this. This is especially important in the severe "croupy" cough of small children (Problem 24, Croup). Drinking large quantities of fluid is helpful for cough, particularly if fever is present to dry out and dehydrate the body. There is serious doubt as to whether any of the oral cough medications help very much in liquefying secretions. Decongestants or nose drops may help nighttime coughs that are caused by postnasal drip.

If cough suppression is needed in order to allow the child to get some rest, dextromethorphan (found in Romilar or Robitussin–DM) is effective. It will not completely eliminate a cough, so do not exceed the recommended dosage.

What to Expect at the Doctor's Office
An examination of the ears, nose, throat, and chest will be made. If a child is suspected of having inhaled a foreign body or if pneumonia is suspected, a chest X-ray will be taken. Antibiotics will be prescribed only for those few cases suspected of being caused by a bacterial infection.

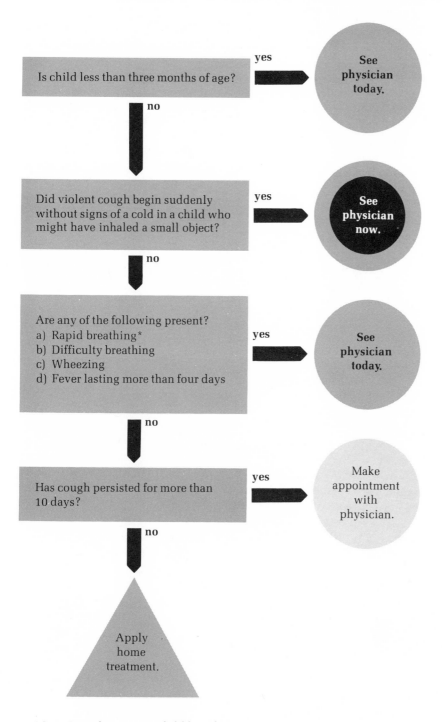

Is child less than three months of age? **yes** → See physician today.

↓ no

Did violent cough begin suddenly without signs of a cold in a child who might have inhaled a small object? **yes** → **See physician now.**

↓ no

Are any of the following present?
a) Rapid breathing*
b) Difficulty breathing
c) Wheezing
d) Fever lasting more than four days

yes → See physician today.

↓ no

Has cough persisted for more than 10 days? **yes** → Make appointment with physician.

↓ no

Apply home treatment.

*See "How fast is your child breathing?" (on p. 142)

25
Croup

Croup is one of the most frightening illnesses that parents will ever encounter. It generally occurs in children under the age of three or four. In the middle of the night a child may sit up in bed gasping for air. Often there will be an accompanying cough that sounds like the barking of a seal. The child's symptoms are so frightening that panic is often the response. However, the most severe problems with croup usually can be relieved safely, simply, and efficiently at home.

Croup is caused by one of several different viruses. The viral infection causes a swelling and outpouring of secretions in the larynx (voice box), trachea (windpipe), and the larger airways going to the lungs. The air passages of the young child are made narrower because of the swelling. This is further aggravated by the secretions, which may become dried out and caked. This combination of swelling and thickened, dried secretions makes it extremely difficult to breathe. There may also be a considerable amount of spasm of the airway passages, further complicating the problem. Treatment is designed to dissolve the dried secretions.

In some children, croup is a recurring problem; these children may have three or four bouts of croup. Seldom does this represent a serious underlying problem, but a physician's advice should be sought. Croup will be outgrown as the airway passages grow larger; it is unusual after the age of seven.

Occasionally, a more serious obstruction caused by a bacterial infection and known as epiglottitis can be confused with croup. Epiglottitis is more common in children over the age of three, but there is considerable overlap in the ages of children affected by these two conditions. Children with epiglottitis often have more serious difficulty breathing. They may have an extremely hard time handling their saliva and will be found to be drooling. Often they assume a characteristic position with their head tilted forward and their jaw pointed out and will be gasping for air. Epiglottitis will not be relieved by the simple measures that bring prompt relief of croup. It must be brought to medical attention immediately.

Home Treatment

Mist is the backbone of therapy for croup, and is supplied efficiently by a cold steam vaporizer. We prefer cold steam vaporizers to hot steam ones because of the possibility of scalding from the hot water.

If the breathing is very hard, you can get faster results by taking the child to the bathroom and turning up the hot shower to make thick clouds of steam. Steam can be created more efficiently if there is some cold air in the room. Remember that steam rises, so sitting on the floor with the child will not offer the child the benefit of the steam. Relief usually occurs promptly and should be noticeable within the first 20 minutes. Not becoming alarmed and keeping the child calm is also important; holding the child may comfort him or her and may help relieve some of the airway spasm. If the child is not showing significant improvement within 20 minutes, you should contact your physician or the local emergency room immediately. They will want to see the child and will make arrangements in advance while you are in transit. Unfortunately, few emergency rooms can provide steam as well as the home shower can.

What to Expect at the Doctor's Office

If the physician feels confident that this is croup, a further trial of mist will be offered. In difficult cases, differentiating croup from epiglottitis can be hard; X-rays of the neck are a reliable way of differentiating croup from epiglottitis. A swollen epiglottis often can be seen in the back of the throat, but this examination has its risks and should not be tried at home. If epiglottitis is found, the child will be admitted to the hospital, an airway will be placed in the child's trachea to enable the child to breathe, and intravenous antibiotics directed at curing the bacterial infection will be started. In the case of croup, the trip to the doctor often cures the problem that was resistant to steam at home; keep the car windows open a bit and let the cool night air in.

216

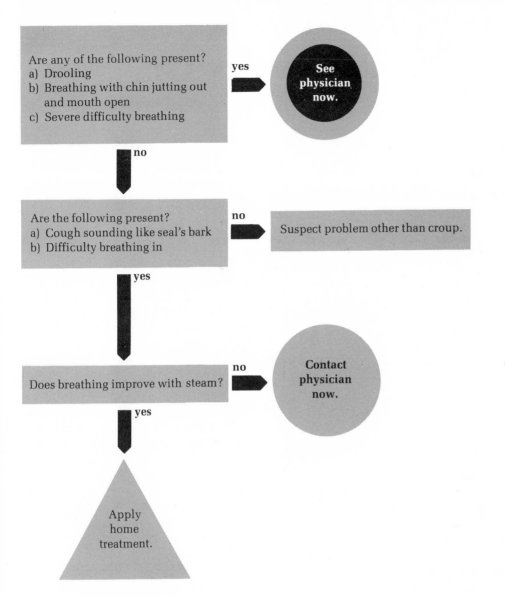

Are any of the following present?
a) Drooling
b) Breathing with chin jutting out and mouth open
c) Severe difficulty breathing

yes → **See physician now.**

no ↓

Are the following present?
a) Cough sounding like seal's bark
b) Difficulty breathing in

no → Suspect problem other than croup.

yes ↓

Does breathing improve with steam?

no → **Contact physician now.**

yes ↓

Apply home treatment.

26
Wheezing

Wheezing is the high-pitched whistling sound produced by air flowing through the narrowed breathing tubes (bronchi and bronchioles). It is most obvious when the child breathes out, but may be present when breathing both in and out. Wheezing comes from the breathing tubes deep in the chest, in contrast to the croupy, crowing, or whooping sounds that come from the area of the voice box in the neck (see Croup, Problem 25). Most often, a narrowing of the breathing tubes in children is due to a viral infection or to an allergic reaction as in asthma. In infants younger than age two, bronchiolitis or narrowing of the smallest air passages can occur due to a viral infection. Pneumonia can also produce wheezing. Wheezing can follow an insect sting or the use of a medicine; these allergic reactions need to be seen by a doctor. Any medication can cause the problem; some individuals even wheeze after taking aspirin. Occasionally a foreign body may be lodged in a breathing tube, causing a localized wheezing that is difficult to hear without a stethoscope.

The importance of wheezing lies in its being an indicator of difficult breathing; it should alert the parent to check carefully for shortness of breath. In a child with a respiratory infection, wheezing may occur before shortness of breath is marked. Therefore, when wheezing appears in the presence of a fever, early consultation with a physician is advisable, even though the illness seldom turns out to be serious.

Treatment of wheezing is symptomatic; there are no drugs that cure viral illnesses or asthma. Home treatment is an important part of this approach. However, the physician's help is needed so that drugs that widen the breathing passages can be used. Intravenous fluids may be required on some occasions.

Home Treatment

Hydration with oral fluids is very important. The use of a vaporizer, preferably one that produces a cold mist, may sometimes help. If a vaporizer is not available, then the shower may be used to produce a mist. Unfortunately, it is hard to get too much vapor down to the small breathing tubes. The child should be encouraged to take as much fluid as possible by mouth. Water is best, but fruit juices or soft drinks may be used if this will increase the amount taken. These measures will be part of the therapy that the doctor recommends and may be begun immediately, even though a visit to the doctor will be necessary.

What to Expect at the Doctor's Office

Physical examination will focus on the chest and neck. Questions will be asked not only about the current illness but also about a past history of allergies either in the child or in the family. The possibility that a foreign body has been swallowed may also be investigated. Drugs to open up the breathing tube, such as adrenalin or aminophylline, may be given by injection, by mouth, or by rectal suppository. (See Asthma, pp. 193–195.) Occasionally hospitalization will be necessary in order to permit fluids to be given through a vein and effective humidification of the air to be achieved. Most important, the child can be closely watched; the hospital is used as a precautionary measure against things getting worse before they get better.

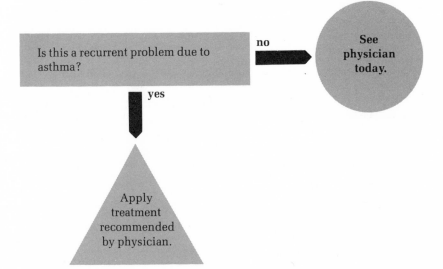

Is this a recurrent problem due to asthma?

no → See physician today.

yes

Apply treatment recommended by physician.

27
Hoarseness

Hoarseness is usually caused by a problem in the vocal cords. In infants under three months of age, this can be due to a serious problem such as a birth defect or thyroid disorder. In young children hoarseness is more often due to prolonged or excessive crying, which puts a strain on the vocal cords.

In older children, viral infections are the most common cause of hoarseness. If the hoarseness is accompanied by either difficulty in breathing or a cough that sounds like a barking seal, the hoarseness is considered a symptom of croup (see Problem 25). Croup is characteristic in children under the age of four, while the symptom of hoarseness by itself is more common in older children.

If hoarseness is accompanied by difficulty breathing, difficulty swallowing, drooling, gasping for air, or breathing with the mouth wide open and the chin jutting forward, a physician must be seen immediately, since this is a medical emergency. This problem is known as *epiglottitis*, and is a bacterial infection that involves the entrance to the airway.

In older children who develop hoarseness or laryngitis without any other symptoms, a virus is most often responsible.

Home Treatment

Hoarseness, unassociated with other symptoms, is very resistant to medical therapy. Nature must heal the inflamed area. Humidifying the air with a vaporizer or taking in fluids can offer some relief. However, the child must wait for healing to occur, and this may take several days. Resting the vocal cords makes sense; crying or shouting makes the situation worse. For the treatment of hoarseness associated with coughs, see Coughs (Problem 24).

What to Expect at the Doctor's Office

If there is severe difficulty in breathing, the first order of business is to ensure that the child has an adequate air passage. This may require placement in the emergency room, hospital, or physician's office of a breathing tube. If X-rays of the neck are taken, a physician should accompany the child at all times.

In uncomplicated hoarseness that has persisted for a long period of time, a physician will look at the vocal cords with the aid of a small mirror. Occasionally hormonal disorders caused by the thyroid or adrenal gland will be found by more extensive physical examination and confirmed by blood tests.

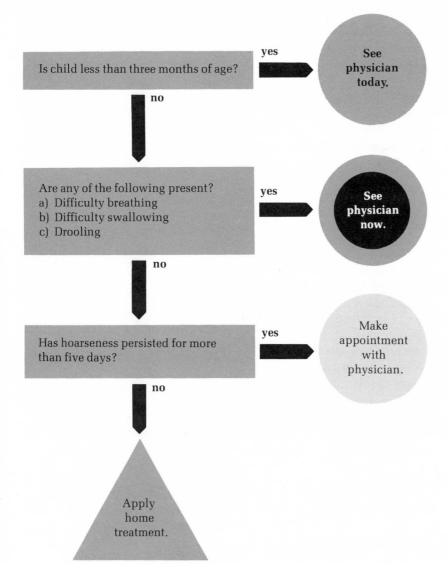

Is child less than three months of age?

yes → See physician today.

no ↓

Are any of the following present?
a) Difficulty breathing
b) Difficulty swallowing
c) Drooling

yes → See physician now.

no ↓

Has hoarseness persisted for more than five days?

yes → Make appointment with physician.

no ↓

Apply home treatment.

27
Hoarseness

28
Swollen Glands

The most common types of swollen glands found in children are swollen lymph glands and swollen salivary glands. The biggest salivary glands are located below and in front of the ears. When they swell, the characteristic swollen jaw appearance of mumps is the result (see Mumps, Problem 52).

Lymph glands are part of the body's defense against infection. They may become swollen even if the infection is trivial or not apparent, although you can usually identify the infection that is causing the swelling. The familiar swollen glands in the neck frequently accompany sore throats or ear infections. Swelling of a gland simply means that it is taking part in the fight against infection. Glands in the groin are enlarged when there is infection in the feet, legs, or genital region; these glands are often swollen when no obvious infection can be found. Sometimes the basic problem may be so minor as to be overlooked (as with athlete's foot).

Swollen glands behind the ears are often the result of an infection in the scalp. If there is no scalp infection, it is possible that your child currently or has recently had German measles (see Rubella, Problem 55). Infectious mononucleosis (mono) can also cause swelling of the glands behind the ears.

If a swollen gland is red and tender, there may be a bacterial infection within the gland itself that requires antibiotic treatment. Swollen glands otherwise require no treatment, since they are merely fighting infections elsewhere. If there is an accompanying sore throat or earache, these should be treated as described in Problems 19 and 20, respectively. However, the swollen glands are usually the result of multiple viral infections that require no treatment. If you have noticed one or several glands progressively enlarging over a period of three weeks, a physician should be consulted. Swollen glands can signal underlying serious problems on very rare occasions.

Home Treatment

Merely observe the glands over several weeks to see if they are continuing to enlarge or if other glands become swollen. The vast majority of swollen glands that persist beyond three weeks are not serious, but a physician should be consulted if the glands show no tendency to become smaller. Soreness in the glands will usually disappear in a couple of days; the pain comes from the rapid enlargement in the early stages of fighting the infection. Getting smaller takes much longer.

What to Expect at the Doctor's Office

The physician will examine the glands and search for infections or other causes of the swelling. Other glands that the parent or child may not have noticed will be examined. Inquiry will be made into fever, weight loss, or other symptoms associated with the swelling of the glands. The physician may decide to simply observe the glands for a period of time or he or she may decide that blood tests are indicated. Eventually, it might be necessary to remove (biopsy) the gland for examination under the microscope, but this is very seldom required.

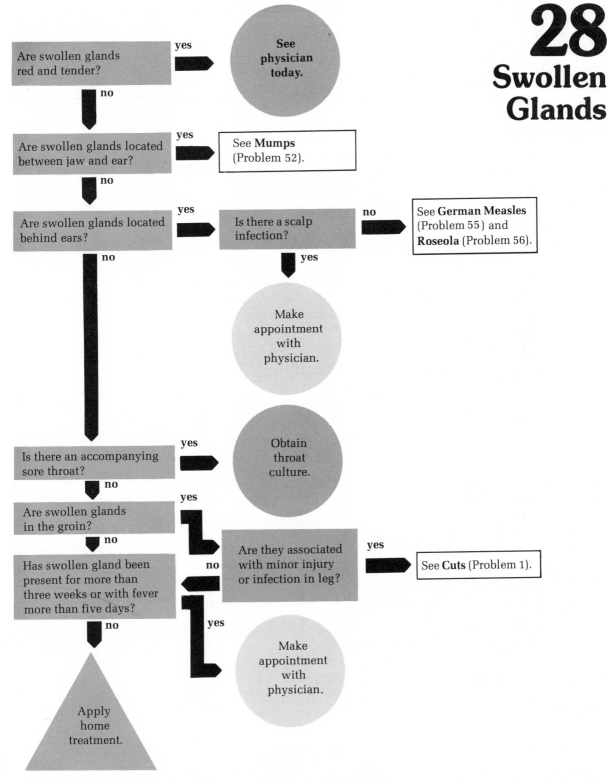

Are swollen glands red and tender? — **yes** → **See physician today.**

no ↓

Are swollen glands located between jaw and ear? — **yes** → See **Mumps** (Problem 52).

no ↓

Are swollen glands located behind ears? — **yes** → Is there a scalp infection? — **no** → See **German Measles** (Problem 55) and **Roseola** (Problem 56).

Is there a scalp infection? — **yes** ↓ Make appointment with physician.

no ↓

Is there an accompanying sore throat? — **yes** → Obtain throat culture.

no ↓

Are swollen glands in the groin? — **yes** → Are they associated with minor injury or infection in leg? — **yes** → See **Cuts** (Problem 1).

Are they associated with minor injury or infection in leg? — **no** →

no ↓

Has swollen gland been present for more than three weeks or with fever more than five days? — **yes** → Make appointment with physician.

no ↓

Apply home treatment.

28
Swollen
Glands

29
Nosebleeds

The blood vessels within the nose lie very near the surface and bleeding may occur with the slightest injury. In children, picking the nose is a common cause. Keeping fingernails cut and discouraging the habit is good preventive medicine. Occasionally, a foreign body in the nose may be the cause of bleeding. Accidents and fights produce their share of nosebleed, but more often than not, the onset is spontaneous.

Nosebleeds are frequently due to irritation by a virus or to vigorous nose blowing. The main problem in this case is the cold, and treatment of cold symptoms will reduce the probability of the nosebleed. If the mucous membrane of the nose is dry, cracking and bleeding is more likely.

These key points should be remembered:

- You can almost always stop the child's nose bleeding yourself.

- The great majority of nosebleeds are associated with colds or minor injury to the nose.

- Treatment such as packing the nose with gauze has significant drawbacks and should be avoided if possible.

- Investigation into the cause of recurrent nosebleeds is not urgent and is best accomplished when the nose is *not* bleeding.

Home Treatment
The nose consists of a bony part and a cartilaginous part: a "hard" portion and a "soft" portion. The area of the nose that usually bleeds lies within the "soft" portion and compression will control the nosebleed. Simply squeeze the nose between thumb and forefinger just below the hard portion of the nose. Pressure should be applied for at least five minutes. The child should be seated. Holding the head back is not necessary. It merely directs the blood flow backward rather than forward. Cold compresses or ice applied across the bridge of the nose may help. Almost all nosebleeds can be controlled in this manner if *sufficient time* is allowed for the bleeding to stop.

Nosebleeds are more common in the winter when both viruses and dry, heated air indoors are common. A cooler house and a vaporizer to return humidity to the air help many children.

If nosebleeds are a recurrent problem, are becoming more frequent, and are not associated with a cold or other minor irritation, then a physician should be consulted on a nonurgent basis. A physician need not be seen immediately after the nosebleed since examination at that time may simply restart the nosebleed.

What to Expect at the Doctor's Office
The child will be seated with head back and nostrils compressed. This will be done even if the child has been doing this at home, and it will usually work. Packing the nose or attempting to cauterize a bleeding point is less desirable. If the nosebleed cannot be stopped, the nose will be examined to see if a bleeding point can be identified. If a bleeding point is seen, coagulation by either electrical or chemical cauterization may be attempted. If this is not successful, then packing of the nose may be unavoidable. Such packing is uncomfortable and may lead to infection; thus the child must be carefully observed.

If a physician is seen because of recurrent nosebleeds, questions about events preceding the bleeds and a careful examination of the nose itself should be expected. Depending on the history and the physical examination, blood-clotting tests may on rare occasions be ordered.

29
Nosebleeds

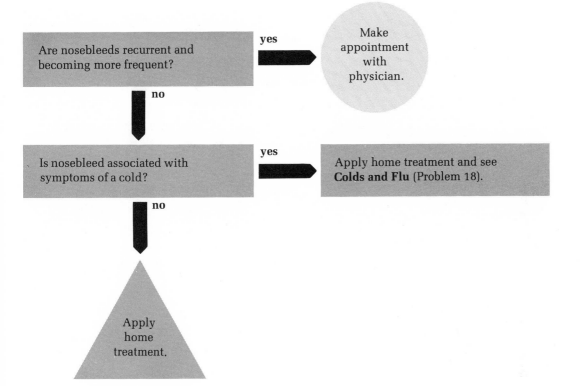

Are nosebleeds recurrent and becoming more frequent? **yes** → Make appointment with physician.

no ↓

Is nosebleed associated with symptoms of a cold? **yes** → Apply home treatment and see **Colds and Flu** (Problem 18).

no ↓

Apply home treatment.

30
Bad Breath

Children seldom have the problem with bad breath in the morning that is so common with adults, and regular tooth brushing should eliminate this problem. Other causes may be more important to identify.

Infections of the mouth as well as sore throats may be the cause of bad breath; because of the possibility of bacterial infection, the physician should be consulted.

A common cause of prolonged bad breath in our experience is a foreign body in the child's nose. This is especially common in toddlers, who have inserted, unnoticed, some small object. Often, but not always, there is a white, yellowish, or bloody discharge from one or both nostrils. A severely decaying tooth may cause bad breath. Finally, unusual problems such as abscesses of the lung or heavy worm infestations have been reported to cause bad breath, although we have not seen these in our practices.

Home Treatment
Proper dental hygiene will prevent most cases of bad breath. If this does not eliminate the odor, then a foreign body in the child's nose is likely and a trip to the doctor will be necessary. Although some foreign bodies may be seen very close to the child's nostril, most are located very deep within the nasal cavity where they are extremely difficult to remove. Do not use mouthwashes to perfume the breath; these cover up, but do not treat, the underlying problem.

What to Expect at the Doctor's Office
A thorough examination of the mouth and the nose will be done. If there is a sore throat or mouth sores a culture may be taken; subsequently, antibiotics may be prescribed. If there is an object in the nose, the physician will use a special forceps to remove the object.

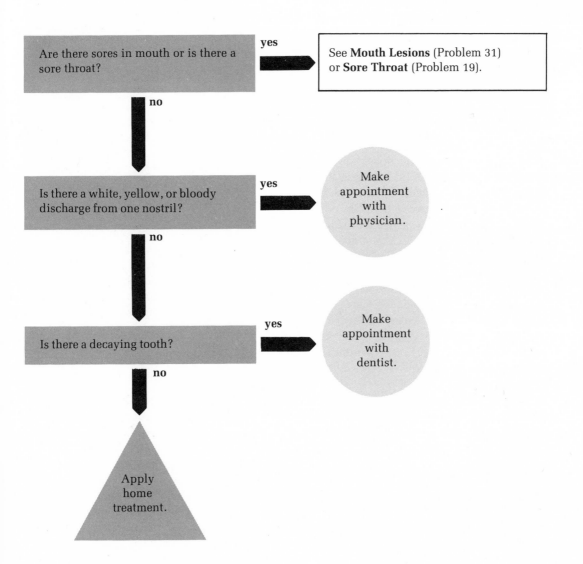

Are there sores in mouth or is there a sore throat?

yes → See **Mouth Lesions** (Problem 31) or **Sore Throat** (Problem 19).

no

Is there a white, yellow, or bloody discharge from one nostril?

yes → Make appointment with physician.

no

Is there a decaying tooth?

yes → Make appointment with dentist.

no

Apply home treatment.

31
Mouth Lesions

Problems in the mouth are very common in children. Doctors frequently use the term *lesion* to describe anything that may be wrong, be it a sore, a patch, or a pimple. In young children large white spots may appear on the roof of the mouth, due to a monilial yeast infection commonly referred to as *thrush*. Thrush can be treated effectively by medication but it often disappears by itself.

Bacteria and viruses can also be responsible for mouth lesions. A bacterial infection more common in older children and adults is commonly known as *trench mouth*; lesions in trench mouth often occur on the gums. Lesions of the gum are more likely to be caused by a herpes virus. Herpes lesions often start as blisters and then change to small spots with white ulcerous centers surrounded by redness. With the first infection they may be found on the gums, inner parts of the lips, cheeks, and even tongue. In repeat infections, it is more usual for the virus to involve only the lips. Because these herpes infections are almost always accompanied by a fever, they are known as fever blisters. The blisters have usually ruptured and generally parents only observe the remaining underlying sore.

A canker sore often follows an injury, such as accidentally biting the inside of the lip or the tongue, or it may appear without obvious cause. These problems are minor and disappear in a short time.

Another virus that can cause mouth lesions is the Coxsackie virus. These lesions are often accompanied by spots on the hands and feet; hence the name "hand-foot-mouth syndrome." Again, this problem will go away by itself.

Allergic reactions to drugs may cause mouth ulcers. In such cases a skin rash may be present on other parts of the body as well, and the physician must be contacted.

Home Treatment

Mouth sores caused by viruses heal by themselves. The goal of treatment is to reduce fever, relieve pain, and maintain adequate fluid intake. Children will seldom want to eat when they have painful mouth lesions. While children can go several days without taking solid foods, it is imperative that they maintain an adequate liquid diet. Cold liquids are the most soothing and Popsicles or iced frozen juices often are helpful. For sores inside the lip and on the gums, a preparation called Orabase, available over the counter, may be applied for protection. For cold sores and fever blisters on the outside of the lips, one of the phenol and camphor preparations (Blistex, Campho-Phenique) may provide relief, especially if applied early. If one of these preparations appears to cause further irritation, then discontinue its use. If the external sores have crusted over, then cool compresses may be applied to remove the crusts. Mouth sores usually resolve in one to two weeks; any sore that persists beyond three weeks should be seen by the physician.

What to Expect at the Doctor's Office

A thorough examination of the mouth will be done. A drug called Nystatin will usually be prescribed for thrush. If a bacterial cause of trench mouth is suspected, an antibiotic may be prescribed. For viral infections, physicians have no more to offer than home remedies. We caution against the use of oral anesthetics such as viscous Xylocaine. This anesthetic can interfere with proper swallowing and can lead to inhalation of food into the lungs.

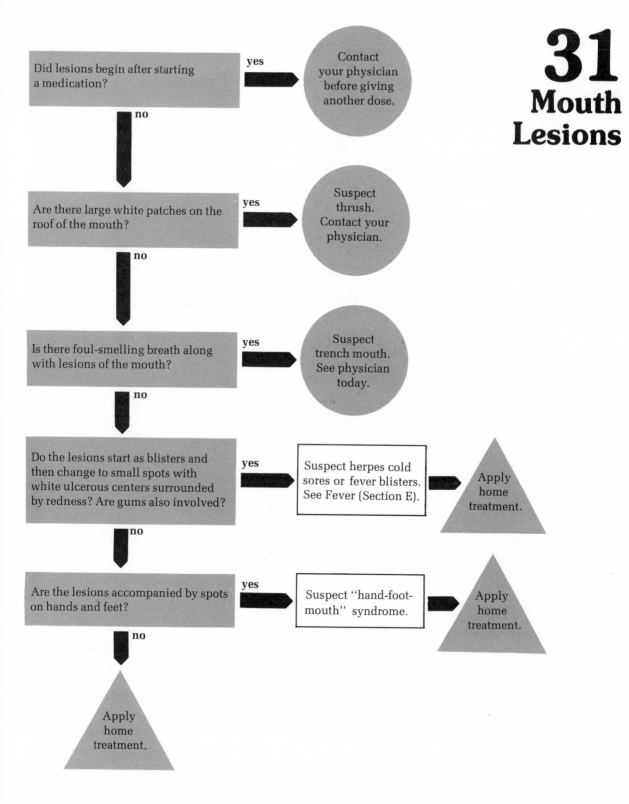

Did lesions begin after starting a medication? — **yes** → Contact your physician before giving another dose.

no ↓

Are there large white patches on the roof of the mouth? — **yes** → Suspect thrush. Contact your physician.

no ↓

Is there foul-smelling breath along with lesions of the mouth? — **yes** → Suspect trench mouth. See physician today.

no ↓

Do the lesions start as blisters and then change to small spots with white ulcerous centers surrounded by redness? Are gums also involved? — **yes** → Suspect herpes cold sores or fever blisters. See Fever (Section E). → Apply home treatment.

no ↓

Are the lesions accompanied by spots on hands and feet? — **yes** → Suspect "hand-foot-mouth" syndrome. → Apply home treatment.

no ↓

Apply home treatment.

32
Toothaches

A toothache is the sad result of a poor program of dental hygiene. Although resistance to tooth decay is partly inherited, the majority of dental problems are preventable. (See the discussion of dental care on pp. 118–121.) Occasionally, it is difficult to distinguish a toothache from other sources of pain. Earaches, sore throats, mumps, sinusitis, and injury to the joint that attaches the jaw to the skull may all be confused with a toothache.

Certainly if you can see a decayed tooth or an area of redness surrounding a tooth, a toothache is most likely. Tapping on the teeth with a wooden Popsicle stick will often accentuate the pain in an affected tooth, even though it appears normal.

If your child appears ill, has a fever, and has swelling of the jaw or redness surrounding the tooth, a tooth abscess is likely and antibiotics will be necessary in addition to proper dental care. In such circumstances a visit to the physician may be in order before seeing the dentist. Alternatively, see the dentist.

If a pain occurs every time your child opens his or her mouth widely, it is likely that the joint of the jaw has been injured; this can occur from a blow or just by trying to eat too big a sandwich.

Home Treatment
Aspirin or acetaminophen may be used for pain when a toothache is suspected and while a dental appointment is being arranged. Aspirin is also helpful for problems in the joint of the jaw.

What to Expect at the Dentist's Office
At the dentist's office, fillings or extractions will be performed. Often in baby teeth, an extraction will be most likely. Root canals as opposed to extraction are generally performed on permanent teeth if the problem is severe. If there is fever or swelling of the jaw, an antibiotic usually will be prescribed.

32
Toothaches

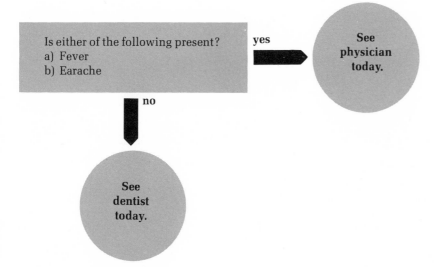

Is either of the following present?
a) Fever
b) Earache

yes → See physician today.

no → See dentist today.

H

Common Skin Problems

Skin Symptom Table   236

33. **Baby Rashes**   238
Usually no treatment needed.

34. **Diaper Rash**   240
Every baby gets it.

35. **Hair Loss**   242
It usually grows back.

36. **Impetigo**   244
Contagious skin infection.

37. **Ringworm**   246
Only skin deep.

38. **Hives**   248
Wheals, itching, and mystery.

39. **Poison Ivy and Poison Oak**   250
The fourteen-day itch.

40. **Skin Lumps, Bumps, and Warts**   252
Mostly minor.

41. **Eczema (Atopic Dermatitis)**   254
When your hands break out.

42. **Boils**   256
A classic pain.

43. **Acne**   258
Infancy and puberty.

44. **Athlete's Foot**   260
Just a fungus.

45. **Jock Itch**   262
And another fungus.

46. **Sunburn**   264
Prevent the pain.

47. **Lice and Bedbugs**   266
In the best of families.

48. **Ticks and Chiggers (Redbugs)**   268
Bites and burrows.

49. **Scabies**   270
Insects in the hands.

50. **Dandruff and Cradle Cap**   272
These can cause a rash.

51. **Patchy Loss of Skin Color**   274
A superficial worry.

Skin problems must be approached somewhat differently from other medical problems. Decision charts that proceed from complaints such as "red bumps" can be developed, but the charts are complicated and somewhat unsatisfactory. This is because most people, including doctors, identify skin diseases by recognizing a particular pattern. This pattern is composed of not only what the skin problem looks like at a particular time, but also how it began, where it spread, and whether it is associated with other symptoms such as itching or fever. Also important are elements of the medical history that may suggest an illness to which the child has been exposed. Fortunately, many times you already have a good idea of the problem, and it is possible to proceed immediately with the question of whether this is or is not poison ivy or ringworm or whatever.

If you are confused about what skin problem is present, we have provided two tables that will help you find a place to start. Each decision chart in this section begins with the question of whether the problem is compatible with the essentials of the pattern for that skin disease. (Note that a more complete description of the pattern is given on the left-hand page.) If it is not, you are directed to reconsider the problem and consult the tables.

Obviously, most cases of a particular skin disease do not look exactly as a textbook says they should, so we have not provided you with pictures. We have tried to allow for a reasonable amount of variation in the descriptions, and you will have to exercise your common sense a good deal. Don't be afraid to ask for other opinions; grandmother or your friends have seen a lot of skin problems over the years and know what the problems we describe in print look like in the flesh. We have listed some of the more common problems, but by no means all. If your problem doesn't seem to fit anything, then common sense as to whether the problem is serious and a call to the doctor if it is will take you a long way.

Finally, because every case is at least a little bit different, even the best doctors will not be able to immediately identify all skin problems. Simple office laboratory methods can help sort these out. The vast majority of skin problems are fortunately minor, are self-limited, and pose no major threat to health.

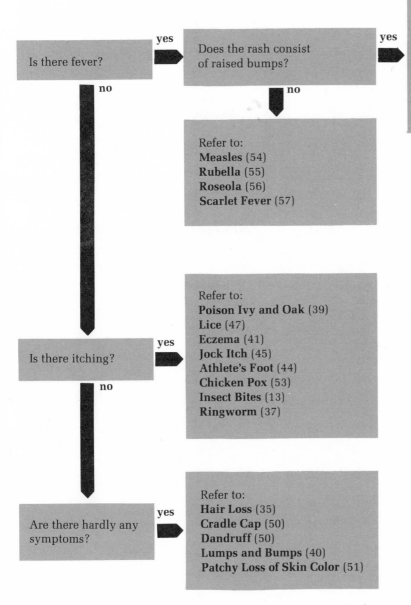

Is there fever?

yes → Does the rash consist of raised bumps?

yes →

Refer to:
Chicken Pox (53)
Mouth Lesions (31)
Impetigo (36)
Boils (42)
Insect Bites (13)
Hives (38)
If none of these,
suspect drug reaction.

no ↓

Refer to:
Measles (54)
Rubella (55)
Roseola (56)
Scarlet Fever (57)

no ↓

Is there itching?

yes →

Refer to:
Poison Ivy and Oak (39)
Lice (47)
Eczema (41)
Jock Itch (45)
Athlete's Foot (44)
Chicken Pox (53)
Insect Bites (13)
Ringworm (37)

no ↓

Are there hardly any symptoms?

yes →

Refer to:
Hair Loss (35)
Cradle Cap (50)
Dandruff (50)
Lumps and Bumps (40)
Patchy Loss of Skin Color (51)

SKIN SYMPTOM TABLE

	Fever	Itching	Elevation
Prickly Heat (33)	No	Sometimes	Slightly raised dots
Diaper rash (34)	No	No	Only if infected
Impetigo (36)	Sometimes	Occasionally	Crusts on sores
Ringworm (37)	No	Occasionally	Slightly raised rings
Hives (38)	No	Intense	Raised with flat tops
Poison ivy (39)	No	Intense	Blisters are elevated
Eczema (41)	No	Moderate to intense	Occasional blisters when infected
Acne (43)	No	No	Pimples, cysts
Athlete's foot (44)	No	Mild to intense	No
Cradle Cap and Dandruff (50)	No	Occasionally	Some crusting
Chicken pox (53)	Yes	Intense during pustular stage	Flat, then raised, then blisters, then crusts
Measles (54)	Yes	None to mild	Flat
German Measles (Rubella) (55)	Yes	No	Flat or slightly raised
Fifth disease (58)	No	No	Flat; lacy appearance
Roseola (56)	Yes	No	Flat, occasionally with few bumps
Scarlet fever (57)	Yes	No	Flat; feels like sandpaper

Color	Location	Duration of Problem	Other
White or red dots; surrounding skin may be red	Trunk, neck, skin folds on arms and legs	Until controlled	
Red	Under diaper	Until controlled	
"Golden crusts on red sores"	Arms, legs, face first; then most of body	Until controlled	
Red	Anywhere, including scalp and nails	Until controlled	Flaking or scaling
Pale raised lesions surrounded by red	Anywhere	Minutes to days	
Red	Exposed areas	7–14 days	Oozing; some swelling
Red	Elbows, wrists, knees, cheeks	Until controlled	Moist; oozing
Red	Face, back, chest	Until controlled	Blackheads
Colorless–red	Between toes	Until controlled	Cracks; scaling; oozing blisters
White to yellow to red	Scalp, eyebrows, behind ears, groin	Until controlled	Fine, oily scales
Red	May start anywhere; most prominent on trunk and face	4–10 days	Lesions progress from flat to tiny blisters, then become crusted.
Pink; then red	First face; then chest and abdomen; then arms and legs	4–7 days	Preceded by fever, cough, red eyes.
Red	First face; then trunk; then extremities	2–4 days	Swollen glands behind ears. Occasional joint pains in older children.
Red	First face; then arms and legs; then rest of body	3–7 days	"Slapped-cheek" appearance. Rash comes and goes.
Pink	First trunk; then arms and neck; very little on face and legs	1–2 days	High fever for 3 days which disappears with rash.
Red	First face; then elbows; spreads rapidly to entire body in 24 hours.	5–7 days	Sore throat. Skin peeling afterwards, especially palms.

33
Baby Rashes

The skin of the newborn child may exhibit a wide variety of bumps and blotches. Fortunately, almost all of these are harmless and clear up by themselves. The most common of these conditions are addressed in this section and only one, heat rash, requires any treatment. If the baby was delivered in a hospital many of these conditions may occur before discharge so that advice will be readily available from nurses or physicians.

Heat rash is caused by blockage of the pores that lead to the sweat glands. It actually can occur at any age, but is most common in the very young child in which the sweat glands are still developing. When heat and humidity rise, these glands attempt to provide sweat as they would normally, but because of the blockage, this sweat is held within the skin and forms little red bumps. It is also known as "prickly heat" or "miliaria."

On the other hand, the "little white bumps of milia" are composed of normal skin cells that have overaccumulated in some spots. As many as 40 percent of children have these bumps at birth. Eventually the bumps break open, the trapped material escapes, and the bumps disappear without requiring any treatment.

Erythema toxicum is an unnecessarily long and frightening term for the flat red splotches that appear in up to 50 percent of all babies. These seldom appear after five days of age and have usually disappeared by seven days. The children involved are perfectly normal, and whether or not any real toxin is involved is not clear.

Because the baby is exposed to the mother's adult hormones, a mild case of acne may develop just as may occur when a child begins to produce adult hormones during adolescence. (The little white dots often seen on a newborn's nose represent an excess amount of normal skin oil, *sebaceous gland hyperplasia,* that has been produced by the hormones.) Acne usually becomes evident at between two and four weeks of age and clears up spontaneously within six months to a year. It virtually never requires treatment.

Home Treatment

Heat rash is effectively treated simply by providing a cooler and less humid environment. Powders carefully applied do no harm, but are unlikely to help. Ointments and creams should be avoided since they tend to keep the skin warmer and block the pores.

Acne should *not* be treated with the medicines used by adolescents and adults. Normal washing usually is all that is required.

None of these problems should be associated with fever and, with the exception of minor discomfort in heat rash, should be painless. If any question should arise about these conditions, a telephone call to the physician's office often will answer your questions.

What to Expect at the Doctor's Office

Discussion of these problems can usually wait until the regular scheduled well-baby visit. The physician can confirm your diagnosis at that time.

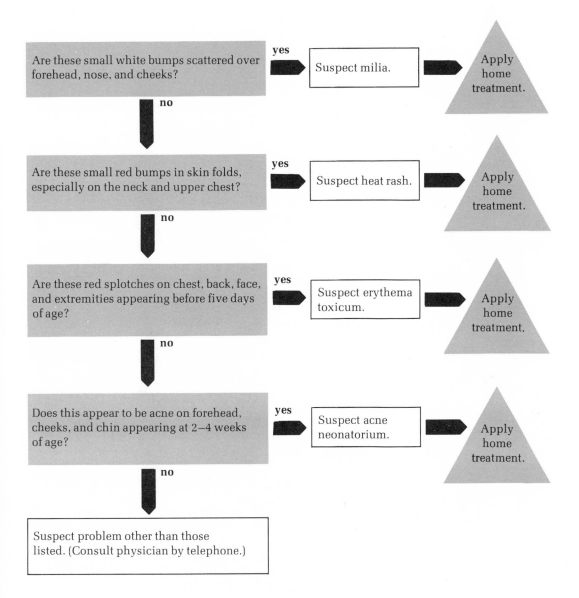

Are these small white bumps scattered over forehead, nose, and cheeks? — **yes** → Suspect milia. → Apply home treatment.

no ↓

Are these small red bumps in skin folds, especially on the neck and upper chest? — **yes** → Suspect heat rash. → Apply home treatment.

no ↓

Are these red splotches on chest, back, face, and extremities appearing before five days of age? — **yes** → Suspect erythema toxicum. → Apply home treatment.

no ↓

Does this appear to be acne on forehead, cheeks, and chin appearing at 2–4 weeks of age? — **yes** → Suspect acne neonatorium. → Apply home treatment.

no ↓

Suspect problem other than those listed. (Consult physician by telephone.)

34
Diaper Rash

The only children who never have diaper rash are those who never wear diapers. An infant's skin is particularly sensitive and likely to develop diaper rash, which is basically an irritation caused by dampness and the interaction of urine and skin. An additional irritant is thought to be the ammonia in urine and often its odor is unmistakably present. Factors that tend to keep the baby's skin wet and exposed to the irritant promote diaper rash and commonly there are three: (1) continuously wet diapers, (2) the use of plastic pants, and (3) the use of disposable diapers, which have a plastic cover. For the most part, treatment consists of reversing these factors.

The irritation of simple diaper rash may become complicated by an infection due to yeast (candida) or bacteria. When yeast is the culprit, small red spots may be seen. Also, small patches of the rash may appear outside the area covered by the diaper, as far away as the chest. Infection with bacteria leads to development of large fluid-filled blisters. If the rash is worse in the skin creases, a mild underlying skin problem known as seborrhea may be present. This skin condition is also responsible for cradle cap and dandruff.

Occasionally parents will notice blood or what appear to be blood spots when boys have diaper rash. This is due to a similar rash at the urinary opening at the end of the penis. This problem will clear up as the rash clears up.

Home Treatment

Treatment of diaper rash is aimed at keeping the skin dry and exposed to air. As implied above, the first things to do are to change the diapers frequently and to discontinue the use of plastic pants or disposable diapers with a heavy plastic coating. Leaving the diapers off altogether for as long as possible will also help. Diapers should be washed in a mild soap and rinsed thoroughly; occasionally the soap residues left in the diapers will act as an irritant. Adding a half cup of vinegar to the last rinse cycle may help counter the irritating ammonia.

While complete clearing of the rash will take several days at least, definite improvement should be noted within the first 48 to 72 hours. If this is not the case or if the rash is extraordinarily severe, the physician should be consulted.

To prevent diaper rash some parents use zinc oxide ointment (Desitin) or petroleum jelly (Vaseline). Others use baby powders (*caution:* talc dust can injure lungs). Caldesene powder is helpful in preventing seborrhea and monilial rashes. Always place powder in your hand first and then pat on baby's bottom. We do not feel that all babies need the use of powders and creams. If a rash has begun, ointments should *not* be used, since they delay healing.

What to Expect at the Doctor's Office

All of the baby's skin should be inspected to determine the true extent of the rash. Occasionally, a scraping from the involved skin will be looked at under the microscope. If a yeast (monilial) infection has complicated the simple diaper rash, the doctor will prescribe home treatment plus the use of a medication to kill the yeast (Mycostatin cream and occasionally oral Mycostatin). If a bacterial infection has occurred, then an antibiotic to be taken by mouth will be recommended. If the rash is very severe or seborrhea is suspected, then a steroid cream may be advised. In any case, home therapy may be begun safely before seeing the doctor.

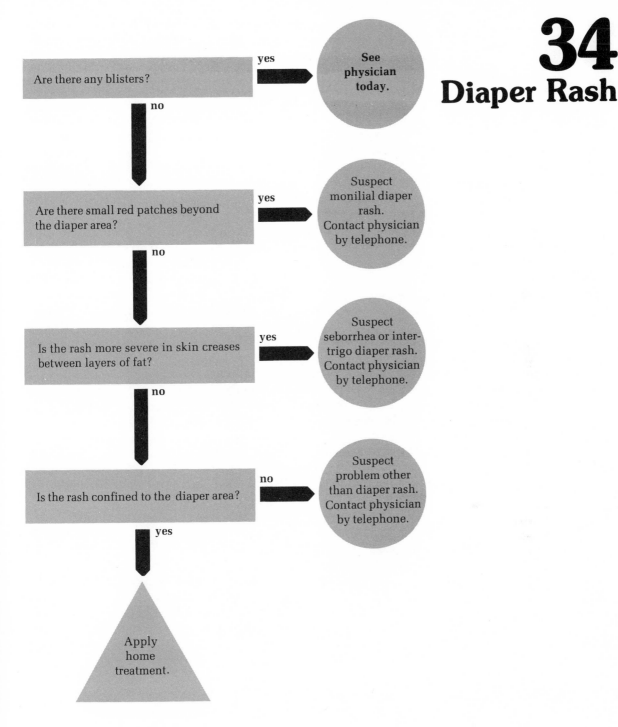

Are there any blisters?

yes → See physician today.

no ↓

Are there small red patches beyond the diaper area?

yes → Suspect monilial diaper rash. Contact physician by telephone.

no ↓

Is the rash more severe in skin creases between layers of fat?

yes → Suspect seborrhea or intertrigo diaper rash. Contact physician by telephone.

no ↓

Is the rash confined to the diaper area?

no → Suspect problem other than diaper rash. Contact physician by telephone.

yes ↓

Apply home treatment.

35

Hair Loss

Hair loss may cause concern in childhood. Often all the hair in one small area will be completely lost, but the scalp underneath will be normal. This problem is called *alopecia areata* and its cause is unknown. Usually the hair will be completely regrown within twelve months, although about 40 percent of children will have a similar loss within the next four to five years. This problem resolves by itself. Cortisone creams will make the hair grow back faster, but the new hair falls out again when the treatment is stopped, so these creams are of little use.

Types of hair loss that may need treatment by a physician are characterized by abnormalities in the scalp skin or the hairs themselves. The most frequent problem in this category is ringworm (see Problem 37). Ringworm may be red and scaly or there may be pustules with oozing. The ringworm fungus infects the hairs so that they become thickened and break easily. Whenever the scalp skin or the hairs themselves appear abnormal, the physician may be able to help.

Hair pulling by the children themselves, or occasionally a friend, often is responsible for hair loss. Tight braids or ponytails may also cause some hair loss. If your child constantly pulls out his or her hair, you should consider this unusual behavior and discuss it with a physician.

Home Treatment
In this instance, home treatment is reserved for presumed alopecia areata and consists of watchful waiting. The skin in the involved area must be completely normal to make a diagnosis of alopecia areata. Should the appearance of scalp or hairs become abnormal, then the physician should be consulted.

What to Expect at the Doctor's Office
An examination of the hair and scalp is usually sufficient to determine the nature of the problem. Occasionally, the hairs themselves may be examined under the microscope. Certain types of ringworm of the scalp can be identified because they fluoresce under a Wood's lamp. Ringworm of the scalp will require the use of an oral drug, griseofulvin, because creams and lotions applied to the affected area will not penetrate into the hair follicles to kill the fungus. We hope that no physician would recommend the use of X-rays today as some did a decade or two ago. If it is offered, it should be flatly rejected and you should find yourself another physician.

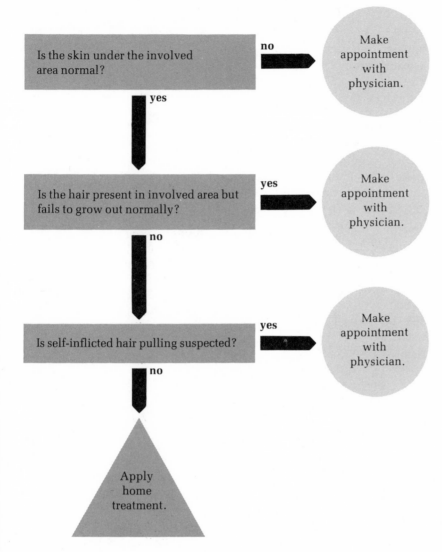

35
Hair Loss

Is the skin under the involved area normal?

no → Make appointment with physician.

yes ↓

Is the hair present in involved area but fails to grow out normally?

yes → Make appointment with physician.

no ↓

Is self-inflicted hair pulling suspected?

yes → Make appointment with physician.

no ↓

Apply home treatment.

36
Impetigo

Impetigo is particularly troublesome in the summer, and especially in warm, moist climates. It can be recognized by the characteristic appearance of the lesions, which begin as small red spots and progress to tiny blisters that eventually rupture, producing an oozing, sticky, honey-colored crust. These lesions are usually spread very quickly by scratching fingers. Another characteristic of impetigo is that it is extremely contagious and children pass it on to their brothers, sisters, and playmates very easily.

Impetigo is a skin infection caused by streptococcal bacteria; occasionally other bacteria may also be found. Impetigo, if it spreads, can be a very uncomfortable problem. There is usually a great deal of itching, and scratching hastens spreading of the lesions. After the sores heal, there may be a slight decrease in skin color at the site. Skin color usually returns to normal, so this need not concern parents.

Of greatest concern is a rare, complicating, kidney problem known as *glomerulonephritis*, which occasionally occurs in epidemics. Glomerulonephritis will cause the urine to turn a dark brown (cola) color and is often accompanied by headache and elevated blood pressure. Although this problem has a formidible name, the kidney problem is short-lived and heals completely in most children.

Unfortunately, antibiotics will not prevent glomerulonephritis, but can prevent the impetigo from spreading to other children, thus protecting them from both impetigo and glomerulonephritis. They are effective in healing the impetigo.

Although there is some debate on this matter, many physicians believe that if only one or two lesions are present and the lesions are not progressing, home treatment may be used for impetigo. The exception to this rule is if an epidemic of glomerulonephritis is occurring within your community.

Home Treatment
Crusts may be soaked off with either warm water or Burrow's Solution (Domeboro, Bluboro). Antibiotic ointments are no more effective than soap and water. The lesions should be scrubbed with soap and water after the crusts have been soaked off. If lesions do not show prompt improvement or if they seem to be spreading, the child should be seen by a physician without delay.

What to Expect at the Doctor's Office
After examining the sores and taking an appropriate medical history, the physician usually will prescribe an antibiotic to be taken by mouth. The drug of choice is penicillin unless there is penicillin allergy, in which case erythromycin will usually be prescribed. Some physicians may check the blood pressure or the urine in order to examine for early signs of glomerulonephritis.

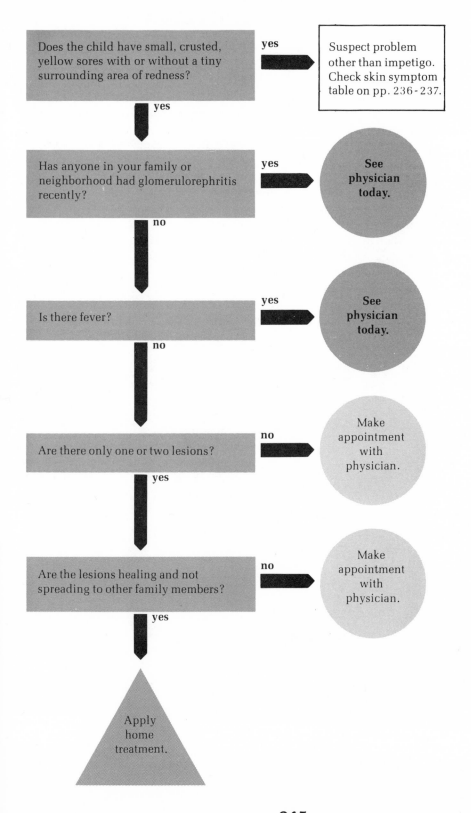

Does the child have small, crusted, yellow sores with or without a tiny surrounding area of redness?

yes → Suspect problem other than impetigo. Check skin symptom table on pp. 236-237.

yes ↓

Has anyone in your family or neighborhood had glomerulorephritis recently?

yes → See physician today.

no ↓

Is there fever?

yes → See physician today.

no ↓

Are there only one or two lesions?

no → Make appointment with physician.

yes ↓

Are the lesions healing and not spreading to other family members?

no → Make appointment with physician.

yes ↓

Apply home treatment.

36
Impetigo

37
Ringworm

Ringworm is a shallow fungus infection of the skin. Worms have nothing whatsoever to do with this condition; the designation "ringworm" is derived from the characteristic red ring that appears on the skin.

Ringworm can generally be recognized by its pattern of development. The lesions begin as small, round, red spots, and get progressively larger. When they are about the size of a pea, the center begins to clear. When the lesions are about the size of a dime, they will have the appearance of a ring. The border of the ring will be red, elevated, and scaly. Often there are groups of infections so close to one another that it is difficult to recognize them as individual rings.

Ringworm may also affect the scalp or the nails. These infections are more difficult to treat, but fortunately are not seen very often. Epidemics of ringworm of the scalp were common many years ago.

Home Treatment

Tolnaftate (Tinactin) applied to the skin is an effective treatment for ringworm. It is available in cream, solution, and powder, and can be purchased over the counter. Either the cream or the solution should be applied two or three times a day. Only a small amount is required for each application. Resolution of the problem may require several weeks of therapy, but improvement should be noted within a week. Selsun Blue shampoo, applied as a cream several times a day, will often do the job just as well and is less expensive. Ringworm that shows no improvement after a week of therapy or that continues to spread should be checked by a physician.

What to Expect at the Doctor's Office

The diagnosis of ringworm can be confirmed by scraping the scales, soaking them in a potassium hydroxide solution, and viewing them under the microscope. Some physicians may culture the scrapings. One of three agents will be prescribed if tinactin has failed: haloprogin (Halotex), clotrimazole (Lotrimin), or miconazole (MicaTin).

In infections involving the scalp, an ultraviolet light (called a Wood's lamp) will cause affected hairs to become fluorescent. The Wood's lamp is used to make the diagnosis; it does not treat the ringworm. Ringworm of the scalp must be treated by griseofulvin, taken by mouth, usually for at least a month; this medication is also effective for fungal infections of the nails. Ringworm of the scalp should never be treated with X-rays.

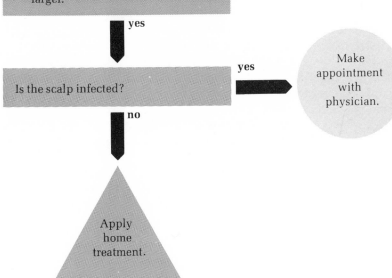

Are all of the following conditions present?
a) Rash begins as a small red, colorless, or depigmented circle that becomes progressively larger.
b) The circular border is elevated and perhaps scaly.
c) The center of the circle begins healing as the circle becomes larger.

no → Suspect problem other than ringworm. Check skin symptom table on pp. 236-237.

yes

Is the scalp infected?

yes → Make appointment with physician.

no

Apply home treatment.

38
Hives

Hives are an allergic reaction. Unfortunately, the reaction can be to almost anything, including cold or heat and even emotional tension. Unless you already have a good idea what is causing the hives or if a new drug has just been taken, the physician is unlikely to be able to determine the cause; most often, a search for a cause is fruitless. Here is a list of some of the things that are frequently mentioned as causes: drugs, eggs, milk, wheat, chocolate, pork, shellfish, freshwater fish, berries, cheese, nuts, pollens, and insect bites. The only sure way to know whether or not one of these is the culprit is to voluntarily expose the child to it. The problem with this approach is that if an allergy does exist, then the allergic reaction may include not only hives but dangerous reactions causing difficulty with breathing or circulation. As indicated by the decision chart, a systemic reaction along with the hives is a potentially dangerous situation and the physician should be consulted immediately. Avoid exposure to a suspected cause to see if the attacks will cease. Such "tests" are difficult to interpret, since attacks of hives are often separated by long periods of time. Actually, most people have only one attack, lasting from a period of hours to weeks.

Home Treatment

Determine whether there has been any pattern to the appearance of the hives. Do they appear after meals? After exposure to the cold? During a particular season of the year? If these seem to be likely possibilities, eliminate these and see what happens. If the reactions seem to be related to foods, an alternative is available. Lamb and rice virtually never cause allergic reactions. The child may be placed on a diet consisting only of lamb and rice until completely free of hives. Foods are then added back to the diet one at a time and the child is observed for the development of hives.

Itching may be relieved by the application of cold compresses, the use of aspirin, or the use of antihistamines such as diphenhydramine (Benadryl) or chlorpheniramine (Chlortrimeton) (see Chapter 9, The Home Pharmacy).

What to Expect at the Doctor's Office

If the child is suffering a systemic reaction with difficulty breathing or dizziness, then injections of adrenalin and other drugs may be given. In the more usual case of hives alone, the physician may do two things for your child. First, he or she can prescribe an antihistamine or use adrenalin injections to relieve swelling and itching. Second, the doctor can review the history of the reaction to try to find an offending agent and advise you as above. Remember that most often the cause of hives goes undetected.

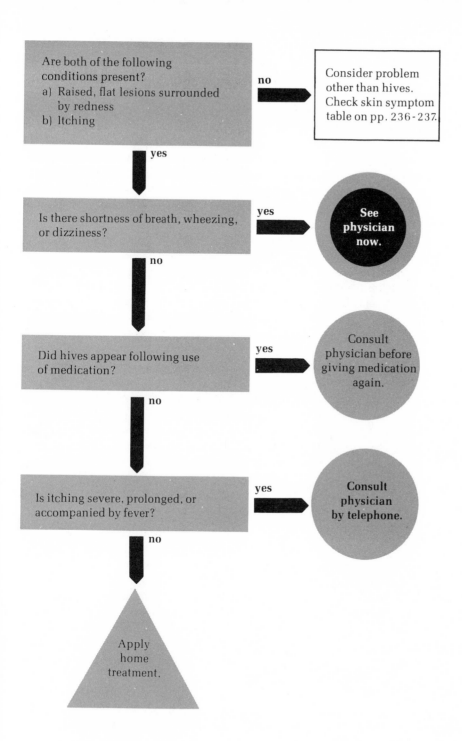

Are both of the following conditions present?
a) Raised, flat lesions surrounded by redness
b) Itching

no → Consider problem other than hives. Check skin symptom table on pp. 236-237.

yes ↓

Is there shortness of breath, wheezing, or dizziness?

yes → See physician now.

no ↓

Did hives appear following use of medication?

yes → Consult physician before giving medication again.

no ↓

Is itching severe, prolonged, or accompanied by fever?

yes → Consult physician by telephone.

no ↓

Apply home treatment.

38
Hives

39
Poison Ivy and Poison Oak

Poison ivy and poison oak need little introduction. The itching skin lesions that follow contact with these and other plants of the Rhus plant family are the most common example of a larger category of skin problems known as *contact dermatitis*. Contact dermatitis simply means that something that has been applied to the skin has caused the skin to react to it. An initial exposure is necessary to "sensitize" the patient; a subsequent exposure will result in an allergic reaction if the plant oil remains in contact with the skin for several hours. The resulting rash begins after 12 to 48 hours delay and persists for about two weeks. Contact may be indirect, from pets, contaminated clothing, or the smoke from burning Rhus plants. It can occur during any season.

Home Treatment
The best approach is to teach your children to recognize and avoid the plants, which are hazardous even in the winter when they have dropped their leaves. Next best is to remove the plant oil from the skin as soon as possible. If the oil has been on the skin for less than six hours, thorough cleansing with ordinary soap, repeated three times, will often prevent reaction. Alcohol-base cleansing tissues, available in prepackaged form (Alco-wipe, etc.) are also effective in removing the oil.

To relieve itching, many physicians recommend cool compresses of Burrow's Solution (Domeboro, BurVeen, Bluboro) or baths with Aveeno or oatmeal (one cup to a tub full of water). Aspirin is also effective in reducing itching. The old standby, calamine lotion, is sometimes of help in early lesions, but may spread the plant oil. (*Caution:* Do not use Caladryl or Zyradryl. They cause allergic reactions in some people. Use only calamine lotion.) Be sure to cleanse the skin, as above, even if you are too late to prevent the rash entirely. Another useful method of obtaining symptomatic relief is the use of a hot bath or hot shower. Heat releases histamine, the substance in the cells of the skin that causes the intense itching. Therefore, a hot shower or bath will cause intense itching as the histamine is released. The heat should be gradually increased to the maximum tolerable and continued until the itching has subsided. This process will deplete the cells of histamine and the child will obtain up to eight hours of relief from the itching. This method has the advantage of not requiring frequent applications of ointments to the lesions and is a good way to get some sleep at night. Poison ivy or poison oak will persist for the same length of time despite any medication. If secondary bacterial infection occurs, healing will be delayed; hence scratching is not helpful. Cut the nails to avoid damage to the skin through scratching.

Poison ivy is not contagious; it cannot be spread once the oil has been absorbed by the skin or removed.

If the lesions are too extensive to be easily treated, if home treatment is ineffective, or if the itching is so severe that the child can't tolerate it, a visit to the physician may be necessary.

What to Expect at the Doctor's Office
After a history and physical examination, the physician may prescribe a steroid cream to be applied four to six times a day to the lesions. This is often of moderate help. Another alternative is to give a steroid (such as prednisone) by mouth for short periods of time. A rather large dose is given the first day and the dose is then gradually reduced. We are reluctant to recommend oral steroids except in children with previous severe reactions to poison ivy or poison oak or extensive exposure. The itching may be treated symptomatically with either an antihistamine (Benadryl, Vistaril) or aspirin. The antihistamines may cause drowziness and interfere with sleep.

39
Poison Ivy and Poison Oak

Are all of the following conditions present?
a) Itching
b) Redness, minor swelling, blisters, or oozing
c) Probable exposure to poison ivy, poison oak, or poison sumac

no → Suspect problem other than poison ivy or poison oak. Check the skin symptom table on pp. 236-237.

yes

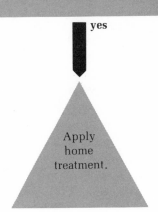

Apply home treatment.

40

Skin Lumps, Bumps, and Warts

Lumps and bumps are common at all ages. The lump may be above the skin as with warts, moles, and insect bites, within the skin as with boils and certain kinds of moles, or under the skin as in the case of swollen lymph glands or small collections of fat called lipomas. If there is only one lump, and it is red, hot, tender, and swollen (inflamed), then it should be considered a boil until proven otherwise. (See Boils, Problem 42). A dark mole that appears to be enlarging or changing color might be a melanoma, a kind of skin cancer, although melanomas are extremely unusual in children.

The most commonly found lumps in children are swollen lymph glands. These are discussed in more detail in Problem 28 (Swollen Glands).

Warts are caused by viral infections, and often spontaneously resolve by themselves. However, warts can occasionally be troublesome, especially if they are on the fingers where they may interfere with writing or on the face where they are cosmetically disturbing.

Home Treatment

Treatment of many lumps and bumps is discussed under Insect Bites (Problem 13), Boils (Problem 42), and Swollen Glands (Problem 28). Warts can be removed with over-the-counter medicines used consistently and carefully. Available preparations include salicylic acid plasters, Compound W, and Vergo. On your child's next visit to the doctor you can ask about any skin lumps or warts that are of concern to you; these are seldom worth a special trip.

What to Expect at the Doctor's Office

The physician may be able to make the diagnosis simply by inspecting the lump or wart and asking you a few questions. In treating warts, a prescription liquid such as Duo-Film, consisting of lactic and salicylic acid, may initially be tried. A wart may be removed by freezing it with liquid nitrogen or by using an electric needle or by chemical cauterization. It is seldom treated surgically since warts are caused by viruses; cutting them out may leave the virus to cause a later recurrence of the wart. A recurrence of warts is common and repeated treatments may be necessary.

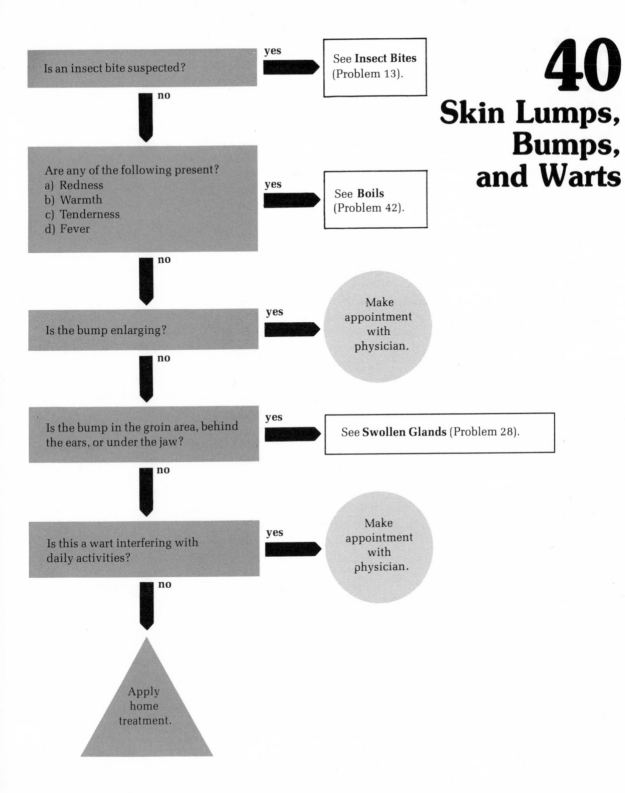

Is an insect bite suspected?

yes → See **Insect Bites** (Problem 13).

no ↓

Are any of the following present?
a) Redness
b) Warmth
c) Tenderness
d) Fever

yes → See **Boils** (Problem 42).

no ↓

Is the bump enlarging?

yes → Make appointment with physician.

no ↓

Is the bump in the groin area, behind the ears, or under the jaw?

yes → See **Swollen Glands** (Problem 28).

no ↓

Is this a wart interfering with daily activities?

yes → Make appointment with physician.

no ↓

Apply home treatment.

40
Skin Lumps, Bumps, and Warts

41
Eczema (Atopic Dermatitis)

Eczema is commonly found in children with a family history of either eczema, hay fever, or asthma. The underlying problem is the inability of the skin to retain adequate amounts of water; the skin of children with eczema is consequently very dry, which causes the skin to itch. Most of the manifestations of eczema are a consequence of scratching.

In young infants who are unable to scratch, the most common manifestation is red, dry, mildly scaling cheeks. Although the infant cannot scratch his or her cheeks, the cheeks can be rubbed by moving against the sheets, and thus become red. In infants, eczema may also be found in the area where the plastic pants meet the skin. The tightness of the elastic produces the characteristic red scaling lesion. In older children, it is very common for eczema to involve the area behind the knees and behind the elbows.

If there is a fair amount of weeping or crusting, the eczema has become infected with bacteria, and a visit to the physician will most likely be required.

The course of eczema is quite variable. Some children only have a brief mild problem; others have manifestations throughout life.

Home Treatment
Attempts must be made to prevent the skin from becoming too dry, and frequent bathings make the skin even dryer. Although the child will feel comfortable in the bath, itching will become more intense after the bath because of the drying effect.

Sweating aggravates eczema; consequently children should not be overdressed so that they perspire. Light night clothing is important. Contact with wool or silk seems to aggravate eczema in some children and should be avoided.

Nails should be kept trimmed short to minimize the effects of scratching. In older children who are helping with household chores, rubber gloves can help prevent drying of the hands after washing dishes or the car.

Washing is best accomplished with a cleansing and moisturizing agent such as Cetaphil lotion.

While fresh water or pool swimming can aggravate eczema by causing loss of skin moisture, ocean swimming does not do so and can be freely undertaken. (Also see Section F, Allergies.)

What to Expect at the Doctor's Office
By history and examination of the lesions, the physician can determine whether the problem is eczema. If home treatment has not improved the problem, steroid creams and lotions may be prescribed. While these are effective, they are not curative; eczema is characterized by repeated occurrences. If crusted or weeping lesions are present, bacterial infection is likely and an oral antibiotic will be prescribed.

Eczema
(Atopic
Dermatitis)

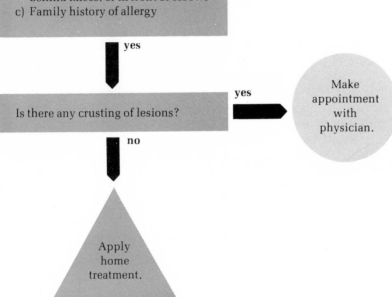

Are the following conditions present (at least two of three)?
a) Itching
b) Flat red areas on cheeks, behind ears, along edge of plastic pants, behind knees, or in front of elbows
c) Family history of allergy

no → Suspect problem other than eczema. Check skin symptom table on pp. 236-237.

yes ↓

Is there any crusting of lesions?

yes → Make appointment with physician.

no ↓

Apply home treatment.

42
Boils

"Painful as a boil" is a familiar term and emphasizes the severe discomfort that can arise from this common skin problem. A boil is a localized infection due to the staphylococcus germ; usually a particularly savage strain of the germ is responsible. When this particular germ inhabits the child's skin, recurrent problems with boils may persist for months or years. Often several family members will be affected at about the same time. Boils may be single or multiple, and they may occur anywhere on the body. They range from the size of a pea to the size of a walnut or larger. The surrounding red, thickened, and tender tissue increases the problem even further. The infection begins in the tissues beneath the skin, and develops into an abscess pocket filled with pus. Eventually, the pus pocket "points" toward the skin surface and finally ruptures and drains. Then it heals. Boils often begin as infections around hair follicles; hence the term *folliculitis* for minor infections. Often areas under pressure (such as the buttocks) are likely spots for boils to begin. A boil that extends into the deeper layers of the skin is called a carbuncle.

Special consideration should be given to boils on the face, since they are more likely to lead to severe complicating infections.

Home Treatment

Boils are handled gently, because rough treatment can force the infection deeper inside the body. Warm, moist soaks are applied gently several times each day to speed the development of the pocket of pus and to soften the skin for the eventual rupture and drainage. Once drainage begins, the soaks will help keep the opening in the skin clear. The more drainage, the better. Frequent thorough soaping of the entire skin helps prevent reinfection. Ignore all temptation to squeeze the boil.

What to Expect at the Doctor's Office

If there is fever or a facial boil, the doctor will usually prescribe an antibiotic. Otherwise, antibiotics may not be used; they are of limited help in abscesslike infections. If the boil feels like fluid is contained in a pocket, but has not yet drained, the physician may lance the boil. In this procedure, a small incision is made to allow the pus to drain. After drainage the pain is reduced and healing is quite prompt. While "incision and drainage" is not a complicated procedure, it is tricky enough that you should not attempt it yourself.

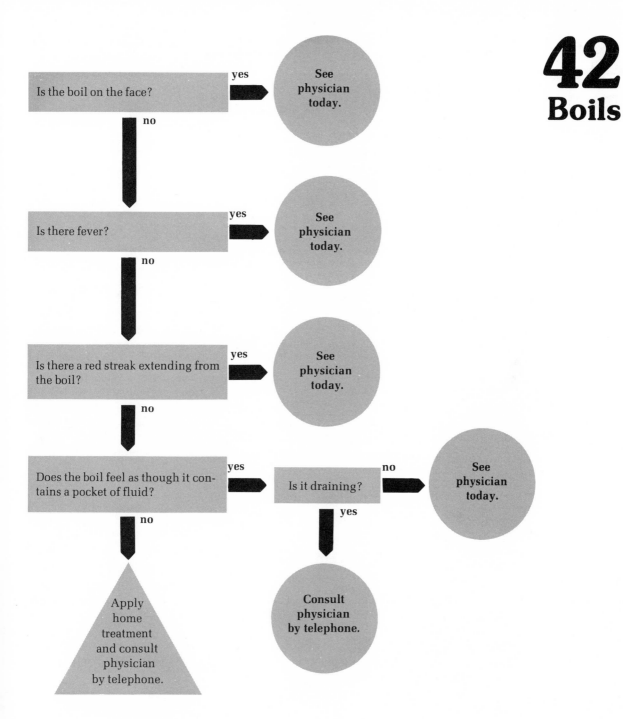

Is the boil on the face? — yes → See physician today.

no ↓

Is there fever? — yes → See physician today.

no ↓

Is there a red streak extending from the boil? — yes → See physician today.

no ↓

Does the boil feel as though it contains a pocket of fluid? — yes → Is it draining? — no → See physician today.

no ↓ (from "Does the boil feel...")

yes ↓ (from "Is it draining?")

Apply home treatment and consult physician by telephone.

Consult physician by telephone.

42
Boils

43
Acne

Acne is a superficial skin eruption caused by a combination of factors. It is triggered by the hormonal changes of puberty and is most common in children with oily skin. The increased skin oils accumulate below keratin plugs in the openings of the hair follicles and oil glands. In this stagnant area below the plug, secretions accumulate and bacteria grow. These normal bacteria cause changes in the secretions that make them irritating to the surrounding skin. The result is usually a pimple, but sometimes may develop into a larger pocket of secretions, or cyst. Blackheads are formed when air causes a chemical change—"oxidation"—of keratin plugs; the irritation of the skin is minimal.

Home Treatment

Cleanliness and good hygiene are important principles for everyone. While excessive dirt will certainly aggravate acne, unfortunately scrupulous cleaning will not always prevent it. With acne, the face should be scrubbed several times daily with a warm washcloth to remove skin oils and keratin plugs. The rubbing and heat of the washcloth help dislodge the keratin plug. Soap will help remove skin oil and will decrease the number of bacteria living on the skin. If there are pimples on the back, a backbrush or washcloth should be used there. Greases and creams on the skin may aggravate the problem. The various patent medicines available over the counter appear to help some people; they are disappointing in others. Diet is not an important factor in most cases, but if certain foods tend to aggravate the problem, avoid them. There is scant evidence that chocolate aggravates acne, despite popular belief.

Several further steps may be taken at home. An abrasive soap, such as Pernox or Brasivol, may be used from one to three times daily to further reduce the oiliness of the skin and to remove the keratin plugs from the follicles.

Steam may help to open clogged pores. Hot compresses are sometimes helpful. Some dermatologists recommend Vlem-Dome as a hot drying compress. A drying agent such as Fostex may be used, but irritation may occur if it is used too often.

Finally, natural sunlight or a sunlamp is effective if used conscientiously. We prefer natural sunlight and do not encourage the use of sunlamps. However, if used, use at a distance of 12 inches, expose three sides of the face in succession (left, center, right), wear goggles or place damp cotton over the eyes, treat two to three times a week, use a timer, and do not read or sleep under a sunlamp. Start at 30 seconds for each surface. Increase the exposure by 30 seconds at each exposure. Should a mild burn occur, discontinue for one week. Restart at one-half the previous time. Do not exceed 10 minutes under the sunlamp.

Should these measures fail to control the problem, make an appointment with the physician.

What to Expect at the Doctor's Office

The physician will advise about hygiene and the use of medications. Several new topical preparations such as retinoic acid (Retin-A) and benzoyl peroxide have been found helpful; they act by fostering skin peeling, which prevents plugging of the hair follicles. This peeling is not noticeable if the medication is used properly.

In resistant cases an antibiotic (tetracycline or occasionally erythromycin) may be prescribed to be taken by mouth. Some physicians use these antibiotics applied to the skin as well.

"Acne surgery" is a term generally applied to the physician's removal of blackheads with a suction device and an eyedropper. Large developing cysts are sometimes arrested with injection of steroids. Such procedures should be required only in severe cases, and are more usually performed on the back than on the face.

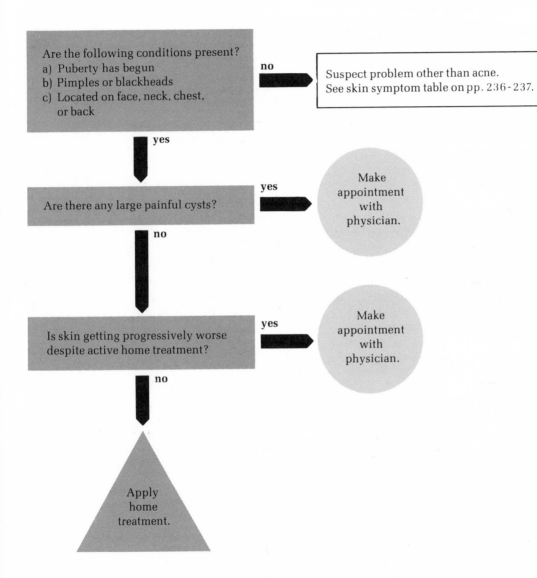

Are the following conditions present?
a) Puberty has begun
b) Pimples or blackheads
c) Located on face, neck, chest, or back

no → Suspect problem other than acne.
See skin symptom table on pp. 236-237.

yes

Are there any large painful cysts?

yes → Make appointment with physician.

no

Is skin getting progressively worse despite active home treatment?

yes → Make appointment with physician.

no

Apply home treatment.

44
Athlete's Foot

Athlete's foot is very common during adolescence, and relatively uncommon before. It is the most common of the fungal infections and is often persistent. When it involves toenails, it can be difficult to treat. Friction and moisture are important in aggravating the problem. In fact, there is evidence that bacteria and moisture cause most of this problem; the fungus is responsible only for getting things started. When many people share locker room and shower facilities, exposure to this fungus is impossible to prevent; and infection is the rule, rather than the exception. But you don't have to participate in sports to contact this fungus; it's all around.

Home Treatment

Scrupulous hygiene, without resorting to drugs, is often effective. *Twice a day,* wash the space between the toes with soap, water, and a cloth; dry the entire area carefully with a towel, particularly between the toes (despite the pain); and put on clean socks. Use shoes that allow evaporation of moisture. Plastic linings of shoes must be avoided. Sandals or canvas sneakers are best. Changing shoes every other day to allow them to dry out is a good idea. Keeping the feet dry with the use of a powder is helpful in preventing reinfection. In difficult cases, over-the-counter drugs such as Desenex powder or cream may be used. The powder has the virtue of helping keep the toes dry. If these are not effective, a more expensive over-the-counter medication, Tinactin (tolnaftate), is available in either cream or lotion. Tinactin powder is better as a preventive then curative preparation. Recently, the twice-daily application of a 30-percent aluminum chloride solution has been recommended for its drying and antibacterial properties. You will have to ask your pharmacist to make up the solution, but it is inexpensive.

What to Expect at the Doctor's Office

Through history and physical examination, and possibly laboratory examination of a skin scraping, the physician will establish the diagnosis. Several other problems, notably a condition called dyshydrosis, may mimic athlete's foot. An oral drug, griseofulvin, may be used for fungal infections of the nails but is not recommended for athlete's foot.

Are both of the following
conditions present?
a) Redness and scaling between toes
   (may have cracks and small blisters)
b) Itching

no

Suspect problem other than athlete's
foot. Check skin symptom table
on pp. 236-237.

yes

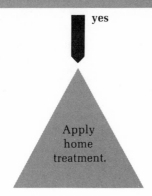

Apply
home
treatment.

45
Jock Itch

We might wish for a less picturesque name for this condition, but "tinea cruris" is a term understood by relatively few. "Jock itch" is a fungus infection of the pubic region. It is aggravated by friction and moisture. It usually does not involve the scrotum or penis nor does it spread beyond the groin area. For the most part, this is a male disease. Frequently the fungus grows in an athletic supporter turned old and moldy in a locker room far from a washing machine. The preventive measure for such a problem is obvious.

Home Treatment

The problem should be treated by removing the contributing factors, friction and moisture. This is done by wearing boxer-type shorts rather than Jockey shorts, by applying a powder to dry the area after bathing, and by frequently changing soiled or sweaty underclothes. It may take up to two weeks to completely clear this problem, and it may recur. The "powder-and-clean-shorts" treatment will usually be successful without any medication. Tinactin (tolnaftate) will eliminate the fungus if the problem persists.

What to Expect at the Doctor's Office

Occasionally a yeast infection will mimic jock itch. By examination and history, the physician will attempt to establish the diagnosis and additionally may make a scraping in order to identify a yeast. Medicines used for this problem are virtually always applied to the affected skin; oral drugs or injections are rarely used. Halotex (haloprigin) and Lotrimin (clotrimazole) are prescription creams and lotions effective against both fungi and certain yeast infections.

45
Jock Itch

Are all of the following conditions present?
a) Involves only groin and thighs
b) Redness, oozing, or some peripheral scaling
c) Itching

no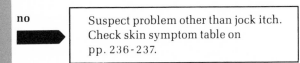

Suspect problem other than jock itch. Check skin symptom table on pp. 236-237.

yes

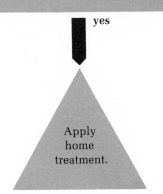

Apply home treatment.

46
Sunburn

Sunburn is common, painful, and avoidable. Very rarely, persons with sunburn have difficulty with vision; if so, they should be seen by a physician. Otherwise, a visit to the doctor is unnecessary unless the pain is extraordinarily severe or unless extensive blistering (not peeling) has occurred. Blistering indicates a second-degree burn, and rarely follows sun exposure. The pain of sunburn is worst between 6 and 48 hours after sun exposure. Peeling of injured layers of skin occurs later—between three and ten days after the burn.

Home Treatment

Cool compresses or cool baths with Aveeno (one cup to a tub full of water) may be useful. Ordinary baking soda (one half cup to a tub) is nearly as effective. Lubricants such as Vaseline feel good to some children, but retain heat and should not be used the first day. Avoid products that contain benzocaine. These may give temporary relief but can cause irritation of the skin and may actually prolong healing. Aspirin by mouth may ease pain and thus help sleep.

Sunburn is better prevented than treated. For protection, effective sunscreens are available. Protection is afforded by Block-out, Pabafilm, Pabonal, and Presun, among others.

What to Expect at the Doctor's Office

The physician will direct the history and physical examination toward determination of the extent of burn and the possibility of other heat-related injuries like sunstroke. If only first-degree burns are found, a prescription steroid lotion may be prescribed. This is not of particular benefit. The rare second-degree burns may be treated with antibiotics in addition to analgesics or sedation. There is no evidence that steroid lotions or antibiotic creams help at all in the *usual* case of sunburn; most physicians prescribe the same therapy that is available at home.

Are any of these conditions present following prolonged exposure to sun?
a) Fever
b) Fluid-filled blisters
c) Dizziness
d) Visual difficulties

yes

Consult physician by telephone.

no

Apply home treatment.

47
Lice and Bedbugs

Lice and bedbugs are found in the best of families. Lack of prejudice with respect to social class is as close as these insects come to having a virtue. At best they are a nuisance and at worst they can cause real disability.

Lice themselves are very small and are seldom seen without the aid of a magnifying glass. Usually it is easier to find the "nits," which are clusters of louse eggs. Without magnification, nits will appear as tiny white lumps on hair strands. The louse bite leaves only a pinpoint red spot but scratching makes things worse. Itching and occasionally small, shallow sores at the base of hairs are clues to the disease. Pubic lice are not a "venereal disease" although they may be spread from person to person during sexual contact. Unlike syphilis and gonorrhea, lice may be spread by toilet seats, infected linen, and other sources. Pubic lice bear some resemblance to crabs; hence the use of the term crabs to indicate a lice infestation of the pubic hair. A different species of lice may inhabit the scalp or other body hair. Lice like to be close to a warm body all the time and will not stay for long periods of time in clotning not being worn, bedding, etc.

Although related to lice, bedbugs present a considerably different picture. The adult is flat, wingless, oval in shape, reddish in color, and about one-quarter inch in length. Like lice, they stay alive by sucking blood. Unlike lice, they feed for only ten or fifteen minutes at a time and spend the rest of the time hiding in crevices and crannies. They feed almost entirely at night, both because that is when bodies are in bed and also because of a real aversion to light. They have such a keen sense of the nearness of a warm body that the Army has used them to detect the approach of an enemy at ranges of several hundred feet! Catching these pests out in the open is very difficult and may require some curious behavior. One technique is to dash into the bedroom at bedtime, flip on the lights, and pull back the bedcovers in an effort to catch them in anticipation of their next meal.

The bite of the bedbug leaves a firm bump; usually there are two or three bumps clustered together. Occasionally, sensitivity is developed to these bites, in which case itching may be severe and blisters may form.

Home Treatment

Over-the-counter preparations are effective against lice; these include A200, Cuprex, and RID. RID has the advantage of supplying a fine tooth comb, a rare item these days. Instructions that come with these drugs must be followed carefully. Linen and clothing must be changed simultaneously. Sexual partners should be treated at the same time.

Since bedbugs don't hide on the body or in clothes, it is the bed and the room that should be treated. A one-percent solution of malathion may be used. (**Caution:** This is a dangerous pesticide and must be kept away from children.) If the infestation is a light one, spray only the bed. Wet the slats, springs, and frame. Change the mattress cover, but spray the mattress only if there are seams or tufts that could harbor the bugs and if the child is older than five years. Use only a very light spray on mattresses. If the mattress is damaged so that stuffing is exposed, then a new mattress is necessary. Never spray a mattress to be used by an infant or young child. Malathion is dangerous if it contacts the skin. If the infestation is a heavy one, then the furniture, walls, and floors of the bedroom should also be sprayed.

What to Expect at the Doctor's Office

If lice are the suspected problem, the doctor will make a careful inspection to see if he can find nits or the lice themselves. Doctors almost always use Kwell for lice. It may be somewhat more effective than the over-the-counter preparations. It is more expensive and has more side effects.

The doctor will be hard-pressed to make a certain diagnosis of bedbug bites without information from you that bedbugs have been seen in the house. However, the bumps may be suggestive and it may be decided to assume that the problem is bedbugs initially. If this is the case, treatment with an insecticide as under Home Treatment will be recommended.

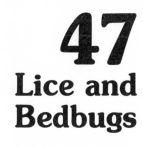

47
Lice and Bedbugs

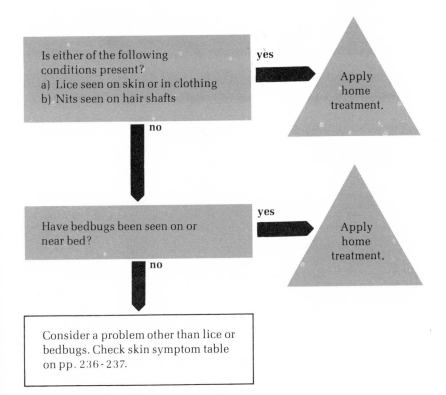

Is either of the following conditions present?
a) Lice seen on skin or in clothing
b) Nits seen on hair shafts

yes → Apply home treatment.

no ↓

Have bedbugs been seen on or near bed?

yes → Apply home treatment.

no ↓

Consider a problem other than lice or bedbugs. Check skin symptom table on pp. 236-237.

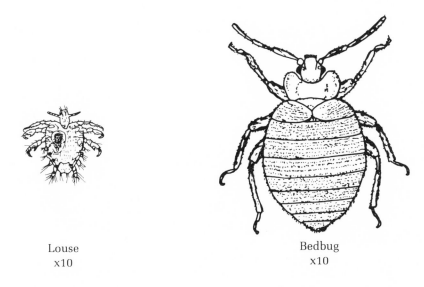

Louse
x10

Bedbug
x10

48
Ticks and Chiggers (Redbugs)

Outdoor living has its dangers. While bears, mountain lions, and vertical cliffs can usually be avoided, shrubs and tall grasses hide tiny insects eager for a blood meal from a passing animal or person. Ticks and chiggers are the most common of the small hazards.

Ticks are rather easily seen, and a tick bite usually has the obvious cause sticking out. Ticks are about one quarter inch long and easy to see. The tick buries its head and crablike pincers beneath the skin, with the body and legs protruding. Ticks feed on passing animals such as dogs or deer or people. In some areas, especially the southeastern United States, they carry other diseases, such as Rocky Mountain spotted fever; if a fever, rash, or headache follow a tick bite by a few days or weeks, the doctor should be consulted. If a pregnant female tick is allowed to remain feeding for several days, under certain circumstances a peculiar condition called tick paralysis may develop. The female tick secretes a toxin that can cause temporary paralysis, clearing shortly after the tick is removed; this complication is quite rare, and can only happen if the tick stays in place many days. In tick-infested areas it is helpful to check your child's hair periodically. You may be able to catch the ticks before they become embedded by checking after hikes. Also check your pets.

Chiggers are small red mites, sometimes called "redbugs." Their bite contains a chemical that eats away at the skin, causing a tremendous itch. Usually the small red sores are around the belt line or other openings in clothes. Careful inspection may reveal the tiny red larvae in the center of the itching sore. They also live on grasses and shrubs.

Home Treatment

Ticks should be removed, although they will eventually "fester" out and the complications are unusual. The trick is to get the tick to "let go" with the pincers before removal and not to kill the tick before getting it out. If the mouth parts and pincers remain under the skin, healing may require several weeks. Make the tick uncomfortable with his new home. Gentle heat from a heated paperclip, alcohol, acetone, or oil will cause the tick to wiggle the legs and begin to withdraw. Grasp the tick (with a tissue if you're squeamish), and remove it quickly with a twisting motion. Tradition says counterclockwise, but we seem to be able to get them out equally well in either direction. If the head is inadvertently left under the skin, soak gently with warm water twice daily until healing is complete. Call the doctor if your child gets fever, a rash, or headache within three weeks.

Chiggers are better avoided than treated. Use of insect repellents, the wearing of appropriate clothing, and bathing after exposure help to cut down on the frequency of bites. Once you get them, they itch, often for several weeks. Keep the sores clean, and soak with warm water twice daily. A200 and Cuprex, applied the first few days, will help kill the larvae, but the itch will persist.

What to Expect at the Doctor's Office

The doctor can remove the tick, but cannot prevent any illness that might have been transmitted. You can do as well. We always seem to be removing them from unusual places, such as armpits and belly buttons, but the scalp is the most common location. The technique is exactly the same, no matter where the tick is.

For chiggers, doctors will usually prescribe Kwell, which is perhaps slightly more effective than A200 or Cuprex, but does not stop the itching either. Antihistamines make the child drowsy and are not frequently used unless intense itching persists despite home treatment with aspirin, warm baths, oatmeal soaks, and calamine lotion.

CHIGGERS

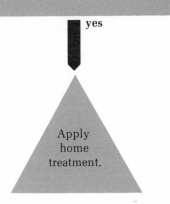

Are any of the following present?
a) Itching red sores around belt line or other opening in clothes
b) Itching red sores following contact with grass or shrubs
c) Small red mites seen on skin or red spot in center of sore

 no → Suspect problem other than chiggers. See skin symptom table on pp. 236-237.

yes

Apply home treatment.

TICKS

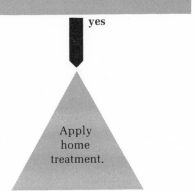

Can tick be seen buried in skin, or is a swollen tick attached to skin?

no → Suspect problem other than ticks. See skin symptom table on pp. 236-237.

yes

Apply home treatment.

49
Scabies

Scabies is an irritation of the skin caused by a tiny mite related to the chigger. No one knows why, but scabies seems to be on the rise in this country. As with lice, it is no longer true that scabies is related to hygiene. It occurs in the best of families and in the best of neighborhoods. The mite is easily spread from person to person or by contact with items that may harbor the mite such as clothing and bedding. Epidemics often spread through schools despite strict precautions against contacts with known cases.

The mite burrows into the skin to lay eggs; favorite locations for this burrowing are given in the decision chart. These burrows may be evident, especially at the beginning of the problem. However, the mite soon causes the skin to have a reaction to it so that redness, swelling, and blisters follow within a short period. Intense itching causes scratching so that there are plenty of scratch marks and these may become infected from the bacteria on the skin. Thus the telltale burrows are often obscured by scratch marks, blisters, and secondary infection. If you can locate something that looks like a burrow, you might be able to see the mite with the aid of a magnifying lens. This is the only way to be absolutely sure that the problem is scabies, but is often not possible. The diagnosis in an individual child is most often made on the basis of a problem that is consistent with scabies and the fact that scabies is known to be in the community.

Home Treatment
Benzyl benzoate (25% solution) is effective against scabies and does not require a prescription. Unfortunately, it is not widely available. If you are able to find it, apply it once to the entire body except for the face and around the urinary opening of the penis and the vaginal opening. Wash it off 24 hours later. This medicine does have an odor that some find unpleasant. If you cannot find benzyl benzoate, you'll have to get a prescription for Kwell from your doctor.

For itching, we recommend cool soaks, calamine lotion, or aspirin. Chlortrimeton, an antihistamine, is available without prescription but often causes drowsiness. Follow the directions that come with the package. As in the case of poison ivy, warmth makes the itching worse by releasing histamine, but if all the histamine is released, then relief may be obtained for several hours. (See Problem 39, Poison Ivy and Poison Oak.)

It will take some time before the skin becomes normal, even with effective treatment, but at least some improvement should be noted within 72 hours. If this is not the case, then a visit to the doctor should be made.

What to Expect at the Doctor's Office
The doctor should examine the entire skin surface for signs of the problem, and may examine the area with a magnifying lens in an attempt to identify the mite. He or she may scrape the lesion to examine under the microscope. Most of the time the doctor will be forced to make a decision based on the probability of various kinds of diseases and then treat much as you would. The proof of the pudding will be whether or not the treatment is successful.

Kwell will often be prescribed. Because of the potency of this medication it should not be used more than two times, a week apart.

Are all of the following
conditions present?
a) Intense itching
b) Raised red skin in a line (represents a burrow) and possibly
   blisters or pustules
c) Located on hands, especially
   between the fingers, elbow crease,
   armpit, groin crease, or behind
   the knees
d) Exposure to scabies

no →

Consider a problem other than scabies.
Check skin symptom table on
pp. 236-237.

yes

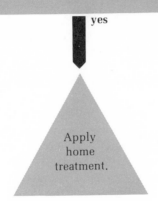

Apply
home
treatment.

50
Dandruff and Cradle Cap

Although they look somewhat different, cradle cap and dandruff are really part of the same problem; its medical term is *seborrhea*. It occurs when the oil glands in the skin have been stimulated by adult hormones, leading to oiliness and flaking of the scalp. This occurs in the infant because of exposure to the mother's hormones and in older children when they begin to make their own adult hormones. However, it does occur between these two ages, and once a child has the problem, it tends to recur.

Seborrhea itself is a somewhat ugly but relatively harmless condition. However, it may make the skin more susceptible to infection with yeast or bacteria. Occasionally this condition is confused with problems such as ringworm of the scalp or psoriasis. Careful attention to the conditions listed in the decision chart will usually avoid this confusion. Remember also that ringworm would be unusual in the newborn and very young child. Psoriasis often stops at the hairline. Furthermore, the scales of psoriasis are on top of raised lesions called "plaques," which is not the case in seborrhea.

Children will frequently have redness and scaling of the eyebrows and behind the ears as well.

Home Treatment

The heavily advertised antidandruff shampoos are helpful in mild to moderate cases of dandruff. For severe and more stubborn cases, there are some less well-known over-the-counter shampoos that are effective. Selsun (available by prescription only) and Selsun Blue are brand names of shampoos that contain selenium sulfide; Selsun Blue is available over the counter and, while weaker, is just as good if you apply more of it more frequently. When using these shampoos, it is important that directions be followed carefully, since oiliness and yellowish discoloration of the hair may occur with their use. Sebulex, Sebucare, Ionil, and DHS are another series of antidandruff preparations that are very effective and also must be used strictly according to directions.

Cradle cap is best treated with a scrub brush. If the cradle cap is thick, then rub in warm baby oil, cover with a warm towel, and soak for 15 minutes. Use a fine tooth comb or scrub brush to help remove the scale; then shampoo with Sebulex or other preparations listed above. Be careful to avoid getting shampoo in the child's eyes.

No matter what you do, the problem will often return, and you may have to repeat the treatment. If the problem gets worse despite home treatment over several weeks, see the doctor.

What to Expect at the Doctor's Office

Severe cases of seborrhea may require more than the medications given above; a cortisone cream is most often prescribed. Most often, a trip is made to the doctor in order to clear up some confusion concerning the diagnosis. The physician usually makes the diagnosis on the basis of the appearance of the rash. Occasionally, scrapings from the involved areas will be looked at under the microscope. Drugs by mouth or by injection are not indicated for seborrhea unless bacterial infection has complicated the problem.

50
Dandruff and Cradle Cap

In an infant, are all of the following conditions present?
a) Thick, adherent, oily, yellowish, scaling or crusting patches
b) Located on the scalp, behind the ears, or (less frequently) in the skin creases of the groin
c) Only mild redness in involved areas

no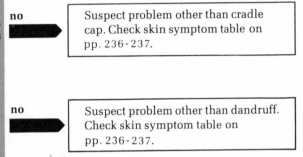

Suspect problem other than cradle cap. Check skin symptom table on pp. 236-237.

In an older child (especially an adolescent), are all of the following conditions present?
a) Fine, white, oily scales
b) Confined to scalp and/or eyebrows
c) Only *mild* redness in involved areas

no

Suspect problem other than dandruff. Check skin symptom table on pp. 236-237.

yes

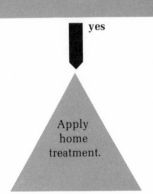

Apply home treatment.

51
Patchy Loss of Skin Color

Children are constantly getting minor cuts, scrapes, insect bites, and other minor skin infections. During the healing process it is common for the skin to lose some of its color. With time, the skin coloring generally returns.

Occasionally, ringworm, a fungal infection discussed in Problem 37, will begin as a small round area of scaling with associated loss of skin color.

In the summertime, many children are noticed to have small round spots on their face in which there is little color. The white spots have probably been present for some time, but the tanning of the skin does not occur in these areas. This condition is known as pityriasis alba; the cause is unknown, but it is a mild condition of cosmetic concern only. It may take many months to disappear and may recur, but there are virtually never any long-term effects.

If there are lightly scaled, tan, pink, or white patches on the neck or back, the problem is most likely due to a fungal infection known as tinea versicolor. This is a very minor and superficial fungal infection.

Home Treatment
Waiting is the most effective home treatment for loss of skin color. Tinea versicolor can be treated by applying Selsun Blue shampoo to the affected area, once every day or so until the lesions are gone.

What to Expect at the Doctor's Office
A history and careful examination of the skin will be performed. Scrapings of the lesions will be taken, since tinea versicolor can be identified from these scrapings. Pityriasis alba should be distinguished from more severe fungal infections that may occur on the face. Again, scrapings will help to identify the fungus.

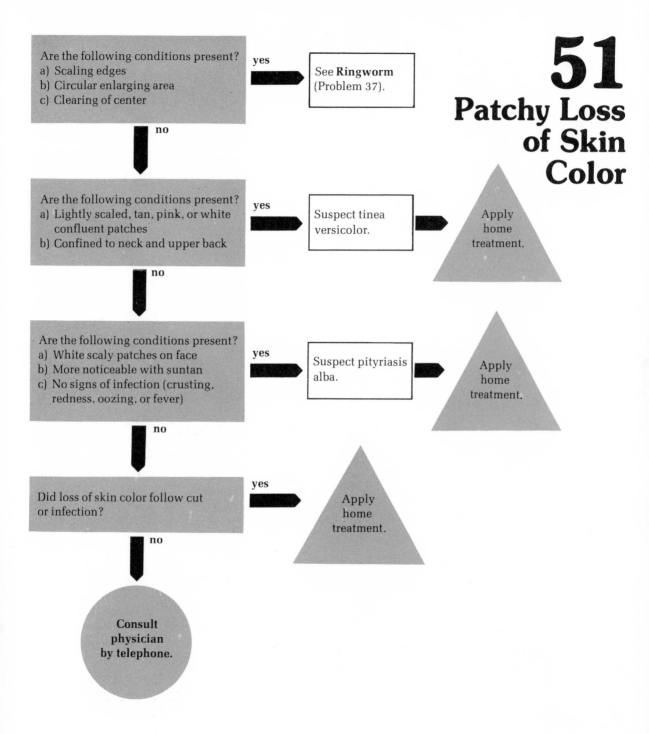

Are the following conditions present?
a) Scaling edges
b) Circular enlarging area
c) Clearing of center

yes → See **Ringworm** (Problem 37).

no

Are the following conditions present?
a) Lightly scaled, tan, pink, or white confluent patches
b) Confined to neck and upper back

yes → Suspect tinea versicolor. → Apply home treatment.

no

Are the following conditions present?
a) White scaly patches on face
b) More noticeable with suntan
c) No signs of infection (crusting, redness, oozing, or fever)

yes → Suspect pityriasis alba. → Apply home treatment.

no

Did loss of skin color follow cut or infection?

yes → Apply home treatment.

no

Consult physician by telephone.

51
Patchy Loss of Skin Color

I

Childhood Diseases

52. Mumps   **278**
Swelling in front of the ear.

53. Chicken Pox   **280**
Small sores and scabs.

54. Measles (Red Measles, Seven- or Ten-Day Measles)   **282**
Serious but preventable.

55. German Measles (Rubella, Three-Day Measles)   **284**
Only three days, but a problem for the pregnant.

56. Roseola   **286**
Fever first, then a rash.

57. Scarlet Fever   **288**
Not so common any more.

58. Fifth Disease   **290**
Last and least.

52
Mumps

Mumps is a viral infection of the salivary glands. The major salivary glands are located directly below and in front of the ear. Before any swelling is noticeable, the child may have a low fever, complain of a headache or an earache, or experience weakness. Fever is variable; it may be only slightly above normal or as high as 104°F. After several days of these symptoms, one or both salivary glands (parotid glands) may swell. It is sometimes difficult to distinguish mumps from swollen lymph glands in the neck; in mumps you will not be able to feel the edge of your child's jaw that is located beneath the ear. With mumps, chewing and swallowing may produce pain behind the ear. Sour substances such as lemons and pickles may make the pain worse. When swelling occurs on both sides, children take on the appearance of chipmunks! Other salivary glands besides the parotid may be involved, including those under the jaw and tongue. The openings of these glands into the mouth may become red and puffy. Approximately one-third of all patients who have mumps do not demonstrate any swelling of glands whatsoever. Therefore, many persons who are concerned about exposure to mumps will already have had the disease without realizing it.

Mumps is quite contagious during the period from two days before the first symptoms to the complete disappearance of the parotid gland swelling (usually about a week after the swelling has begun). Mumps will develop in a susceptible exposed person approximately 16 to 18 days after exposure to the virus. In children, it is generally a mild illness. The chart is directed toward detection of the rare complications, which include encephalitis (viral infection of the brain), pancreatitis (viral infection of the pancreas), kidney disease, deafness, and involvement of the testicles or the ovaries. Complications are far more frequent in adults than they are in children.

Home Treatment

The pain may be reduced with either aspirin or acetaminophen. There may be difficulty eating, but adequate fluid intake is important. Sour foods should be avoided, including orange juice. Adults who have not had mumps should avoid exposure to the child until complete disappearance of the swelling. Many adults who do not recall having mumps as a child may have had an extremely mild case and consequently are not at risk of developing mumps.

What to Expect at the Doctor's Office

If a complication is suspected, then a visit to the physician's office may be necessary. The history and physical examination will be directed at confirming the diagnosis or the presence of a complication. The rare complication of a right ovarian infection may be confused with appendicitis and blood tests may be required. Since mumps is a viral disease, there is no medicine that will directly kill the virus. Supportive measures may be necessary for some of the complications; fortunately these occur rarely and permanent damage to hearing or other functions is unusual. Mumps very rarely produces sterility in men or women even with complicating involvement of the testes or ovaries. Mumps vaccination is discussed on p. 116.

278

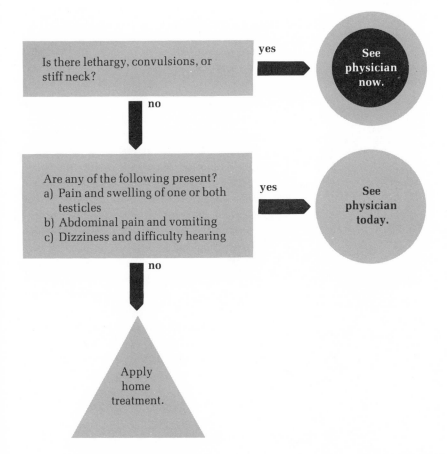

Is there lethargy, convulsions, or stiff neck?

yes → See physician now.

no ↓

Are any of the following present?
a) Pain and swelling of one or both testicles
b) Abdominal pain and vomiting
c) Dizziness and difficulty hearing

yes → See physician today.

no ↓

Apply home treatment.

53
Chicken Pox

How to recognize the chicken pox:

Before the rash: Usually there are no symptoms before the rash appears, but occasionally there is fatigue and some fever in the 24 hours before the rash is noted on the child.

The rash: The typical rash goes through the following stages.

1. First it appears as flat red splotches.
2. They become raised and may resemble small pimples.
3. They develop into small blisters, called vesicles, which are very fragile. They may look like drops of water on a red base. The tops are easily scratched off.
4. As the vesicles break, the sores become "pustular" and form a crust. (The crust is made of dried serum, not true pus.) This stage may be reached within several hours of the first appearance of the rash. The crust falls away between the 9th and 13th day. Itching is often severe in the pustular stage.
5. The vesicles tend to appear in crops with two to four crops appearing within two to six days. All stages may be present in the same area. They often appear first on the scalp and in the mouth, and then spread to the rest of the body, but they may begin anywhere. They are most numerous over shoulders, chest, and back. They are seldom found on the palms of the hands or the soles of the feet. There may be only a few sores, or there may be hundreds.

Fever: After most of the sores have formed crusts, the fever usually subsides.

Chicken pox spreads very easily—over 90 percent of brothers and sisters catch it! It may be transmitted from 24 hours before the appearance of the rash up to about six days after. It is spread by droplets from the mouth or throat or by direct contact with contaminated articles of clothing. It is not spread by dry scabs. The incubation period is from 14 to 17 days. Chicken pox leads to lifelong immunity to recurrence with rare exceptions. However, the same virus that causes chicken pox also causes shingles and the individual with a history of chicken pox may develop shingles (herpes zoster) later in life.

Most of the time, chicken pox should be treated at home. Complications are rare and far less common than with measles. The specific questions on the chart deal with two severe complications that may require more than home treatment: encephalitis (viral infection of the brain) and severe bacterial infection of the lesions. Encephalitis is rare.

Home Treatment
The major problem in dealing with chicken pox is control of the intense itching and reduction of the fever. Warm baths containing baking soda (½ cup to a tubful of water) frequently help. The use of antihistamines is sometimes necessary and may require contact with your physician; check by phone before exposing other children in a doctor's office. Aspirin and acetaminophen are effective itch relievers.

Cut the fingernails or use gloves to prevent skin damage from intensive scratching. When lesions occur in the mouth, gargling with salt water (½ teaspoon salt to an eight-ounce glass) may help comfort. Hands should be washed three times a day and all of the skin should be kept gently but scrupulously clean in order to prevent a complicating bacterial infection. Minor bacterial infection will respond to soap and time; if it becomes severe and results in return of fever, then see the physician. Scratching and infection can result in permanent scars.

What to Expect at the Doctor's Office
Do not be surprised if the physician is willing and even anxious to treat the case "over the phone." If it is necessary to bring the child to the doctor's office, then attempts should be made to keep him or her separate from the other children. In healthy children chicken pox has few lasting ill effects, but in children with other serious illnesses it can be a devastating or even fatal disease. A visit to the physician's office may not be necessary unless a complication seems possible.

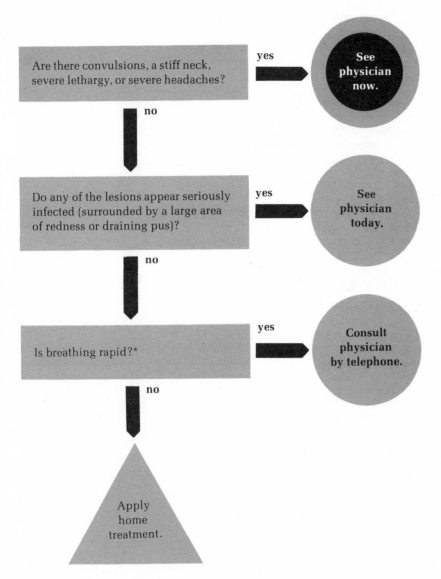

53 Chicken Pox

Are there convulsions, a stiff neck, severe lethargy, or severe headaches?

yes → See physician now.

no

Do any of the lesions appear seriously infected (surrounded by a large area of redness or draining pus)?

yes → See physician today.

no

Is breathing rapid?*

yes → Consult physician by telephone.

no

Apply home treatment.

*See "How fast is your child breathing?" (on p. 142)

54

Measles
(Red
Measles,
Seven- or
Ten-Day
Measles)

Measles is a preventable disease. Unlike some of the other "childhood" illnesses, measles can be quite severe. It is tragic that more than 13 years after the licensing of the measles vaccine, thousands of children still contract this disease annually, and some of these die. We should like to be able to eliminate this section in the next edition of this book. Only immunization of your children can make this possible.

Measles is a viral illness that begins with fever, weakness, a dry "brassy" cough, and inflamed eyes that are itchy, red, and sensitive to the light. These symptoms begin three to five days before the appearance of the rash. Another early sign of measles is the appearance of fine white spots on a red base inside the mouth opposite the molar teeth (Koplik's spots). These fade as the skin rash appears.

The rash begins on about the fifth day as a pink, blotchy, flat rash. The rash first appears around the hairline, on the face, on the neck, and behind the ears. The spots, which fade on pressure early in the illness, become somewhat darker and tend to merge into larger red patches as they mature. The rash spreads from head to chest to abdomen and finally to the arms and legs. It lasts from four to seven days and may be accompanied by mild itching. There may be some light brown coloring to the skin lesions as the illness progresses.

Measles is a highly contagious viral disease. It is spread by droplets from the mouth or throat and by direct contact with articles freshly soiled by nose and throat secretions. It may be spread during the period from three to six days before the appearance of the rash to several days after. Symptoms begin in an exposed susceptible person approximately 8 to 12 days after exposure to the virus.

There are many complications of measles; sore throats, ear infections, and pneumonia are all common. Many of these complicating infections are due to bacteria and will require antibiotic treatment. The pneumonias can be life-threatening. A very serious problem that can lead to permanent damage is measles encephalitis (infection of the brain); life-support measures and treatment of seizures are necessary when this rare complication occurs.

Home Treatment

Symptomatic measures are all that is needed for uncomplicated measles. Aspirin or acetaminophen should be used to keep the fever down, and a vaporizer can be used for cough. Dim lighting in the room often makes the child feel more comfortable because of the eye's sensitivity to light. In general, the child feels "measley." He or she should be isolated until the end of the contagious period. All unimmunized children in contact should be brought to be immunized immediately after symptoms begin in one child.

What to Expect at the Doctor's Office

The history and physical examination will be directed at determining the diagnosis of measles and the nature of any complications. Bacterial complications, such as ear infections and pneumonia, can usually be treated with antibiotics. The child with symptoms suggestive of encephalitis (lethargy, stiff neck, convulsions) will be hospitalized and a spinal tap will be performed. Very rarely, there may be a problem with blood clotting so that bleeding occurs, usually first apparent as dark purple splotches in the skin. It is best to avoid all of these problems with measles immunization, which is discussed on pp. 113–114.

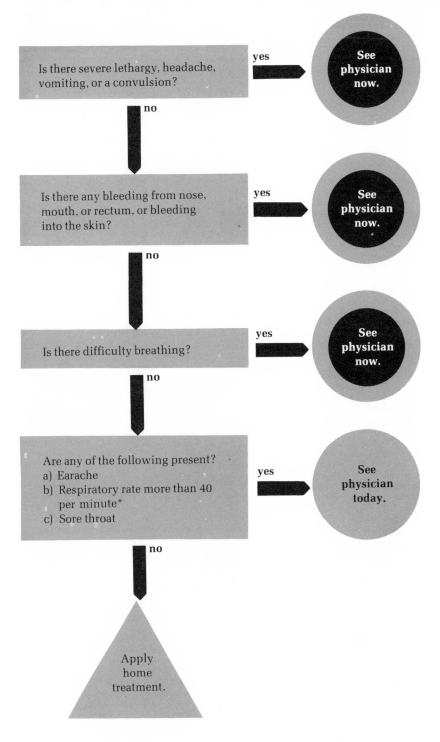

Is there severe lethargy, headache, vomiting, or a convulsion?

yes → See physician now.

no ↓

Is there any bleeding from nose, mouth, or rectum, or bleeding into the skin?

yes → See physician now.

no ↓

Is there difficulty breathing?

yes → See physician now.

no ↓

Are any of the following present?
a) Earache
b) Respiratory rate more than 40 per minute*
c) Sore throat

yes → See physician today.

no ↓

Apply home treatment.

*See "How fast is your child breathing?" (on p. 142)

55

German Measles (Rubella, Three-day Measles)

How to recognize the German measles:

Before the rash: There may be a few days of mild fatigue. Lymph nodes at the back of the neck may be enlarged and tender.

Rash: The rash first appears on the face as flat or slightly raised red spots. It quickly spreads to the trunk and the extremities and the discrete spots tend to merge into large patches. The rash of rubella is highly variable and is difficult for even the most experienced parents and physicians to recognize. Often, there is *no* rash.

Fever: The fever rarely goes above 101°F and usually lasts less than two days.

Joint pains occur in about 10 to 15 percent of older children and adolescents. The pains usually begin on the third day of illness.

German measles is a mild virus infection that is not as contagious as measles or chicken pox. It is usually spread by droplets from the mouth or throat. The incubation period is from 12 to 21 days with an average of 16 days. The specific questions on the chart are addressed to possible complications. These are extremely rare.

The main concern with German measles is an infection in an unborn child. If three-day measles occurs during the first month of pregnancy, there is a 50 percent chance that the fetus will develop an abnormality such as cataracts, heart disease, deafness, or mental deficiency. By the third month of pregnancy, this risk decreases to less than 10 percent and it continues to decrease throughout the pregnancy. Because of the problem of congenital defects, a vaccine for German measles has been developed; rubella immunization is discussed on pp. 114–116.

Home Treatment

Usually no therapy is required. Occasionally fever will require the use of aspirin or acetaminophen. Isolation is usually not imposed. Avoid any exposure of the child to women who could possibly be pregnant. If a question of such exposure arises, the pregnant woman should discuss the risk with her physician. Blood tests are available that will indicate whether a pregnant woman has had rubella in the past and is immune, or whether problems with the pregnancy might be encountered.

What to Expect at the Doctor's Office

Visits to the physician's office are seldom required for uncomplicated German measles. Questions about possible infection of pregnant women are more easily and economically discussed over the telephone.

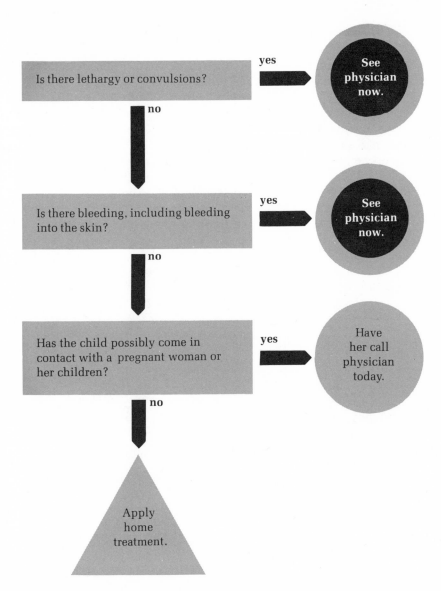

Is there lethargy or convulsions?

yes → See physician now.

no

Is there bleeding, including bleeding into the skin?

yes → See physician now.

no

Has the child possibly come in contact with a pregnant woman or her children?

yes → Have her call physician today.

no

Apply home treatment.

55
German Measles (Rubella, Three-day Measles)

56
Roseola

How to recognize roseola: Before the rash appears there usually are several days of sustained high fever, and sometimes this fever can trigger a convulsion or seizure in a susceptible child. Otherwise, the child appears well. The rash appears as the fever is decreasing or shortly after it is gone. It consists of pink, well-defined patches that turn white on pressure and first appear on the trunk. It may be slightly bumpy. It spreads to involve the arms and neck but is seldom prominent on the face or legs. The rash usually lasts less than 24 hours. Occasionally, there is a slight runny nose, throat redness, or swollen glands at the back of the head, behind the ears, or in the neck. Most often, there are no other symptoms.

Roseola is most common in children under the age of three but may occur at any age. Its main significance lies in the sudden high fever, which may cause a convulsion. Such a convulsion is due to the high temperature and does not indicate that the child has epilepsy. Prompt treatment of the fever is essential (see Section E, Fever).

This disease is probably caused by a virus and is contagious. The child should be kept from contact with other children until the fever has passed. The incubation period is from 7 to 17 days.

Encephalitis (infection of the brain) is a very rare complication of roseola; roseola is basically a mild disease.

Home Treatment

Home treatment is based on two principles. The first is effective treatment of the fever, discussed in Section E. The second is careful watching and waiting. This depends on the fact that the child should appear reasonably well and have no other significant symptoms when the fever is controlled. To be watched for especially are symptoms of ear infection (a complaint of pain or tugging at the ear), cough (see Problem 24, Cough), or lethargy. If these occur, then the appropriate sections of this book should be consulted. If the problem still is not clear, a phone call to the physician may be necessary. Remember that roseola should not last more than four or five days; you should consult your physician about a persistent problem.

What to Expect at the Doctor's Office

Children are usually seen soon after the onset of the illness because of the high fever. As noted, at this stage there is little else to be found in roseola. The ears, nose, throat, and chest should be examined. If the fever remains the only finding, then the physician will recommend home treatment (control of the fever with careful waiting and watching to see if the rash of roseola will appear). There is no medical treatment for roseola other than that available at home.

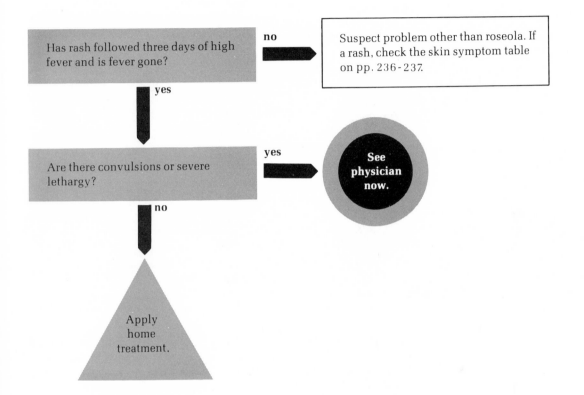

Has rash followed three days of high fever and is fever gone?

no → Suspect problem other than roseola. If a rash, check the skin symptom table on pp. 236-237.

yes

Are there convulsions or severe lethargy?

yes → See physician now.

no

Apply home treatment.

57
Scarlet Fever

Scarlet fever derived its name over 300 years ago from its characteristic red rash. The illness is caused by a streptococcal infection, usually of the throat. Strep throats are discussed in Problem 19 (Sore Throat).

You can recognize the illness by its characteristic features. A fever and weakness usually precede the rash. The fever is often accompanied by a headache, stomachache, and vomiting. A sore throat is usually but not always present. The rash appears 12 to 48 hours after the illness begins.

The rash begins on the face, trunk, and arms and generally covers the entire body by the end of 24 hours. It is red, very fine, and covers most of the skin surface. The area around the mouth is pale. With your eyes closed, it has the feeling of fine sandpaper. Skin creases, such as in front of the elbow and the armpit, are more deeply red. Pressing on the rash will produce a white spot lasting several seconds. The intense redness of the rash lasts for about five days, although peeling of skin can go on for weeks. It is not unusual for peeling, especially of the palms, to last for more than a month.

Examination often reveals a red throat, spots on the roof of the mouth (soft palate), and a fuzzy white tongue, later becoming swollen and red. There may be swollen glands in the neck.

Home Treatment
Since scarlet fever is due to a streptococcal infection, a medical visit is required for antibiotic treatment. Streptococcal infections are quite contagious, and other children within the home should also have throat cultures. In addition to antibiotics you will wish to reduce the fever with aspirin or acetaminophen, keep up with fluid requirements, and give plenty of cold liquids to help soothe the throat.

What to Expect at the Doctor's Office
There are several rashes that can be confused with scarlet fever, including those of measles and drug reactions. If the rash is sufficiently typical of scarlet fever the physician will probably begin antibiotics, usually penicillin (or erythromycin if the child is allergic to penicillin), and take throat cultures from the rest of the family. If the physician is uncertain of the cause of the rash, a throat culture may be taken before beginning treatment. Treatment that is delayed by a day or two while waiting for culture results will still prevent the complication about which we are most concerned: rheumatic fever.

Are both of the following present?
a) Fever
b) Fine, red rash on trunk and extremities which feels like sandpaper

 no

Suspect a problem other than scarlet fever. If there is a skin rash, check the skin symptom table on pp. 236-237.

yes

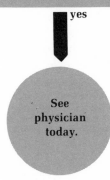

See physician today.

58
Fifth Disease

Consider the strange case of the fifth disease, whose only claim to fame is that it might be mistaken for another disease. It is so named because it is always listed last (and least) when the five very common contagious rashes of childhood are listed. Its medical name, erythema infectiosum, is easily forgotten.

It comes very close to not being a disease at all. It has no symptoms other than rash, has no complications, and needs no treatment. It can be recognized because it causes a characteristic "slapped cheek" appearance in children. The rash often begins on the cheeks and is later found on the backs of the arms and legs. It often has a very fine, lacy, pink appearance. It tends to come and go and may be present one moment and absent the next. It is prone to recur for days or even weeks, especially as a response to heat (warm bath or shower) or irritation. In general, however, the rash around the face will fade within four days of its appearance and the rash on the rest of the body within three to seven days of its appearance. Its only significance is that it could worry you or cause you to make an avoidable trip to the doctor's office. It is very contagious; epidemics of fifth disease have resulted in unnecessary school closings. The agent responsible for this "non-disease" is not known; a virus is suspected. The incubation period is thought to be from 6 to 14 days.

Home Treatment
There is none. Just watch and wait to make sure you are dealing with fifth disease. Check that there is no fever; fever is very unusual with fifth disease. No restrictions on activities are necessary.

What to Expect at the Doctor's Office
The physician may be able to distinguish fifth disease from other rashes. If the rash fits the description given in this section, the physician is going to make the same diagnosis that you might have. Taking the child's temperature and looking at the rash can be expected. Since there are no tests for the unknown cause, laboratory tests are unlikely. Waiting and watching is the means of dealing with fifth disease.

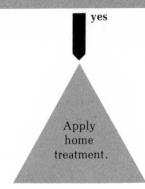

Are all of the following
conditions present?
a) No fever.
b) Rash is the first and only symptom.
c) Palms and soles are not involved.

 no

Suspect problem other than fifth
disease. If a rash, check the skin
symptom table on pp. 236-237.

yes

Apply
home
treatment.

J

Bones, Muscles, and Joints

59. Pain in the Muscles or Joints   **294**
If a joint is swollen, take it seriously.

60. Low-back Pain   **296**
A curse of the upright posture.

61. Bowlegs and Knock-knees   **298**
Cowboy or comedy star.

62. Pigeon Toes and Flat Feet   **300**
Too much ado.

59
Pain in the Muscles or Joints

Pains in the joints are not to be confused with muscle aches and pains or with "growing pains." Growing pains are found in the mid-portion of the upper and lower legs, generally at night, in children from six to twelve years of age. The cause is unknown, but millions of children have had them and they are of absolutely no medical significance. Muscle aches and pains are common after strenuous exercise or during mild viral illness.

In children, very seldom does pain in the joint mean arthritis. The word arthritis comes from "arth" meaning "joint," and "itis," denoting that the joint is red, warm, swollen, and painful to move. The word arthralgia means pain in the joint *without* redness, warmth, or swelling. Since injuries are so common in children, they are the most common cause of joint pain, and are discussed under the specific injury.

Most true arthritis in children is caused by infection. Occasionally, arthralgia may precede the arthritis by a day or two. This is often true in gonococcal arthritis, which may occur in adolescents.

Arthritis accompanied by a fever occurs in rheumatic fever. Arthritis accompanied by abdominal pain and a blotchy, dark rash most prominent on the legs can be part of a rare illness in children that temporarily affects small blood vessels. Arthritis may also occur in children with sickle-cell disease. In addition, arthritis somewhat similar to the rheumatoid arthritis of adults occurs occasionally in children.

Arthralgia (pain without swelling) is a common temporary complaint in many viral illnesses. It can occur with German measles (rubella) and may be accompanied by swollen lymph glands behind the ears as well as the rash. If rubella is suspected, special attention must be taken to prevent exposure of pregnant women.

A cause of knee pain in active adolescents is Osgood-Schlatter's disease. This problem is caused by a strong set of thigh muscles pulling at their insertion on the tibial bone in the knee. Resting the leg is the treatment of choice. Some diseases of children and adolescents that cause pain in the knees actually may have their origins in the hips. Persistent arthralgia should therefore be attended to by a physician.

Home Treatment
Heat will often relax sore muscles caused by strenuous exercise. Aspirin or acetaminophen is often effective in relieving the muscle pain of viral illness. A combination of the above remedies may be of comfort in severe "growing pains." Home treatments for various injuries are discussed in those particular sections. All arthritis in children must be seen by a physician immediately because of the potential serious consequences of the underlying infections. In the arthralgia that accompanies viral illnesses such as rubella, or that follows rubella immunization, aspirin may afford relief of pain.

What to Expect at the Doctor's Office
A history and physical examination of the joints will be made. A more complete examination will depend on the specific history. Depending on the nature of the condition, blood tests and X-rays will often be obtained. If a joint contains fluid, the fluid may be removed and tested. Treatment of serious infections will very often require hospital administration of antibiotics.

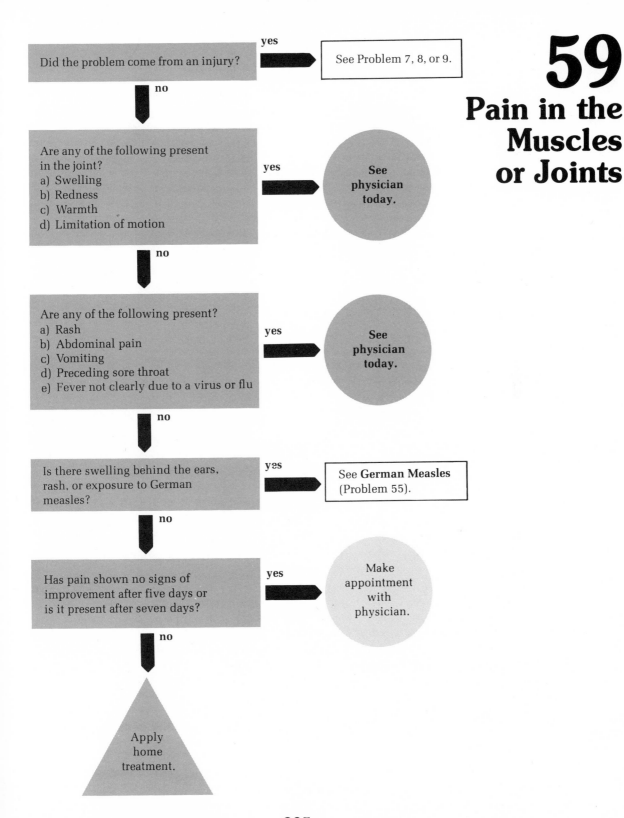

Did the problem come from an injury? — **yes** → See Problem 7, 8, or 9.

no

Are any of the following present in the joint?
a) Swelling
b) Redness
c) Warmth
d) Limitation of motion

— **yes** → See physician today.

no

Are any of the following present?
a) Rash
b) Abdominal pain
c) Vomiting
d) Preceding sore throat
e) Fever not clearly due to a virus or flu

— **yes** → See physician today.

no

Is there swelling behind the ears, rash, or exposure to German measles? — **yes** → See **German Measles** (Problem 55).

no

Has pain shown no signs of improvement after five days or is it present after seven days? — **yes** → Make appointment with physician.

no

Apply home treatment.

59
Pain in the Muscles or Joints

60
Low-back Pain

Low-back pain is an uncommon complaint before adolescence. If a young child complains of back pain and there is accompanying fever or pain on urination, a urinary tract infection is often to blame. Falls on the tailbone are another fairly frequent cause of this symptom. While children's bones are far more resilient than those of adults, spinal injuries do occur; persistent pain or weakness in the lower extremities should alert parents to this possibility. Weakness without pain is unusual. However, if it is clearly present, see the doctor.

Some developmental disorders of the hip may present themselves first as back complaints; often these children will have a limp or other problems as well. Another cause of back complaints is a developmental (congenital) abnormality of the spine. A spine that appears crooked either in a side-to-side or back-to-front direction should be discussed with a physician during a regularly scheduled visit.

Low-back pain in adolescents is similar to that in adults and usually results from muscular strain. The strain causes spasm of the supportive muscles alongside the spine. Any injury to the back may produce such spasms, resulting in severe pain and stiffness. Pain may be immediate or may occur some hours after the exertion or injury; often the cause is not clear.

Muscular problems of the back that are linked to some exertion or lifting must heal naturally; give them time. The pain due to muscular back strain is usually in the low back; if it extends beyond the low-back area, a more serious problem may exist. Pain that travels down one leg (sciatica) is very different from pain confined to the low back, and suggests pressure on the nerves as they leave the spinal cord. Such complications require medical attention.

Backache may also be caused by the daily strain of supporting an obese body, by the rupture of small fat sacs, or by the loose ligaments following rapid weight reduction. Obesity is not good for the back. Low-back ache is common during the menstrual period. This is discussed further in Problem 91 (Menstrual Problems).

Home Treatment

When a muscle strain is present, resting the injured part will help healing; the spasm of the muscles itself helps rest the part. When the pain first appears, having the child rest flat on his or her back for at least 24 hours may help. After the complete bed rest a gradual increase in activity, carefully avoiding reinjury, is begun. Severe muscle spasm pain usually lasts for 48 to 72 hours and is followed by days or weeks of less severe pain. Complete recovery will generally take six weeks; strenuous activity during that six weeks can bring the problem back and delay complete recovery. Slow improvement is the rule with back pain. But if there is no improvement within 48 hours, see the doctor.

After healing, an exercise program can help prevent reinjury. No drug will hasten healing; they only reduce symptoms. The child should sleep pillowless on a very firm mattress, with a bedboard under the mattress. Some individuals report being most comfortable on the floor. A folded towel beneath the low back may increase comfort.

Heat applied to the affected area will provide some relief. Two aspirin every four hours (in children over ten) may be continued for as long as there is significant pain.

When standing or sitting, at least one foot can be elevated and placed on an adjacent chair with the knee flexed. This position helps to straighten the lower back and to increase comfort.

What to Expect at the Doctor's Office

The physical examination will be directed toward determining whether the problem has its origins in the urinary tract, the skeleton, or the muscular system. The examination will center on the back, the abdomen, and the arms and legs, with special attention to testing the nerve function of the legs. If the injury is the result of a fall or blow to the back, or if there is a limp present, X-rays are indicated; otherwise, usually not. X-rays do not show injuries to muscles,

Is pain associated with any of the following?
a) Abdominal pain
b) Nausea or vomiting or diarrhea
c) Pain, bleeding, or frequency of urination
d) Menstrual period
e) Flu-like symptoms

yes →

See **Acute Abdominal Pain** (Problem 84), **Recurrent Abdominal Pain** (Problem 85), **Nausea/Vomiting** (Problem 82), **Diarrhea** (Problem 83), **Painful, Frequent or Bloody Urination** (Problem 88), **Vaginal Bleeding and Menstrual Problems** (Problem 91), **or Colds and Flu** (Problem 18).

no ↓

Is there fever or does pain travel down one or both legs below the knee, or is there weakness of the legs?

yes →

See physician today.

no ↓

Apply home treatment.

only to bones. If the history and physical examination are consistent with low-back strain, the physician's advice will be similar to that described above. Urinary tract infections will require antibiotics. Infections of the bones are very rare but quite serious; they can be diagnosed by X-ray and will be treated with antibiotics and hospitalization. Developmental problems of the hip or spine may require special braces.

Muscle relaxants have not been demonstrated to be superior to heat and aspirin for relief of pain due to muscle spasm.

61

Bowlegs and Knock-knees

These problems are quite common and almost never need treatment. Practically all normal infants and toddlers have some bowing of the legs. The bowing is its worst at about one year of age and usually disappears by age two. The strengthening of the leg muscles that occurs in the first year of walking appears to be responsible for correcting the leg bowing. Bowed legs are often more apparent than real, and may disappear merely by placing the ankles together.

Knock-knee usually develops a year or so later. It appears the worst at about age three and is often accompanied by pigeon toeing, which is actually a compensating balancing response. Knock-knee tends to correct itself without any treatment by age six.

Many years ago vitamin D deficiency (rickets) sometimes caused bowleg, but this is virtually never the case in an adequately nourished child in this country today. In some parts of the eastern United States, a hereditary form of rickets still occurs. Rarely, there are cases of bowleg that require medical treatment, but in these the bowing is severe and tends to get even worse as time goes by. Knock-knee that requires medical treatment is also rare. A proper decision to treat is made after careful measurements indicate that the problem is getting worse and that the deformity is more than mild. This problem can almost always be discussed incidental to another examination and seldom requires a separate appointment with the doctor.

Home Treatment

Watching is usually all that is required. Remember that bowleg tends to be most apparent during the first year of life and tends to resolve thereafter. Adequate walking and other exercise that will strengthen the leg muscles are important for the overall health of your child, as well as for proper leg development.

What to Expect at the Doctor's Office

Careful examination will be made of the back, hips, and legs with appropriate measurements. Observation of the child's gait will be made. If there is excess bowing, an X-ray may be taken and a referral to an orthopedic surgeon may be made. Treatment usually consists of using a nighttime brace (Dennis-Browne splint). Surgery is rarely needed. Surgical intervention in a severe case of knock-knee is seldom recommended before age eight or nine.

Bowlegs and Knock-knees

Bowleg:

With the ankles touching, is the distance between the knees more than 1½ in. or 4 cm?

Knock-knee:

With the knees touching, is the distance between the ankles more than 2 in. or 5 cm?

yes → Make appointment with physician.

no ↓

Apply home treatment.

62

Pigeon Toes and Flat Feet

As a nation, we have had a fetish of foot fascination. Many readers may remember shoe-stores with fluoroscopes where you could stare with wonder at the bones in your feet. The radiation was dangerous and, of course, not necessary for shoe fitting; yet it was tolerated for some time.

Most concerns about foot development can be allayed by understanding normal foot development. When children are born, their feet often are turned in because of the cramped uterine environment. You should be able to straighten the foot easily by manipulating it gently with your own fingers. If it cannot be easily straightened, discuss this with the physician. Occasionally, the bones of the foot may not be aligned perfectly, causing a problem known as *metatarsus adductus*. This problem is simple to correct if detected early in the newborn. All infants have fat feet, not to be confused with flat feet. Unless there is an obvious bony deformity of the foot, with ankle bones protruding on the inside of the foot, you need not be concerned.

In the older child a flat foot can be checked for by examining the shoe. A worn inner edge of the heel indicates a possible flat foot. Children with severe flat feet may complain of foot pain and have no visible arch even if they stand on their toes. Most flat feet are more imagined than real.

When children begin to walk, they keep their legs far apart and have their feet pointing out. This "duck-walking" provides the most stable base for the new, unsteady walker.

Many toddlers appear to have bowed legs and later walk with their toes pointing in—"pigeon toes." Rarely, toeing in can be caused by the leg being set into the hip at the wrong angle; with the child lying on his or her back, the feet should be able to be turned outward.

(If this is not possible, check it with your doctor on the next visit.) Toeing in can also be caused by one of the bones in the lower leg being twisted in excessively; as the child grows, the bone naturally twists outward. Excessive twisting can be detected by checking the child's ankle bones when the child is sitting on a table. If the outer ankle bone is in front of the inner, this condition is present. Pigeon toeing can also be caused by metatarsus adductus.

Most children outgrow their pigeon toeing by the age of four. A severe problem causing frequent tripping or any of the findings discussed in the previous paragraph suggest the need for discussion with a physician.

Home Treatment

Most children will grow up to have straight feet and legs, and most of the variations are normal developmental occurrences. The best home treatment is to encourage physical activities, since muscles assist in the growing and straightening process. You need *not* spend large sums on shoes; the purpose of a shoe is to protect the bottom of the child's foot from scrapes and cuts. Except for the first few months of walking when high top shoes may assist the walking process, sneakers are a good choice. They are inexpensive (which is especially important for a rapidly growing foot), have a straight last, and won't cramp the toes.

What to Expect at the Doctor's Office

A thorough examination of the foot, ankle, knee, and hips will be done, and the physician will observe the child's gait. If a foot deformity such as metatarsus adductus is suspected, X-rays may be ordered. Treatment will depend on the child's age and the extent of the problem. Finally, you should be reassured that perfectly straight feet and legs, although cosmetically more satisfying, do not offer any functional advantages. Many sports are played with greater ease by people with feet that are slightly turned in (tennis) or out (fencing).

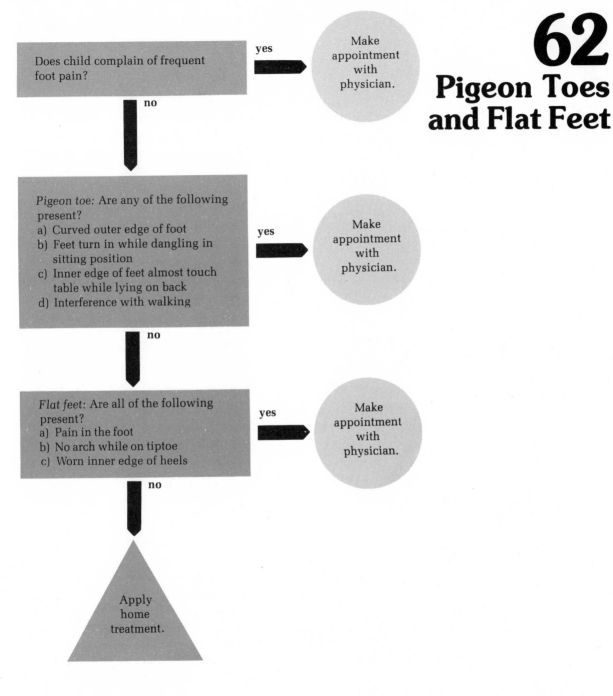

Does child complain of frequent foot pain?

yes → Make appointment with physician.

no ↓

Pigeon toe: Are any of the following present?
a) Curved outer edge of foot
b) Feet turn in while dangling in sitting position
c) Inner edge of feet almost touch table while lying on back
d) Interference with walking

yes → Make appointment with physician.

no ↓

Flat feet: Are all of the following present?
a) Pain in the foot
b) No arch while on tiptoe
c) Worn inner edge of heels

yes → Make appointment with physician.

no ↓

Apply home treatment.

62
Pigeon Toes and Flat Feet

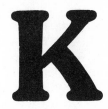

K

Common Concerns

63. Headache   **304**
Most common and seldom serious.

64. Hyperactivity   **306**
Seldom a disease.

65. Bedwetting   **308**
Wait and wait again.

66. Constipation and Soiling   **310**
Diet and emotion.

67. Overweight   **312**
Forget the glands.

68. Underweight   **314**
Thin is in, but check the chart.

69. Stress, Anxiety, and Depression   **316**
Life as we live it.

70. Weakness and Tiredness   **318**
Not enough sleep?

71. Dizziness and Fainting   **320**
Common and uncommon causes.

72. Seizures (Convulsions, Fits, Falling-out Spells)   **322**
Check them out with the doctor.

73. Swallowed Foreign Objects   **324**
Amazing things pass through.

74. Frequent Illnesses   **326**
Nature's immunizations.

See also

86. Colic   **358**

63
Headache

More than 40 percent of all children have had a headache by the age of seven, and four percent of seven-year-olds are troubled by frequent headaches. By the age of 15, 75 percent of children have had a headache and 20 percent will have experienced frequent headaches.

An isolated headache is often due to an earache, sore throat, toothache, or eye infection. Young children have poorly developed sinuses so sinusitis is uncommon. When a child has a neck so stiff that the chin cannot be touched to the chest, marked irritability, a soft spot (fontanel) that is bulging, or vomiting with a fever, meningitis should be suspected.

In younger children, the cause of head pain is frequently stress. Stress and tension can cause headaches even in five-year-olds; in older children *most* headaches are due to stress. Muscle spasms in the neck and scalp cause these pains, aggravated possibly by a widening of blood vessels inside the brain. Tension headaches can occur in any part of the head, produce a dull or swollen feeling inside the head, and usually come on slowly. Headaches are often the first symptom of stressful problems at school, at home, or with friends. A child who is functioning poorly in any of these areas needs help.

Many medications, including decongestants and antihistamines, can cause headaches. Headache is also common just before menstruation. Eyestrain is often blamed but is seldom a cause of headache; usually it is tension.

Migraine headaches may start in childhood. Many toddlers who vomit frequently have migraine; as they become older they can tell you that their head aches. Children with migraine usually have at least two of the following: (1) headaches on one side of the head only, (2) nausea, (3) visual disturbances before an attack, (4) other family members with migraines. These headaches often begin suddenly and are throbbing in character.

Occasionally, headaches will be the only sign of a seizure disorder. These headaches usually begin suddenly and are followed by a period of drowsiness or sleep.

Many parents are concerned about brain tumors. Headaches associated with brain tumors are often persistent and progressive, present in the morning, and accompanied by other problems such as difficulty walking, personality changes, vomiting, visual problems, limb weakness, and speech difficulties. Fortunately, brain tumors are very rarely the cause of a headache, even a severe headache. Only one child in 40,000 is found to have a tumor of the brain or nervous system.

Home Treatment

Headaches due to ear infections, toothaches, strep throats, acute sinusitis, or other serious infections require medical help. For headache associated with colds, flu, or stress, aspirin (or acetaminophen) is quite effective. Headache may frequently be relieved by massage or heat to the back of the neck. Children with hay fever often have headaches during the pollen season and antihistamines and decongestants may help; but remember that these drugs *cause* headaches in some children!

Persistent headaches that do not respond to such measures should be called to the attention of a physician. Headaches associated with weakness of the arms or legs or with slurring of speech, as well as those that are rapidly increasing in frequency and severity, also require a visit to the physician. Remember, tension is the usual cause of head pain. Whenever possible, identify the causes of the stress and work with your children in relieving them.

What to Expect at the Doctor's Office

The physician will check the blood pressure, head, eyes, ears, nose, throat, and neck and also test nerve function. The child's temperature will be taken. Any laboratory tests ordered will depend on what is found in the history and physical examination; usually none are needed. With an acute headache, a source of infection may be found. Even with most recurring headaches, a history and physical examination are probably all that is required. Occasionally, brain wave tests are performed if a seizure disorder is suspected.

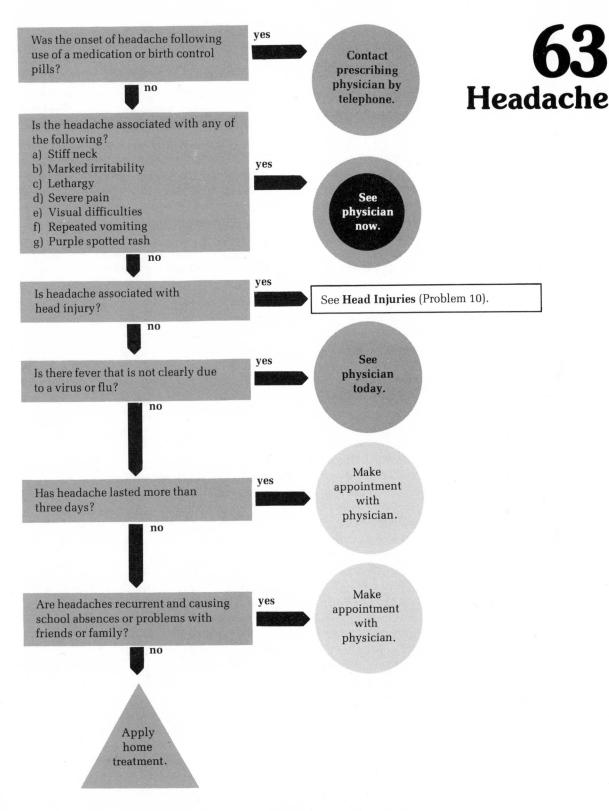

Was the onset of headache following use of a medication or birth control pills?

yes → Contact prescribing physician by telephone.

no

Is the headache associated with any of the following?
a) Stiff neck
b) Marked irritability
c) Lethargy
d) Severe pain
e) Visual difficulties
f) Repeated vomiting
g) Purple spotted rash

yes → See physician now.

no

Is headache associated with head injury?

yes → See **Head Injuries** (Problem 10).

no

Is there fever that is not clearly due to a virus or flu?

yes → See physician today.

no

Has headache lasted more than three days?

yes → Make appointment with physician.

no

Are headaches recurrent and causing school absences or problems with friends or family?

yes → Make appointment with physician.

no

Apply home treatment.

63
Headache

64
Hyper-activity

Controversy and confusion are the rule when it comes to the problem of hyperactivity; the word means "more than normal activity." The problem here is in knowing what is "normal." The normal activity level of a three-year-old is certainly much greater than that of most 40-year-olds. Is this hyperactivity? Children's activity levels change as they become older, as they are placed in new situations, or when they are excited. In addition, activity that would be considered normal in the schoolyard may be considered abnormal in the classroom or dining room. The term hyperactivity can only be used in the context of the child's age and appropriateness of activities. Hyperactivity merely indicates the child's activity in relationship to normal activities as compared to other children of the same age.

Hyperactivity is a symptom, not a disease. It may be found in most normal children (especially ages two to four); older children of above average intelligence with inquisitive behavior; children reacting to problems in school, at home, with friends or siblings; children unable to adjust to different standards of behavior and performance at home and in school; children who do not speak English in schools that are not bilingual; and children with hearing difficulties, drug reactions, or visual difficulties. Medical causes of hyperactivity include seizure disorders, retardation, hyperthyroidism, and psychiatric disorders.

Very often teachers will be the first to point out hyperactive behavior in a child. A learning problem may be the basis for hyperactive behavior in school. If a child is not able to comprehend what is going on in the classroom, boredom and ultimately hyperactive behavior may result. If there is a discrepancy between your child's behavior in school and at home, a learning problem should be suspected.

Finally, there is a small group of children to whom the word hyperactive has been applied as the name of a syndrome. In medical terminology, a syndrome is a group of symptoms that occur together; often there is no known cause. The hyperactivity syndrome, sometimes called minimal brain dysfunction (MBD), consists of greatly increased activity, easy distractability, wide mood changes from moment to moment, poor impulse control, explosive moods, and often learning problems. Some of these children may be clumsy, with difficulties controlling fine movements. The underlying cause for this syndrome is not known. A variety of causes have been suggested, ranging from genes, to birth trauma, to reactions to food dyes. Probably a number of different causes may be found.

Common drugs may cause hyperactivity; these include Dimetapp, Actifed, Sudafed, Triaminic, and many other decongestants and antihistamines.

Home Treatment

Observation of the neighborhood children is the best guide to your own child's activity levels. You will notice that there are many extremely active children of all ages. Some seem to be on constant "seek-and-destroy" missions. If there are problems developing in school, a conference should be held with the teacher to determine the precise nature of the problem. Medical assistance in dealing with this type of problem can often be helpful. If your child's hyperactivity began following the use of a medication, discontinue using this medication immediately and contact the prescribing physician.

What to Expect at the Doctor's Office

Most often the consultation with the physician can be conducted in conjunction with a visit for another reason. If a problem is suspected, a lengthy evaluation will be scheduled. Most physicians evaluating school-aged children will wish to review a copy of the child's school records; you can save time by arranging to have these at the time of the visit. The history and physical examination will put special emphasis on the child's nervous system, and the physician will be most interested in your observations with respect to the child's behavior. Tests of muscle coordination, reading, spelling,

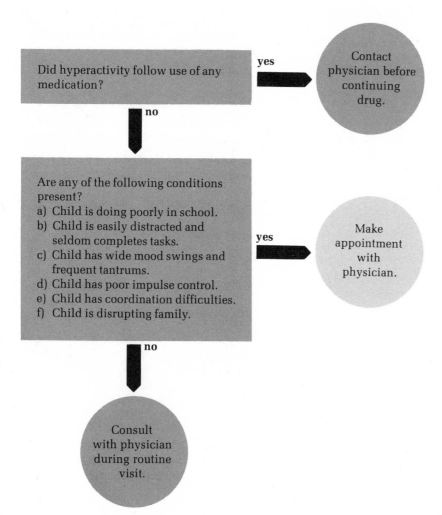

Did hyperactivity follow use of any medication?

yes → Contact physician before continuing drug.

no ↓

Are any of the following conditions present?
a) Child is doing poorly in school.
b) Child is easily distracted and seldom completes tasks.
c) Child has wide mood swings and frequent tantrums.
d) Child has poor impulse control.
e) Child has coordination difficulties.
f) Child is disrupting family.

yes → Make appointment with physician.

no ↓

Consult with physician during routine visit.

and so on may be conducted in the doctor's office. Hearing and vision will be tested.

If a seizure disorder is suspected, brain wave tests (electroencephalogram or EEG) may be performed. The decision to begin any form of therapy (such as use of the drug Ritalin or institution of diets free of food additives and salicylates) should be reached only after careful consideration and discussion. Behavioral techniques may be used in management. A proper therapeutic approach requires coordination between physician, parents, school, and child.

65
Bedwetting

Achieving nighttime bladder control has already been discussed (see pp. 59–60). A number of maturational factors determine when a child will become dry. While many children are dry at night by the age of four, others are not. With each successive year, many more children will naturally develop control.

Children who have been dry for many months or even years may suddenly wet the bed, often in response to a stressful event. Children may regress because of the arrival of a new brother or sister, a move, or a severe illness. Only occasionally is a urinary tract infection the cause, and then there are usually other symptoms such as increased frequency of urination, burning, abdominal pain, or fever. For symptoms such as these, the physician should be seen.

Home Treatment

Most important is your attitude. First, you must expect it to happen. Bedwetting should not be considered unusual until beyond the age of six and it is still normal for children to occasionally lose control during stressful events for the next year or so. A reaction of disgust or anger may make it more difficult for the child to gain control. Second, the child often cannot help it. Bladder control is a complex developmental and neurological task that requires a mature child. Making the child feel guilty about bedwetting will only delay resolution of the problem; you should think in terms of supporting rather than punishing the child. Because constant sheet changing is often tiresome for parents, placing a short sheet on top of a rubber pad placed on top of the regular sheet will cut down on laundering.

Most of the time, your best course is to ignore the problem and wait it out. After the age of six, you and your child may want to make a "team effort" to solve this problem. First, encourage fluids during the morning and early afternoon and discourage them during the several hours before bedtime. Have the child void just before going to bed. Fluids during the day help ensure that the bladder is big enough and voiding ensures that it is as empty as possible at bedtime. Second, develop a chart or use a calendar to indicate when the child has achieved control by awarding a gold star. When your child gets tired of gold stars, you may try drawing smiling faces or sad faces on your calendar. Try these measures alone for several weeks or months. If progress is not being made, consider the addition of an awakening routine, by simply getting the child up within the first three hours of sleep for voiding, thus emptying the bladder again. If the child is already wet, awaken for voiding a little sooner. Older children can participate in the laundering process in order to learn that they are responsible for their actions and some of the consequences.

Although many claims have been made for nighttime alarms that sound when the child begins to void in bed, we feel this is seldom indicated and quite possibly detrimental.

If a child continues to wet the bed after the age of six, a consultation with the physician can be helpful.

What to Expect at the Doctor's Office

The medical history is the most important part of the office visit. The physician will inquire at what time of night the child wets the bed, as well as how often and under what circumstances. A physical examination with attention to the genitalia will be performed. A urinalysis will be done. You should think of this visit as adding the physician to the team. The implication that the child is being punished should be avoided. The physician will need to get to know your child; this may best be accomplished without your presence. Don't be offended. In rare instances, a drug, imipramine (Tofranil), will be added to the regimen of home treatment. Extensive tests such as X-rays of the kidneys and bladder are seldom necessary. Bedwetting is almost never due to a surgical condition and several physicians should be consulted for additional opinions if surgery is suggested.

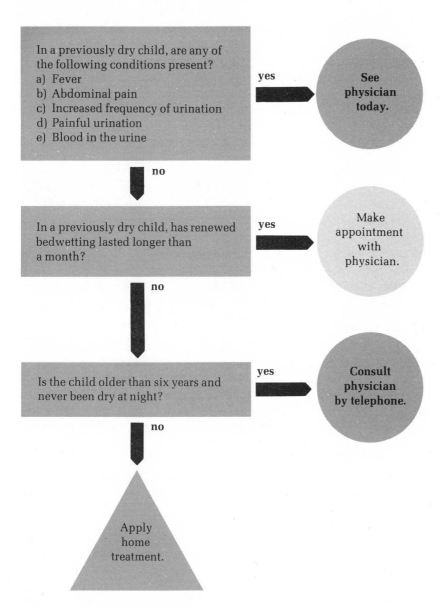

In a previously dry child, are any of the following conditions present?
a) Fever
b) Abdominal pain
c) Increased frequency of urination
d) Painful urination
e) Blood in the urine

yes → **See physician today.**

no ↓

In a previously dry child, has renewed bedwetting lasted longer than a month?

yes → Make appointment with physician.

no ↓

Is the child older than six years and never been dry at night?

yes → **Consult physician by telephone.**

no ↓

Apply home treatment.

66
Constipation and Soiling

It is not necessary to have a bowel movement every day. Many children have bowel movements only once every three or four days, and they are perfectly normal. Most parents are concerned about constipation when the stool (feces) is very hard or when a child experiences pain when passing stool. Sometimes the pain is due to a tear in the rectum (rectal fissure). It is often unclear whether the hard fecal material is responsible for the tear or whether the tear is responsible for the child holding back the bowel movement in order to avoid the pain. In any event, treatment is directed toward softening the stool.

Frequently infants with a severe diaper rash will withhold bowel movements to avoid pain. If so, work to clear the rash rather than to soften the stool. (See Problem 34, Diaper Rash.)

Infants and older children will frequently be constipated during illnesses. Adequate fluid intake is very important in this case.

Constipation can have emotional causes; for example, it may begin at the time of toilet training. In the struggle of will between child and parent, the child may decide to retain control by holding on to a bowel movement.

If a child retains stool for long enough, liquid material will escape around the hardened bowel plug. This liquid material is apt to leak out and soil underpants; hence the term "soiling." Soiling in an older child is a sign of longstanding constipation and should be treated by a physician.

Home Treatment

Dietary changes are usually all that is necessary and are superior to medicines. Prune juice is remarkable in its efficiency. You might eliminate rice cereal for a while, as it tends to be constipating. In infants, Karo syrup (one tablespoonful to four ounces of water or milk) is helpful. In older children, encouragement of bran products and fiber (celery, whole oranges) often helps. Adequate fluid intake is essential; water is fine. On rare occasions, a laxative may be needed. Glycerin suppositories are safe and effective, and Colace, Metamucil, and Maltsupex are acceptable. Infants should never be given mineral oil, since it can cause a serious pneumonia if it finds its way to the lungs. However, in older children it is quite effective. Enemas are virtually never needed and are potentially dangerous.

What to Expect at the Doctor's Office

An examination of the abdomen and rectum will be done in some instances. In the case of soiling, the physician will assess whether the child has developed to the point where bowel control can be expected, and, if so, whether stresses might be causing the problem. The child will need your support if a serious soiling problem is to be treated successfully. Rarely, X-rays of the lower bowel are necessary. Constipation is an example of a case in which the best physician may well do few or no tests and perform little or no examination, and the less competent physician may make a nonproblem into a big deal. Soiling is a more serious problem, and will be investigated more thoroughly.

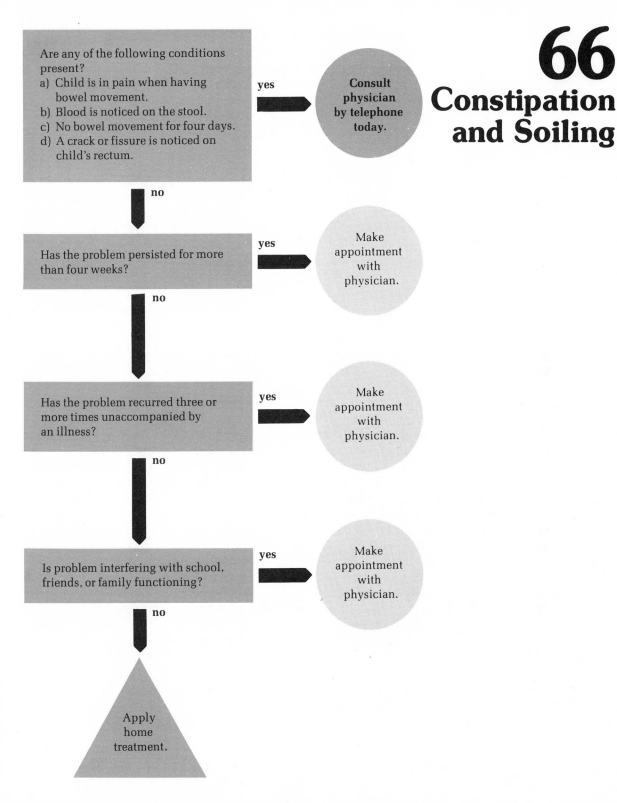

Are any of the following conditions present?
a) Child is in pain when having bowel movement.
b) Blood is noticed on the stool.
c) No bowel movement for four days.
d) A crack or fissure is noticed on child's rectum.

yes → Consult physician by telephone today.

no

Has the problem persisted for more than four weeks?

yes → Make appointment with physician.

no

Has the problem recurred three or more times unaccompanied by an illness?

yes → Make appointment with physician.

no

Is problem interfering with school, friends, or family functioning?

yes → Make appointment with physician.

no

Apply home treatment.

66 Constipation and Soiling

67
Overweight

We hope that you read this about the time that your child is born. The number of fat cells in the body is probably determined in the first year of life. Too many calories during this time will cause too many fat cells and these fat cells never go away. Even with the strictest of diets in later life, it will be possible only to reduce the size but not the number of fat cells. The fat cells will be around for the rest of the child's life, attempting to turn every available calorie into fat. This helps explain why fat babies have more difficulty maintaining normal weight as an adult.

There are a number of ways to detect obesity but none beats the human eye. Fat is easy to see if you don't try to fool yourself. Weight and height charts often have such a wide range of "normal" weights that there is ample opportunity for self-deception.

Obesity is almost always due to too many calories and not enough exercise. Trying to find a way around this simple truth is one of America's favorite pastimes. The problem is complicated by the peculiar notion that a fat baby is happy and healthy. Along with our traditional attitudes toward cleaning up the plate ("think of the starving orphans in Asia"), this can be a tragic combination of concepts, and can lead to social problems and premature death as an adult.

There are certain hormone disorders that cause what appears to be obesity, but glands get blamed for a lot more problems than they actually cause. Even to the untrained eye, children with these problems do not appear the same as a typical chubby child. One of the most constant findings of gland problems (thyroid) in younger children is that growth is retarded so that height is not normal. Often weight is gained in a relatively short period of time and is associated with other symptoms. In other words, this type of weight gain is part of an illness and is not an isolated happening. Such illnesses are not common. Steroid medications can also be responsible for weight gain.

Home Treatment

With an infant, you must overcome the feeling that too much is better than not enough and that a fat baby is a healthy baby. Forcing food is not necessary. Infants have a pretty good idea of how much they need; they will not starve in the presence of food. Fat babies cannot make themselves that way without the help of their parents.

Older children and adolescents are a different story. As youngsters become adults, they take on the adult patterns of obesity. While older children may be initially discouraged in trying to slim down after years of being overweight, they should realize that proper nutrition and exercise at any age will eventually be rewarded.

Since eating is one way of handling stress and is enjoyable, the psychology of obesity is complex. The psychological problems need not be solved before the problem of obesity can be solved. Unhappiness is sometimes used as an excuse for not doing anything about obesity when in fact working on the obesity may help with the unhappiness.

To help with the basics of losing weight, keep a diary or chart of calorie intake, exercise, and weight on a daily basis. Charting progress (or lack of it) is central to any method of weight control. It is important to eat meals only at the table. The battle of the bulge is most often lost snacking at the refrigerator. Rewarding even minor weight loss is important. Weight reduction is a family problem; childrens' eating patterns largely are determined by those of their parents. Teenagers can participate in group efforts at weight control; these methods are often helpful. Whatever method is used, its success will depend on both you and your child. Do not expect the physician to solve the problem for you. If all else fails, then a visit to the doctor or nutritionist and a fresh look from a different perspective may be needed. However, don't go to the doctor for diet pills; these do not work and can hurt.

What to Expect at the Doctor's Office

An extensive dietary history and physical examination will be conducted. Height charts are

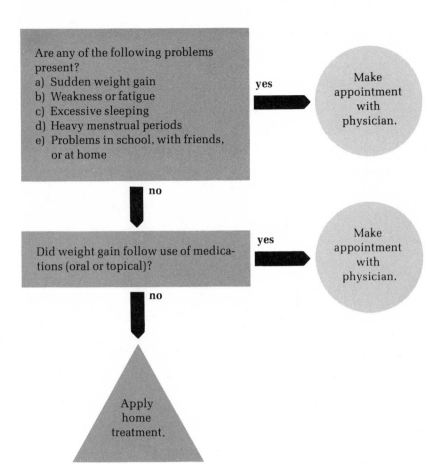

Are any of the following problems present?
a) Sudden weight gain
b) Weakness or fatigue
c) Excessive sleeping
d) Heavy menstrual periods
e) Problems in school, with friends, or at home

yes → Make appointment with physician.

no ↓

Did weight gain follow use of medications (oral or topical)?

yes → Make appointment with physician.

no ↓

Apply home treatment.

more important for infants than for adolescents. Blood tests may also be done but, as in adults, tests for thyroid function as a cause of obesity are usually not needed. The physician may know of a group approach to weight control and be willing to refer your child to that group. Nutritional or behavioral counseling is often recommended. Most often the physician will elaborate on the principles of controlling food intake and increasing exercise as a home treatment.

68
Underweight

Parents are naturally concerned that their children grow and put on weight properly. Proper growth and weight gain are determined by adequate nutrition as well as genetic factors. Of course, it is only over nutrition that we have any control. Often parents of a breast-fed baby will be concerned that their child is not as fat as the baby next door, or the baby in the food ads; this is because many breast-fed babies gain weight at a slower rate than bottle-fed babies. There are, of course, feeding problems in both breast- and bottle-fed infants that can cause a child to be underweight. Inadequate intake, excessive vomiting, or long-lasting diarrhea can all lead to inadequate weight gain in infants. Children with underlying heart failure or long-standing urinary tract infections may also gain weight poorly; this may occur with other serious medical problems as well. Malabsorption is an intestinal disturbance that produces terrible-smelling, greasy-looking bowel movements. Food is absorbed poorly, resulting in insufficient weight gain.

Physicians are as concerned about weight gain as are the parents. They will take height and weight measurements in the office during well-baby visits. A child who is more than two "weight lines" away from the height line is seriously underweight. You can check your child on the charts in Part III. For example, if your daughter is one year old and is 29 inches or 74 centimeters tall, this is on the 50th percentile line. If the weight is only 17 pounds or 8 kilograms, this is only the 5th percentile and is more than two lines away from the 50th percentile. This child is underweight and should be seen by a physician.

Children who are on the lean side (not markedly underweight) have many health advantages. They often feel better about themselves and find physical activities much easier. In addition, "thin is in" these days.

Sometimes older children will refuse to eat. While a short diet with a few pounds of weight loss is fine, prolonged or excessive weight loss can be dangerous. Such children frequently will insist that they feel fat and don't wish to eat, even after they have become emaciated and have developed other health problems. If prolonged, this problem, called anorexia nervosa, can be life-threatening. Children with this problem have a real aversion to food and sometimes even induce vomiting after they do eat. Anorexia nervosa requires medical help.

In general, if nutrition is adequate and weight loss has not been marked, it is far better to be on the lean side than the fat side. During periods of rapid growth children often get gangly and "string out." This is not a cause for concern.

Home Treatment
Children will eat a sufficient amount if it is presented to them. Do not be concerned if your child refuses to eat a meal or two or is a picky eater. Children become underweight only if inadequate amounts of foods are available.

What to Expect at the Doctor's Office
A complete history and physical examination will be done. Special attention will be paid to the dietary and bowel patterns. Height and weight will be carefully measured, and further investigations will depend on what is found. If an intestinal problem is suspected, stool analysis and possibly bowel X-rays will be done. If a heart problem is suspected, X-rays or an EKG will be performed; if infection is likely, a blood test and urinalysis will be done.

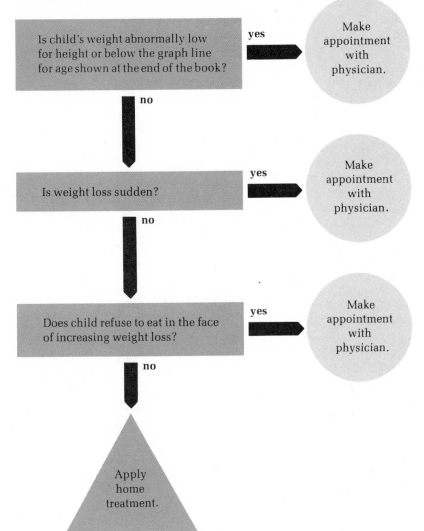

68
Underweight

Is child's weight abnormally low for height or below the graph line for age shown at the end of the book?

yes → Make appointment with physician.

no

Is weight loss sudden?

yes → Make appointment with physician.

no

Does child refuse to eat in the face of increasing weight loss?

yes → Make appointment with physician.

no

Apply home treatment.

69
Stress, Anxiety, and Depression

Stress is a normal part of our lives. It is not necessarily good or bad. It is not a disease. All children are subject to stress. Toddlers must learn to communicate. Preschoolers need to know how to interact in a socially acceptable fashion. School-aged children have peer and teacher pressures. Adolescents must begin to think about future careers. In addition, they will find and often lose meaningful relations with members of the opposite sex. Leaving home is one of the greatest stresses children encounter. In addition to the daily stresses of their own lives, children absorb the stresses of their parents as well. It is difficult to hide from a child your own concerns about problems at work, problems with your spouse, serious illness in relatives, etc.

With all these stresses, it is not unusual for children to become seriously affected. Frequently this will appear first as anxiety and often progress to depression. The degree of anxiety or depression is much more a function of the individual than of the degree of stress. A child who feels a great deal of family support will be able to deal with minor stresses far more easily. Major stresses, such as parental separation or a move, will affect all children. The length of the recovery period will be a function of the child's strength and parental guidance during this time. If the stress or its consequent anxiety or depression is severe enough, children can develop significant physical and emotional problems. Failure to go to school, difficulty falling asleep, excessive sleeping, nightmares or night terrors, refusal to eat, significant weight loss or weight gain, constantly being sad are all symptoms that must be taken seriously if they persist for more than a few days.

Anxiety can often lead to the hyperventilation syndrome. Hyperventilation means excessive breathing. In this condition, an anxious older child or adolescent may rapidly develop a feeling of inability to get enough air into the lungs. Sometimes this is associated with a feeling of chest pain or chest constriction. The sensation of being out of breath leads to further overbreathing, the exhaling of too much carbon dioxide, and the lowering of the carbon dioxide level in the blood (carbon dioxide is present in exhaled air). The lower level of carbon dioxide gives symptoms of numbness and tingling of the hands, feet, and mouth, as well as dizziness. Any of these varied symptoms can be the major one for a particular person.

Home Treatment
The best approach is to be open and to discuss stressful occurrences with your children as they are growing up. Children who feel they can talk over their anxieties with their parents have support in working through their problems when they are young. This hopefully leads to a better ability to work through stressful situations independently as an adult. Identification of the source of anxiety or depression can be difficult and may require the help of a professional; most communities have resources that can help. Social workers, ministers, mental health centers, and medical professionals can help if friends and family cannot.

With the hyperventilation syndrome, open recognition that this is a stress reaction will usually stop the attacks. During an attack, place a paper bag loosely over the nose and mouth so that the child can rebreathe the carbon dioxide in the expelled air. This will raise the blood level of carbon dioxide and the attack will pass after ten minutes or so. After an attack, seat the child on a couch and have him or her take 50 or 100 deep breaths. Usually they will notice the same kinds of symptoms that they had during an attack, and this will convince them that overbreathing was the problem; it is difficult to so convince a child during the panic of a hyperventilation attack.

What to Expect at the Doctor's Office
The physician will attempt to identify the source of the problem. School records and records from other health professionals will help. Seldom can the problem be solved in one visit. Many physicians will rely on social workers, clinical psychologists, or psychiatrists to help with the problem.

Are any of the following conditions present for longer than one week?
a) School problems
b) Problems with friends
c) Excessive sleeping
d) Withdrawal
e) Excess irritability
f) Unusual aggression

yes → Make appointment with physician.

no ↓

Are any of the following conditions present for longer than one month?
a) Bedwetting in a previously dry child
b) Soiling
c) Abdominal pain
d) Headaches

yes → Make appointment with physician.

no ↓

Is problem disruptive to either parent or to siblings?

yes → Make appointment with physician.

no ↓

Apply home treatment.

70
Weakness and Tiredness

Children often have periods of being extremely tired or feeling weak; these symptoms may appear quite suddenly. In younger and older children alike, the sudden development of weakness most often signifies the beginnings of a cold or other infection. Weakness may precede a fever or occur simultaneously with the fever in the early stages of many infections. Weakness is a signal that the body should receive some rest in order to recover most quickly from the infection. In younger children, colds, sore throats, earaches, and stomach flu are the most frequent reasons for weakness. In older children, infectious mononucleosis, a prolonged but seldom serious viral infection, or influenza is often the cause.

The fatigue that is associated with an infection will usually develop quickly and last only for a short period of time; exceptions are in the case of hepatitis, mononucleosis, and a poorly understood syndrome called *neurasthenia,* which may follow other viral infections on rare occasions. Even in these cases there is nothing to do but wait it out. Children have an extraordinary amount of energy and it is unusual for them to complain of being tired for long periods of time. However, we often see young children who seem to have no energy during the day and can trace the problem to late-night watching of television in their rooms. It is not surprising that a young child who is awake until the wee hours of the morning will have little energy for usual daytime activities. Thin walls, noisy neighbors, and late-night talks with brothers or sisters are among factors that can easily disturb the sleep of children.

Normally, parents can let nature tell the child when sleep is needed, but if the child is droopy and sleepy late in the day, action may be needed to ensure that adequate amounts of sleep are received.

Anemia (low blood) is a very occasional cause of chronic weakness or tiredness, often suspected but seldom present. The most common anemia is iron deficiency anemia. Iron is abundant in meat products, cereal, nuts, lima beans, lentils, peas, soybeans, spinach, and many other products. Cow's milk is low in iron and a diet consisting exclusively of cow's milk is dangerous in its ability to produce anemia in infants. Exclusive ingestion of goat's milk can lead to another type of anemia in infants. Restrictive diets, such as the Zen macrobiotic diet, are inadequate for children. Variety of diet, including all the major food groups, is the most important principle, rather than sets of rigid rules. Given enough varied raw materials, the body is very good at selecting out what is needed and eliminating the rest.

Hypoglycemia (low blood sugar) is another commonly discussed but rarely found medical problem. True hypoglycemia causes other symptoms such as sweating, nervousness, headaches, and irritability, as well as fatigue. Children do not usually have this combination of symptoms unless they are undereating severely or having prolonged vomiting. Treatment is, of course, to control vomiting and maintain an adequate dietary intake.

Long-standing weakness and tiredness in children may result from depression. It is a common mistake to assume that only adults are subject to emotional stresses and therefore capable of becoming depressed. Children may react severely to a move, the loss of a pet or friend, an inability to keep up in school, an inability to be successful with friends, or an inability to compete in sports, by withdrawing. Depressed children often have little energy, feel tired all the time, refuse to eat or eat too much, have trouble falling asleep at night or sleep too much, and may complain of a number of physical ailments. These symptoms should be treated seriously. The longer a child spends away from school or from normal everyday activities, the harder it is to begin functioning normally again. If you are having difficulty dealing with a problem that is disturbing your child, you should seek professional help for the child.

Home Treatment

Watching and waiting is all that is called for in the case of weakness that accompanies a mild

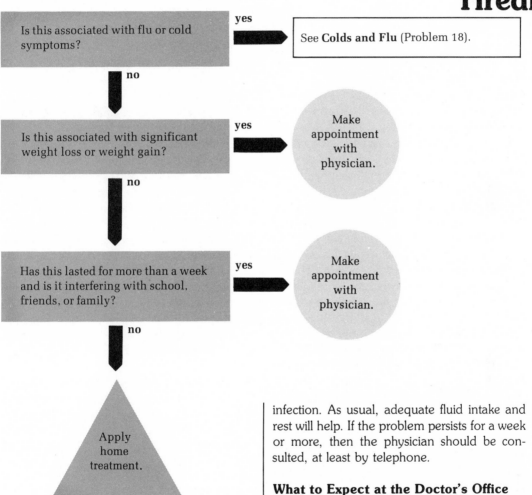

Is this associated with flu or cold symptoms?

yes → See **Colds and Flu** (Problem 18).

no ↓

Is this associated with significant weight loss or weight gain?

yes → Make appointment with physician.

no ↓

Has this lasted for more than a week and is it interfering with school, friends, or family?

yes → Make appointment with physician.

no ↓

Apply home treatment.

infection. As usual, adequate fluid intake and rest will help. If the problem persists for a week or more, then the physician should be consulted, at least by telephone.

What to Expect at the Doctor's Office

A careful history and physical examination with measurement of height and weight will be performed. For some types of infections, specific laboratory tests will be ordered; infectious mononucleosis and hepatitis can be detected by a blood test. Most physicians will check for anemia and hypoglycemia only if the dietary history or symptoms are suggestive of these problems.

71
Dizziness
and Fainting

These complaints are frustrating to children, parents, and physicians alike. They are common, worrisome, and occasionally frightening, but most often they go unexplained. Some children have a special interest in fainting, it seems, even to the point of inventing games to make themselves pass out. Young children may be subject to the frightening but generally harmless phenomenon of breath-holding spells. Altogether a problem with dizziness or fainting can be a pretty confusing situation. Defining the terms correctly will help in understanding the problem.

The term fainting may be used to describe a lightheaded and woozy episode without loss of consciousness or it may signify a complete collapse with loss of consciousness. Lightheadedness frequently accompanies viral illnesses. It may also occur if a child suddenly stands up from a reclining or sitting position; it takes a few seconds for the body to adjust to this new position, so that there is temporarily a decrease in flow of blood to the head. Low blood sugar is commonly talked about but hardly ever is responsible. For lightheadedness, the attention of a physician is needed only if it persists for several weeks. If the child has lost consciousness completely, however, the physician should be seen without delay.

The exception to this last rule occurs with breath-holding spells. These spells are described on p. 68. Breath-holding may lead to complete unconsciousness and even a seizure. Try to prevent injury from falling or from a seizure by observation and support. If you are certain that loss of consciousness occurred because of a breath-holding spell, then apply home treatment and discuss the situation with your physician on the phone.

Dizziness refers to a situation in which the room seems to spin about the child; this is also called vertigo, and may be accompanied by nausea and vomiting. Except for the case when children spin themselves in a circle rapidly, vertigo indicates that the balance mechanism in the inner ear has been disturbed. This most often occurs because of minor viral infections called *labyrinthitis*. Sometimes it occurs with ear infections; if there is an earache, see your physician.

Some medications can cause vertigo. Telephone your physician if this is a possibility.

Home Treatment
If the problem is one of lightheadedness upon arising suddenly from a sitting or reclining position, then simple avoidance of such sudden changes in position is all that is necessary. This problem is called postural hypotension and does not need the help of the physician unless it has suddenly become worse. Otherwise, it may wait and be discussed at the next routine visit. If it is caused by a virus it will go away within a few days.

Breath-holding spells are difficult problems. Drugs will not help. In the meantime, one tries to prevent damage from falls or seizures by alerting teachers and friends so that they may be aware of the possibility and ready to help. The child will outgrow them eventually.

What to Expect at the Doctor's Office
The history of the episodes provides the most important piece of information in deciding what to do. Physical examination will include examination of the eyes and ears and blood pressure measurements. Sometimes tests on the blood and the urine may be done. X-rays and brain wave tests (EEG) are rarely of use. Tests of the inner ear may be performed. Vertigo may be treated with drugs.

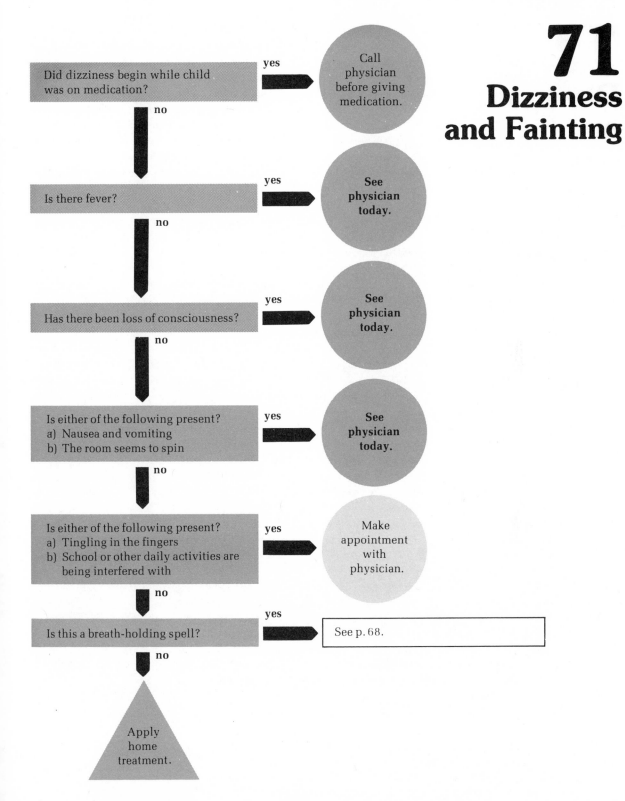

Did dizziness begin while child was on medication?

yes → Call physician before giving medication.

no ↓

Is there fever?

yes → **See physician today.**

no ↓

Has there been loss of consciousness?

yes → **See physician today.**

no ↓

Is either of the following present?
a) Nausea and vomiting
b) The room seems to spin

yes → **See physician today.**

no ↓

Is either of the following present?
a) Tingling in the fingers
b) School or other daily activities are being interfered with

yes → Make appointment with physician.

no ↓

Is this a breath-holding spell?

yes → See p. 68.

no ↓

Apply home treatment.

72
Seizures (Convulsions, Fits, Falling-out Spells)

About five percent of all children will have one or more seizures (convulsions, fits, falling-out spells) before the age of fifteen. The most common cause is a high fever; such seizures are often referred to as "fever fits" or "febrile seizures." These occur most often in children between the ages of six months and four years, and are associated with very high fevers. Anyone would have a seizure if his or her body temperature were raised high enough, let us say to 107° to 109°F. Children, who may even have seizures at temperatures as low as 103°F, are thought to have a lower threshold for seizing. Part of this lowered threshold may be due to the immaturity of the nervous system in young children. More than half of the children who have a febrile seizure will never have a second. Yet in some children who have a febrile seizure, this is the first sign of recurrent seizures of epilepsy, and later seizures may be spontaneous and not associated with fever. Less than one half of one percent of the population is diagnosed as having epilepsy. Almost all of these individuals are leading normal lives because of the remarkable effectiveness of currently available medications.

Seizures occur because of a disruption of the normal electrical impulse pattern of the brain. This disruption can occur spontaneously, it may be triggered by fevers, poisons, or infection (meningitis), or occasionally it may occur after a breath-holding spell. There are many types of seizures, but parents will have no trouble recognizing the abnormal condition in their child. Some children will become stiff and roll their eyes backward. Others will exhibit rhythmic jerking of their arms and legs. Some may have staring spells or suddenly collapse. All of these will naturally cause great alarm. Fortunately most seizures end in a few minutes without permanent damage to the child.

Home Treatment

In this instance, home treatment consists of things that you should do before you see the doctor. Seizures are very frightening experiences and it is easy to panic during your first experience with one. Panic can be avoided if you can keep a few simple principles in mind. First, most childhood seizures stop by themselves within a few minutes and it is rare for the seizure itself to do any lasting harm to the child. While the seizure is occurring, you should be concerned with preventing injury to the child from a fall and preventing a blow to the head. Tongue chewing or swallowing does not often occur. Jamming objects into the child's mouth can do more harm than good.

It is important for the child to have a good air passage. Extending the child's neck (chin as far from the chest as possible) while gently pulling on the jaw will best accomplish this. Second, if the seizure has stopped and the child has vomited, clear the mouth. Third, if the seizure has stopped and there is a fever, begin temperature-lowering procedures. You cannot give medicine by mouth, but a rectal aspirin suppository can be used. Sponging with cool water will help. Beware of attempting to give a full bath to a semiconscious child. Sponging the child can continue during the trip to the doctor. Do not bundle the child up; both you and the child must keep cool. If there is a considerable distance to be traveled, temperature lowering en route becomes important; remember that you can lower a fever as effectively as the doctor can. Breath-holding spell seizures are seldom serious but your physician should be consulted by phone.

Following a seizure, the child will be drowsy or may seem to be in a deep sleep. This is called the post-ictal state, and is not harmful. You need not attempt to arouse the child from this state.

What to Expect at the Doctor's Office

If the seizure has not stopped, then drugs will be given by injection to bring this about. Following control of the seizure, the physician will perform a thorough physical examination and

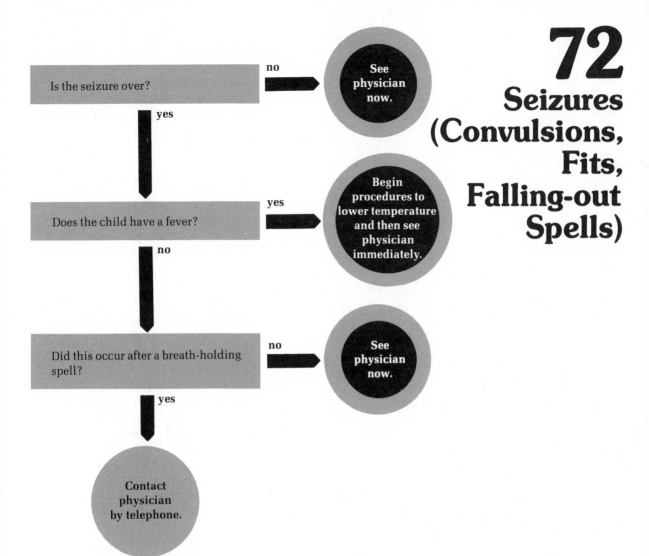

Is the seizure over? — no → **See physician now.**

yes ↓

Does the child have a fever? — yes → **Begin procedures to lower temperature and then see physician immediately.**

no ↓

Did this occur after a breath-holding spell? — no → **See physician now.**

yes ↓

Contact physician by telephone.

will want to talk to you in depth concerning the circumstances of the seizure. If a fever is present, then search will be made for the source of the infection. Most often these are the common infections of childhood (colds, roseola, gastroenteritis, and ear infections). A spinal tap will be necessary to investigate the possibility of infection in the brain or spinal cord, if this is the first seizure. Hospitalization is sometimes required for observation, treatment, or further evaluation. Children under six months of age will almost always be admitted to the hospital. A brain wave test (electroencephalogram or EEG) will usually be done. Often it is better to wait a week or ten days before doing this test; brain wave tests do not necessarily require a hospital admission.

Although there has been a great deal of controversy over this subject, a recent study demonstrates the value of phenobarbital in preventing recurrences of febrile seizures in children. Because phenobarbital does have side effects and must be taken for a long time, and because most children will not have a second febrile seizure, discussion will undoubtedly continue about the desirability of using this drug. Be sure to discuss the facts fully with your physician.

73
Swallowed Foreign Objects

Babies and small children delight in swallowing any and all things that they can get their hands on and that are small enough to go down. In this section we are concerned with things that will not dissolve in the stomach. Anything that *will* dissolve is a potential poison and Problem 16 (Oral Poisoning) should be consulted. The children's favorites among nondissolving objects are coins, buttons, the eyes from teddy bears and dolls, safety pins, and fruit pits. Nature seems to have prepared the digestive tract well, since even very sharp objects such as open safety pins, pieces of glass, needles, and straight pins regularly pass through the bowels with the greatest of ease. Therefore the best strategy is to do nothing unless you're forced to do something.

Of immediate concern is the possibility that an object has become lodged in the windpipe. Violent coughing or difficulty in breathing suggests that the object may be lodged in the windpipe. As long as the child is able to breathe, proceed immediately to the doctor or emergency room. Attempting to dislodge an object that is partially obstructing breathing may lead to complete obstruction. If the windpipe is completely obstructed, a rapidly applied bear hug to the child's chest may force the object loose.

Pain and/or vomiting indicate that help is needed for an abdominal problem. If the object swallowed is very sharp and could possibly puncture the intestine, then you should call your physician. The purpose of this call is to let the doctor know that assistance could be needed in the next few days on rather short notice. The doctor can make appropriate arrangements. If the object should perforate the intestine, then surgery will be needed, and these prior arrangements can make the surgery go more smoothly. Be prepared, but do not panic. Even razor blades have been passed through the entire digestive system without noticeable effect.

Home Treatment
If the object is smooth, then you may want to look at the bowel movements for the next few days to reassure yourself that it has passed. If you don't see it, it is a far better bet that you missed it than that it did not pass.

If the object is sharp, then the physician will likely ask you to look for the object to pass and to be on the alert for the symptoms of abdominal pain or vomiting. He or she, in turn, should make sure that surgical help will be available if needed.

What to Expect at the Doctor's Office
If the object is lodged in the throat, the physician may be able to remove it in the office. Otherwise, a visit to the hospital may be necessary. If the problem is shortness of breath, wheezing, pain in the chest or abdomen, or vomiting, then a history and physical examination along with X-rays will be performed. Remember that nonmetallic objects may not be seen on an X-ray. In this instance, special X-rays (such as a barium swallow) may show the object but may be unwise if puncture of the intestine is suspected.

If puncture of the intestine has occurred, then surgery will be necessary. If the object is in the respiratory tract it must be removed. This can often be accomplished through an instrument known as a bronchoscope, which enables physicians to visualize and remove foreign objects.

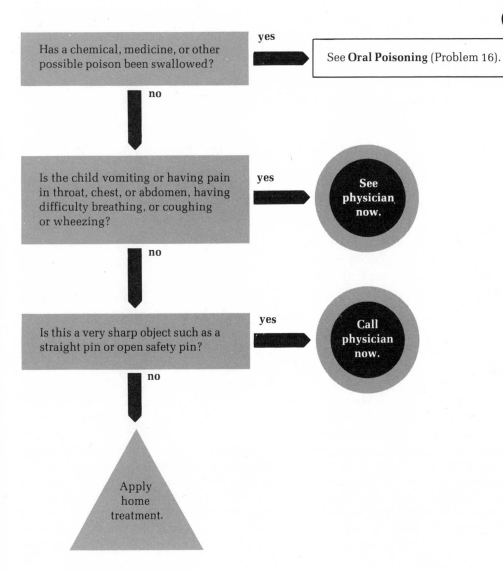

Has a chemical, medicine, or other possible poison been swallowed?

yes → See **Oral Poisoning** (Problem 16).

no ↓

Is the child vomiting or having pain in throat, chest, or abdomen, having difficulty breathing, or coughing or wheezing?

yes → See physician now.

no ↓

Is this a very sharp object such as a straight pin or open safety pin?

yes → Call physician now.

no ↓

Apply home treatment.

74
Frequent Illnesses

Frequent illnesses are the rule and not the exception for most children. Recent studies have revealed that the average child has between six and nine viral illnesses per year. In some children, these viral illnesses are so mild that the parent will not notice any symptoms. Other children will have a cough or runny nose or some other minor symptom. We do not think of these viral infections as illnesses, but rather as immunizations that serve to protect children against the more serious consequences of these illnesses at a later age.

In addition to the frequent minor colds that most children have, the majority of children will also experience one or more ear infections in a lifetime. Similarly, we expect most children to have several bouts of diarrhea while they are young and at least one or two strep throats in the school years. When you start adding up the number of illnesses we expect in children, it is a wonder that they spend so much time free of symptoms.

Abnormalities of the body's immune defense mechanisms, of concern to many parents, virtually never present themselves as frequent minor infections. Children with immune deficiencies often have repeated severe infections of the lungs or skin. These children seldom grow normally, and are often quite underweight because of the repeated infections. For any of these problems, a medical evaluation is important. Similarly, if there is history of a family relative dying at a young age because of an overwhelming infection, you should discuss your concern with your physician.

Allergies are often confused with illnesses. Children with allergic rhinitis or hay fever will usually have sneezing, eye itching, and runny noses at a particular time of year, usually in the spring and in the fall. These children will often be rubbing their noses constantly.

While the younger children in a family often seem to have more colds than their older brothers and sisters did at the same age, they are just as healthy as their older counterparts. The younger child merely gets many of the common viral illnesses at an earlier age because of exposure to older brothers and sisters. Similarly, while some studies have shown that children in day-care centers or nursery schools seem to get a few more colds early on, there is no evidence that these children are not every bit as healthy as their peers who remain at home. There are at least 60 different viral strains against which most adults are partly immunized because of childhood illnesses. The sooner the child develops these immunities, the sooner the relatively illness-free years of the adult can begin.

Home Treatment
Home treatment of the minor problems of childhood are discussed throughout this book. Frequent illnesses that are troublesome enough to interfere with schoolwork should be evaluated by a physician.

What to Expect at the Doctor's Office
A careful history and physical examination will be performed. Cataloguing of the nature and severity of the frequent illnesses will be done. Particular attention will be paid to the child's height and weight development. Depending on the nature of the problem, various laboratory tests may be performed.

True immune deficiency states in children are very rare, and these children need special treatment. Frequent colds or recurrent earaches do *not* warrant the use of gamma-globulin shots. Gammaglobulin deficiency must be confirmed by blood testing.

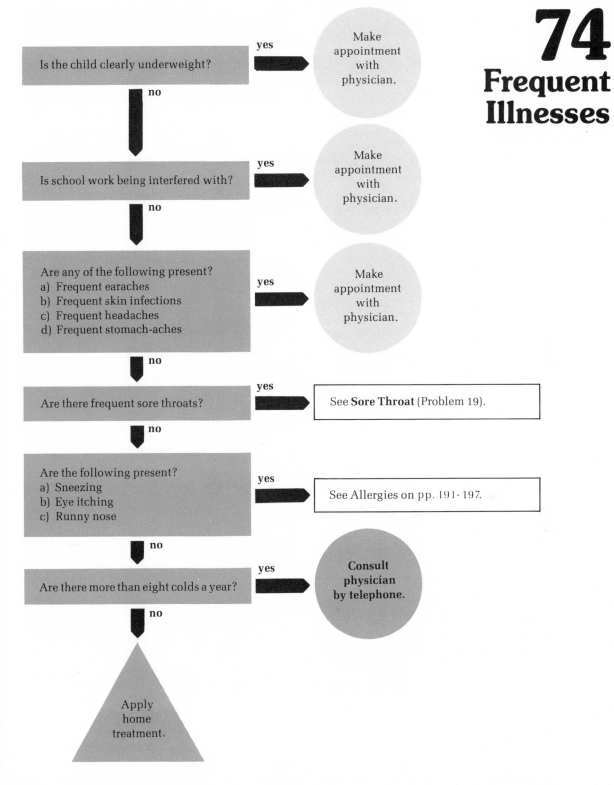

Is the child clearly underweight?

yes → Make appointment with physician.

no ↓

Is school work being interfered with?

yes → Make appointment with physician.

no ↓

Are any of the following present?
a) Frequent earaches
b) Frequent skin infections
c) Frequent headaches
d) Frequent stomach-aches

yes → Make appointment with physician.

no ↓

Are there frequent sore throats?

yes → See **Sore Throat** (Problem 19).

no ↓

Are the following present?
a) Sneezing
b) Eye itching
c) Runny nose

yes → See Allergies on pp. 191-197.

no ↓

Are there more than eight colds a year?

yes → **Consult physician by telephone.**

no ↓

Apply home treatment.

L

Chest Pains, Shortness of Breath, and Palpitations

75. Chest Pain   **330**
Almost never the heart.

76. Shortness of Breath   **332**
The lungs or the nerves?

77. Palpitations   **334**
Pounding of the heart.

75
Chest Pain

Chest pain in children frequently results from severe coughing, which leads to a pain or burning sensation underneath the breastbone (sternum). Pain can also come from the chest wall (including muscles, ligaments, ribs, and rib cartilage), the lungs, the outside covering of the heart (pericardium), the gullet (esophagus), the diaphragm, the spine, the skin, and the organs in the upper part of the abdomen. Often it is difficult even for a physician to determine the precise origin of the pain. In general, pains that are made worse by breathing, coughing, or movement of the chest are due to problems of the chest wall, the lungs, or the covering of the heart. Other pains may be due to problems with the heart or abdominal organs.

A shooting pain lasting a few seconds is common in healthy young people and means nothing. It is probably due to a trapped gas bubble of the stomach. A sensation of a "catch" at the end of a deep breath is also trivial and does not need attention. Heart pain almost never occurs under 30 years of age. You can check for chest-wall pain by pressing a finger on the chest at the spot of discomfort and reproducing or aggravating the pain; it usually becomes worse with movement of the chest. The hyperventilation syndrome (see Problem 69, Stress, Anxiety, and Depression) is a frequent cause of chest pain, particularly in adolescents. If there is dizziness accompanied by a tingling in the fingers, suspect this problem.

One of the serious problems that can present itself as chest pain is a *pneumothorax*. A pneumothorax is a problem in which the outside lining of the lung has ruptured and air begins to accumulate around the outside of the lung, compressing it. This problem often occurs in patients with a history of asthma, but can occur spontaneously in patients without any prior lung problems. Breathing becomes progressively difficult; if chest pain is accompanied by shortness of breath, the physician should be consulted immediately.

A heart attack in a family member can be a frightening experience for everyone. It is not uncommon for children to become concerned about their own hearts at such a time. Children will often be very concerned about minor chest problems and fear that they may also be having a heart attack. These complaints should be taken seriously by parents; reassurance is usually all that is required.

Finally, excessive hard exercise in someone not accustomed to prolonged exercise can produce chest pain. These pains are usually temporary and disappear with a few moments of rest.

Home Treatment
Pains arising from the chest wall can usually be managed at home with aspirin or acetaminophen. Heat sometimes helps. With chest-wall injuries, wrapping the chest loosely with an Ace bandage will limit the movement of the chest wall, which often aggravates the pain. If a persistent cough is responsible for the chest pain, time will heal this problem. In particularly severe chest pain due to coughs, a cough suppressant with dextromethorphan (Romilar or Robitussin-DM) will help.

What to Expect at the Doctor's Office
A thorough history and examination of the chest wall, lungs, heart, and abdomen will be made. Only if a serious underlying problem such as pneumonia, pneumothorax, or inflammation of the heart is suspected will X-rays and an electrocardiogram be ordered.

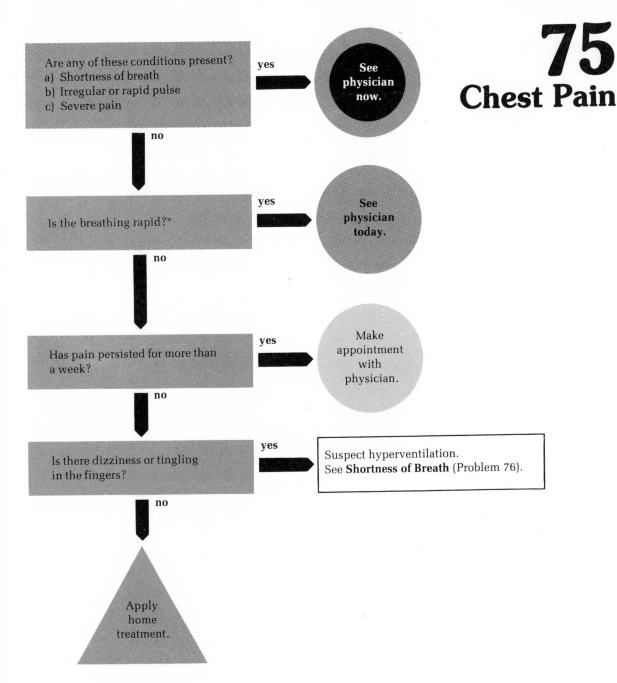

Chest Pain

Are any of these conditions present?
a) Shortness of breath
b) Irregular or rapid pulse
c) Severe pain

yes → See physician now.

no ↓

Is the breathing rapid?*

yes → See physician today.

no ↓

Has pain persisted for more than a week?

yes → Make appointment with physician.

no ↓

Is there dizziness or tingling in the fingers?

yes → Suspect hyperventilation.
See **Shortness of Breath** (Problem 76).

no ↓

Apply home treatment.

*See "How fast is your child breathing?" (on p. 142)

76
Shortness of Breath

When children run hard and long they become short of breath; this symptom is certainly normal under such circumstances. Medical use of the term shortness of breath does not include shortness of breath after such heavy exertion.

Shortness of breath can be due to several different problems. Your child may experience difficulty breathing in. This symptom is common in croup (Problem 25), where it is usually accompanied by a barking cough. If a child is having difficulty breathing and at the same time is gasping for breath, drooling, or breathing with the head tilted forward, a serious obstruction of the airway passages is likely and the child should immediately be brought to the physician.

If a child is having difficulty breathing out, the expiration will take longer than normal. Often difficulties in breathing out are accompanied by wheezing. More often, difficulty breathing out is accompanied by wheezing that cannot be heard unless you place your ear to your child's chest. Wheezing is discussed further in Problem 26.

The term shortness of breath is frequently used to mean rapid breathing. Respiratory rates in infants are usually high; breathing rates of 50 to 60 times per minute are common. As infants grow older, the normal respiratory rate declines. By about one year of age the respiratory rate of a child is between 25 and 35 while resting, although in an active but not exercising child it may be as high as 45. It is therefore important to assess the breathing rate when the child is resting. A rate of 40 at rest is of concern except in children under a year of age. In children over the age of six, rates greater than 30 are of concern.

The most common reasons for elevated respiratory rates are fevers and pneumonia. One of the body's mechanisms for lowering temperature is to increase the respiratory rate. If you reduce the fever with aspirin or cool baths and the child's respiratory rate is still elevated, you should be concerned about possible pneumonia.

Another cause for an elevated respiratory rate is an overdose of aspirin; if you suspect this, call the doctor.

More unusual causes of an elevated respiratory rate include diabetes and metabolic disturbances that may accompany severe diarrhea. These need the doctor's attention.

Home Treatment

Most causes of shortness of breath require medical attention. Mist will usually relieve croup (see Problem 25). Children with asthma will already be under medical supervision and the usual regimen should be begun. All other cases should be brought to the physician.

What to Expect at the Doctor's Office

A thorough history and examination of the lungs, heart, and upper airway passages will be done. Depending on the nature of the problem, chest and neck X-rays may be ordered. Severe obstruction of the airway will almost always require hospitalization. Pneumonia, asthma, and croup can usually be managed without hospitalization.

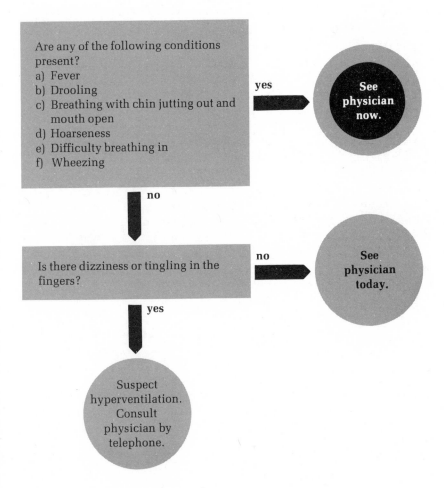

Are any of the following conditions present?
a) Fever
b) Drooling
c) Breathing with chin jutting out and mouth open
d) Hoarseness
e) Difficulty breathing in
f) Wheezing

yes → See physician now.

no ↓

Is there dizziness or tingling in the fingers?

no → See physician today.

yes ↓

Suspect hyperventilation. Consult physician by telephone.

77
Palpitations

Pounding of the heart is brought on by strenuous exercise or intense emotion and is seldom associated with serious disease. Most of us have experienced what is known as "bent-bumper syndrome"; after a near collision with another car, the heart seems almost to stop, and then pounds with such force that you feel as though you're being punched in the chest. Simultaneously, the knees become wobbly and the palms sweaty. These events are due to a large discharge of adrenalin from the adrenal glands. Almost no one is concerned by such pounding of the heart. But if there is no obvious exertion or frightening event, many people become worried.

Most people who complain of palpitations do not have heart disease but are overly concerned about the possibility of such disease and thus overly sensitive to normal heart actions. Often this is because of heart disease in parents, other relatives, or friends.

An irregular or very fast pulse may be more serious. There is a normal variation in the pulse with respiration (faster when breathing in, slower when breathing out). Even though the pulse may speed or slow, the normal pulse has a regular rhythm. Occasional extra heartbeats occur in nearly everyone. Consistently irregular pulses, however, are usually abnormal. The pulse can be felt on the inside of the wrist, in the neck, or over the heart itself. Ask the nurse to check you out on taking pulses on your next visit. Take your own pulse and those of your children, noting the variation with respiration.

The most common time for palpitations to occur is just before going to sleep. If the pulse rate is under 120, relax.

Hyperventilation may also cause pounding and chest pain, but the heart rate also remains less than 120 beats per minute. Refer to Problem 76, Shortness of Breath.

In older children and adolescents, a resting heart rate greater than 120 beats per minute (without exercise) is a cause to check with the physician. Young children may have normal heart rates in that range, but they rarely complain of the heart pounding. If one should, check the situation with your physician. Keep in mind that the most frequent causes of rapid heartbeat (other than exercise) are anxiety and fever. The presence of shortness of breath (Problem 76) or chest pain (Problem 75) increases the chances of a significant problem.

Home Treatment

If a child seems stressed or anxious, focus on this rather than on the possibilities of heart disease. If anxiety does not seem likely and the child has none of the other symptoms on the chart, discuss it with the physician at your next visit.

What to Expect at the Doctor's Office

Tell the doctor the exact rate of the pulse and whether or not the pulse rhythm was regular. Usually, the symptoms will have disappeared by the time the doctor is consulted, so that your accuracy is important. The doctor will examine the heart and lungs. An electrocardiogram (EKG) is unlikely to help if the problem is not present when it's being done. A chest X-ray is seldom needed.

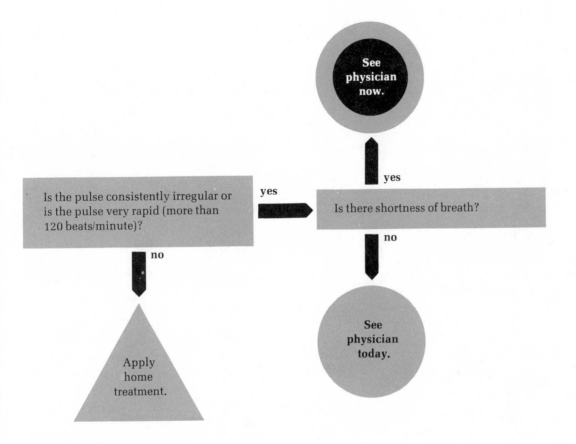

M

Eye Problems

78. Eye Burning, Itching, and Discharge   **338**
   Pink eye and other problems.

79. Foreign Body in Eye/Eye Pain   **340**
   Check it out.

80. Styes and Blocked Tear Ducts   **342**
   Some moist heat first.

81. Decreased Vision and Crossed Eyes   **344**
   See the doctor.

78
Eye Burning, Itching, and Discharge

These symptoms usually signal *conjunctivitis* or *pink eye*; this is an inflammation of the membrane that lines the eye and the inner surface of the eyelids. The inflammation may be due to an irritant in the air, an allergy to something in the air, a viral infection, or a bacterial infection. In the newborn there may be a discharge in the first two days of life because of irritation from medication given to protect against gonococcal infection. This discharge seldom lasts more than two days. Discharges after the third day are usually due to an infection or blocked tear duct (see Problem 79).

Environmental pollutants in smog can produce burning and itching, which sometimes seem as severe as the symptoms experienced in a tear-gas attack. These symptoms represent a chemical conjunctivitis, and affect anyone exposed to enough of the chemical. The smoke-filled room, the chlorinated swimming pool, the desert sandstorm, or sun glare on snow can give similar physical or chemical irritation.

In contrast, allergic conjunctivitis affects only those certain people who are allergic. Almost always the allergen is in the air, and grass pollens are probably the most frequent offender. Depending on the season for the offending pollen, this problem may occur in spring, summer, or fall, and usually lasts from two to three weeks.

A minor conjunctivitis frequently accompanies a viral cold. Epidemics of conjunctivitis are most often caused by a virus. The eye discharge is not as thick as in more severe bacterial infections. Often a small swollen lymph gland will be found in front of the ear in epidemic conjunctivitis. Conjunctivitis is also common in the first day or so of measles (Problem 54). Some viruses, such as herpes, may cause deep painful ulcers in the cornea and may interfere with vision. Bacterial infections cause pus to form, and a thick, plentiful discharge runs from the eye. Often the eyelids are crusted over and "glued" shut upon awakening. These infections require antibiotic treatment.

Some major diseases affect the deeper layers of the eye—those layers that control the operation of the lens and the size of the pupillary opening. This condition is termed *iritis* or *uveitis* and may cause irregularity of the pupil or pain when the pupil reacts to light. It is unusual in children. Medical attention is required.

Home Treatment
If a physical, chemical, or allergic exposure is the cause of the symptoms, there is nothing to do but avoid the exposure. Special glasses that keep out pollen are available for severe cases. Antihistamines obtained either over the counter or by prescription may help slightly if the problem is an allergy, but don't expect total relief and drowsiness may occur. Similarly, a viral infection related to a cold or flu will run its course in a few days, and it is best to be patient. Avoiding light affords relief in conjunctivitis due to measles.

If it doesn't clear up, if the discharge gets thicker, or if there is eye pain or a problem with vision, see your physician. Do not expect a fever with a bacterial infection of the eye; it may be absent. Since the infection is superficial, washing the eye gently will help remove some of the bacteria, but the physician should still be seen. Murine, Visine, and other eyedrops are seldom helpful in affording more than very temporary relief.

What to Expect at the Doctor's Office
The physician will check vision, eye motion, the eyelids, and the reaction of the pupil to light. Antihistamines may be prescribed for allergy. If a bacterial infection is likely, a culture may be taken. Antibiotic eyedrops or ointments are frequently given. Cortisone-like eye ointments should be prescribed very infrequently; certain infections (herpes) will get worse with these medicines. If herpes is diagnosed, usually by an ophthalmologist, special eyedrops and other medicines will be needed.

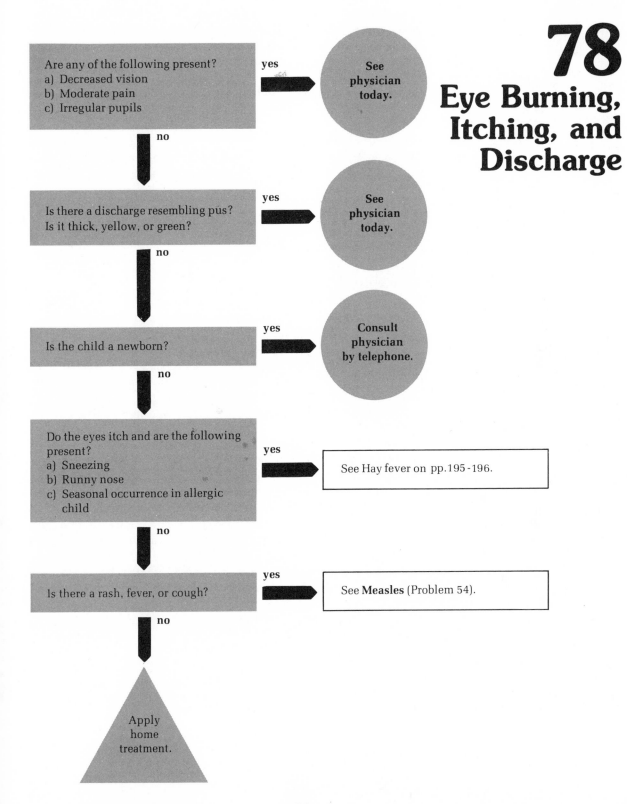

Are any of the following present?
a) Decreased vision
b) Moderate pain
c) Irregular pupils

yes → **See physician today.**

no ↓

Is there a discharge resembling pus?
Is it thick, yellow, or green?

yes → **See physician today.**

no ↓

Is the child a newborn?

yes → **Consult physician by telephone.**

no ↓

Do the eyes itch and are the following present?
a) Sneezing
b) Runny nose
c) Seasonal occurrence in allergic child

yes → See Hay fever on pp. 195-196.

no ↓

Is there a rash, fever, or cough?

yes → See **Measles** (Problem 54).

no ↓

Apply home treatment.

78
Eye Burning, Itching, and Discharge

79
Foreign Body in Eye/ Eye Pain

All *eye* injuries should be taken seriously; if there is any question, a visit to the physician is indicated. The stakes are too high. A foreign body must be removed, or the threat of infection and loss of sight in that eye is present. Be particularly careful if the foreign body was caused by the striking of metal on metal; this can cause a small metal particle to strike the eye with great force and to penetrate the eyeball.

Under a few circumstances, you may treat the injury at home. If the foreign body is minor, such as sand, and did not strike the eye with great velocity, it may feel as though it is still in the eye even when it is not. Small round particles like sand rarely stick behind the upper lid for long.

If it feels as though a foreign body is present but it is not, then the covering of the eye (cornea) has been scraped or cut. A minor corneal injury will usually heal quickly without problems; a major one requires medical attention.

Even if you think the injury to be minor, run through the questions on the decision chart daily. If any symptoms at all are present after 48 hours and are not clearly resolving, see the physician. Minor problems will heal within 48 hours; the *eye* repairs injury quickly.

Eye pain is an unusual symptom that may signify a serious inflammation of the eye (iritis) or a serious infection with herpes virus. A physician should be consulted.

Home Treatment

Be gentle. Wash the *eye* out; water is fine. Inspect the *eye* and have someone else check it as well. Use a good light and shine it from both the front and the side. Pay particular attention to the cornea—this is a clear membrane that covers the colored portion of the eye. Do not rub the eye; if a foreign body is present you will abrade or scratch the cornea. An eye patch will relieve pain, and usually it is needed for 24 hours or less. Make the patch with several layers of gauze and tape firmly in place. Check vision each day and compare the two eyes. If you are not sure that all is going well, see the doctor.

What to Expect at the Doctor's Office

The physician will perform a vision check, inspection of the *eye*, and inspection under the upper lid; this is not painful. Usually, a fluorescent stain will be dropped into the eye and the eye then examined under ultraviolet light; this too is not painful or hazardous. A foreign body, if found, will be removed. In the office, this may be done with a cotton swab, an eyewash solution, a small needle, or an "eye spud." Strong magnets are sometimes used to remove metallic objects. If these measures do not suffice, an ophthalmologist (a surgeon specializing in diseases of the eye) may be consulted. An antibiotic ointment is sometimes applied and an eye patch may be provided. If a foreign body is possibly inside the globe of the eye, X-rays may be taken. If an iritis is present, steroid drops (as well as special drops to dilate the pupil) may be used.

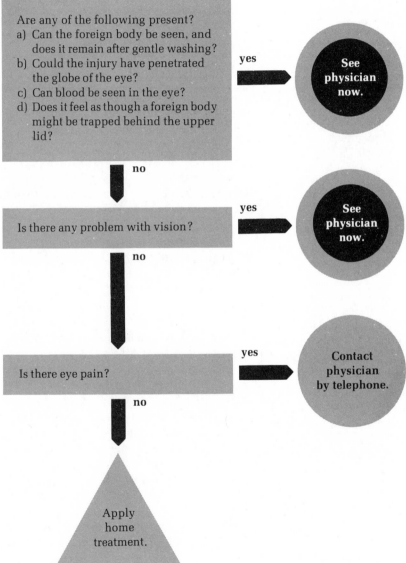

Are any of the following present?
a) Can the foreign body be seen, and does it remain after gentle washing?
b) Could the injury have penetrated the globe of the eye?
c) Can blood be seen in the eye?
d) Does it feel as though a foreign body might be trapped behind the upper lid?

yes → See physician now.

no

Is there any problem with vision?

yes → See physician now.

no

Is there eye pain?

yes → Contact physician by telephone.

no

Apply home treatment.

80
Styes and Blocked Tear Ducts

We might have called this problem "bumps around the eyes," since that is how they appear. Styes are infections (usually with staphylococcal bacteria) of the tiny glands in the eyelids. They are really small abscesses and the bumps are red and tender. They grow to full size over a day or so. Another type of bump in the eyelid called a chalazion appears more slowly over many days or even weeks and is not red or tender. A chalazion often requires drainage by a doctor, whereas most styes will respond to home treatment alone. However, there is no urgency to the treatment of a chalazion and home treatment will not cause any harm.

Tears are the lubricating system of the eye. They are continually produced by the tear glands and then drained away into the nose by the tear ducts. These tear ducts are often incompletely developed at birth so that the drainage of tears is blocked. When this happens, the tears may collect in the tear duct and cause it to swell, appearing as a bump along the side of the nose just below the inner corner of the eye (see figure). This bump is not red or tender unless it has become infected. Most blocked tear ducts will open by themselves in the first month of life and most of the remainder will respond to home treatment. Tears running down the cheek are seldom noted in the first month of life because the infant produces only a small volume of tears.

The eyeball itself is *not* involved in a stye or a blocked tear duct. Problems with the eyeball, and especially with vision, should not be attributed to these two relatively minor problems.

Home Treatment
Stye: Apply warm, moist compresses for ten to fifteen minutes at least three times a day. As with all abscesses, the objective is to drain the abscess. The compresses help the abscess to "point," which means that the tissue over the abscess becomes quite thin and the pus in the abscess is very close to the surface. After an abscess points, it often will drain spontaneously. If this does not happen, then it is ready to be lanced by the physician. Most styes will drain spontaneously; they may drain inwardly toward the eye or outwardly onto the skin. Sometimes the stye goes away without coming to a point and draining. Chalazions usually do not respond to warm compresses but neither will they be harmed. If no improvement is noted with home treatment after 48 hours, then see the doctor.

Blockage of the tear ducts: Simply massage the bump downward with warm, moist compresses several times a day. If the bump is not red and tender (indicating infection), this may be continued for up to several months. If the problem exists for this long, discuss it with your physician. If the bump becomes red and swollen, antibiotic drops will be needed.

What to Expect at the Doctor's Office
If the stye is pointing and ready to be drained, the physician will open it with a small needle. If it is not pointing, then compresses usually will be advised and antibiotic eyedrops sometimes will be added. Attempting to drain a stye that is not pointing is usually not very satisfactory. If the physician feels that the problem is a chalazion, then it may be removed with minor surgery. Whether to have the surgery will be up to you; chalazions are not dangerous and the operation may be disturbing to the child.

If the child is over six months of age and is still having problems with blocked tear ducts, they can be opened in almost all cases with a very fine probe. This probing is successful on the first try in about 75 percent of all cases and on subsequent attempts in the remainder. Only rarely is a surgical procedure necessary to establish an open tear duct. For red and swollen ducts, antibiotic drops as well as warm compresses usually will be recommended.

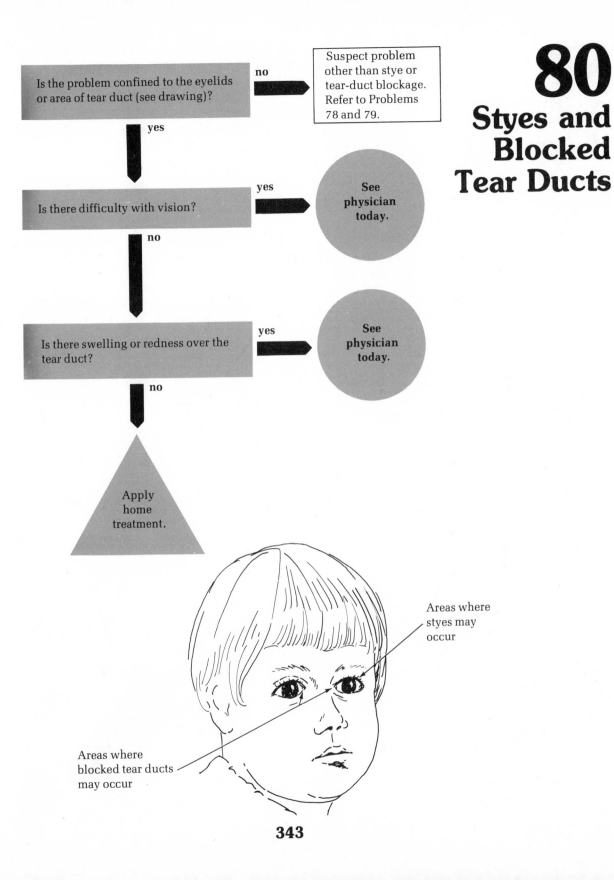

Is the problem confined to the eyelids or area of tear duct (see drawing)?

no → Suspect problem other than stye or tear-duct blockage. Refer to Problems 78 and 79.

yes ↓

Is there difficulty with vision?

yes → See physician today.

no ↓

Is there swelling or redness over the tear duct?

yes → See physician today.

no ↓

Apply home treatment.

Areas where styes may occur

Areas where blocked tear ducts may occur

81

Decreased Vision and Crossed Eyes

Although children can see at birth, the eye is not fully developed. The eye completes its development by about six months of age, and coordination between the two eyes is complete at about one year of age. It is difficult to determine how clearly the child sees (visual acuity) before the age of three or four. Problems with vision may be suggested by the child not reaching for objects or failing to follow a moving object with his or her eyes. Remember that the child's vision is still developing in the first months of life; do not be too quick in your judgment. Even in older children, significant problems with vision may not be detected without the use of eye tests, and eye tests are important for the school-age child.

Crossed eyes may be striking in the newborn child. This occurs simply because muscle coordination between the eyes is not yet fully developed; the problem usually corrects itself by the sixth month of life. If crossed eyes persist beyond this age, then you should discuss this at a regular checkup.

Strabismus is a problem of the eye muscles also known as "lazy eye"; one or both eyes may be involved. If the lazy eye is allowed to remain lazy, vision may be lost in that eye. Strabismus should be suspected in a child in which one or both eyes turn in or out after the age of four months. Ordinarily, a light shining from several feet in front of the child's eyes should reflect in the same location in each eye.

Fortunately, sudden loss of vision is less frequent in children than in adults. When it does occur, a quick trip to the doctor is obviously warranted.

An optometrist and ophthalmologist are often involved in the care of these problems. Before referral, however, you should have the opportunity to discuss the problem with your doctor; this may help sort out the problem and will result in a referral if necessary.

Home Treatment

Home treatment is reserved for children under the age of six months who have crossed eyes. This problem is usually present at birth and gets better as the child gets older. Full correction may take as long as a year. Home treatment consists merely of observation to make sure that the problem corrects itself. Crossed eyes occurring at any other age should be discussed with your physician.

What to Expect at the Doctor's Office

Visual acuity, eye movements, and pupils will be examined. With children too young to read, eyecharts with pictures are used. The physician will alternately cover each eye while asking the child to look at a distant object. Eye movement in a suddenly uncovered eye is a sign of strabismus. The inside of the eye will be examined with a hand-held instrument called an ophthalmoscope. A special kind of microscope, called a slit lamp, may be used to examine the front portion of the eye. If necessary, corrective lenses will be prescribed (this can be done even in very small children). Sometimes surgery will be required to correct crossed eyes, and will be necessary in occasional cases of decreased vision. Most often, strabismus will be treated with an eye patch. The younger the age at which this condition is detected, the better the chances for saving the vision in the eye. Make sure that your physician always checks for visual acuity while your child is young.

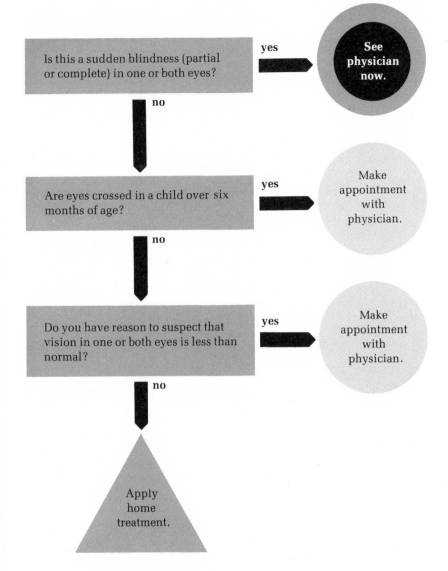

Is this a sudden blindness (partial or complete) in one or both eyes?

yes → See physician now.

no ↓

Are eyes crossed in a child over six months of age?

yes → Make appointment with physician.

no ↓

Do you have reason to suspect that vision in one or both eyes is less than normal?

yes → Make appointment with physician.

no ↓

Apply home treatment.

N

The Digestive Tract

82. Nausea/Vomiting   **348**
A little patience at first.

83. Diarrhea   **351**
Fluid loss and fluid replacement.

84. Acute Abdominal Pain   **354**
Every pain is not the appendix.

85. Recurrent Abdominal Pain   **356**
Common and not usually serious.

86. Colic   **358**
About three months of age.

87. Rectal Pain, Itching, or Bleeding   **360**
Pinworms and minor tears.

See also

66. Constipation and Soiling   **310**

82
Nausea/
Vomiting

Most newborns and infants will spit up a small amount of food after feeding. Even with proper belching, small amounts of vomitus can be expected at this age. Often, feeding with the child held at a 45-degree angle will be helpful. Persistent or violent vomiting or the failure to gain weight are signs that this may be more than simple spitting up. Fever is unusual in the newborn. If it is present along with vomiting, the child should be brought to the physician immediately.

Infants and toddlers will often vomit with viral infections of the gastrointestinal tract. When abdominal pain is present, parents are often concerned about the possibility of appendicitis or other serious abdominal problems. These are discussed further in Problem 84 (Acute Abdominal Pain).

With many gastrointestinal infections, diarrhea accompanies the vomiting. The younger the child, the more serious this combination can be. Children under six months of age can become dehydrated very easily, especially in the warm summer months or in the presence of a fever. If your child's eyes appear sunken, if the skin feels dry or wrinkles easily, if the urine output is scant or deep yellow, or if the mouth is dry, see the doctor immediately.

If vomiting is accompanied by flecks of blood in the stool (feces) and/or intermittent abdominal pain is present, intestinal blockage is possible and professional medical care is necessary.

In younger children, the possibility of accidental poisoning or medication intake should not be overlooked. In older children, excess alcohol ingestion can cause vomiting.

Hepatitis may begin with nausea and vomiting; often children with hepatitis will have dark urine. Yellow jaundice is not always present in hepatitis but abdominal tenderness over the liver (the upper right quarter of the abdomen underneath the rib cage) usually is. If you suspect hepatitis, a visit to the doctor is important.

Other members of the family can obtain gamma globulin shots, which will reduce the severity of the symptoms in the event that they come down with the disease.

Nausea and vomiting can also accompany urinary tract infections. Fever, problems with urination, and occasionally abdominal or back pain will also be present. See Problem 88 (Painful, Frequent, or Bloody Urination).

A serious infection that produces vomiting, and one that is fortunately not very common, is meningitis. This infection of the covering of the brain and spinal cord will also produce either irritability or lethargy, and fever is almost always present. In young children the soft spot (fontanel) will be bulging while older children will have a stiff neck that prevents them from touching their chin to their chest. Meningitis is a medical emergency that must be attended immediately.

Head injuries can cause vomiting and are discussed in further detail in Problem 10.

Excessive excitement or emotional stress can also cause vomiting in young children. Vomiting, when it accompanies headaches, may be a sign of migraine in children, discussed further in Problem 63 (Headache).

Nausea usually precedes or accompanies vomiting in children with mild gastrointestinal infections. Often, it occurs by itself, especially in children who have problems with motion sickness. Car sickness is aggravated by looking out the side windows of a moving vehicle, which forces the children to continuously focus on objects rapidly moving past them. The eye movements required bring about the car sickness.

Many medications can cause nausea. Remember also that if your child is taking a medication for another purpose, the vomiting will interfere with the absorption of the medicine. Call the doctor.

Home Treatment

Avoid solid foods. Frequent, small feedings of clear liquids should be given instead. A tablespoon of clear fluid every few minutes will usually stay down. Often, Popsicles or iced fruit

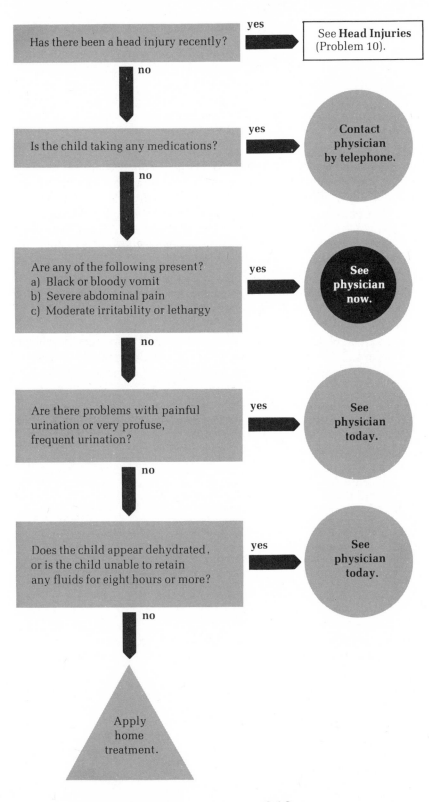

Has there been a head injury recently? — **yes** → See **Head Injuries** (Problem 10).

no

Is the child taking any medications? — **yes** → Contact physician by telephone.

no

Are any of the following present?
a) Black or bloody vomit
b) Severe abdominal pain
c) Moderate irritability or lethargy

yes → See physician now.

no

Are there problems with painful urination or very profuse, frequent urination? — **yes** → See physician today.

no

Does the child appear dehydrated, or is the child unable to retain any fluids for eight hours or more? — **yes** → See physician today.

no

Apply home treatment.

82
Nausea/
Vomiting

bars will work if nothing else will stay down. As the condition improves, larger amounts of fluids and then jello and applesauce may be given. Sometimes, sucking on hard candy or chewing ice chips helps.

What to Expect at the Doctor's Office
A history and physical examination will direct attention to whether the child is dehydrated and to the abdomen. With girls, a urinalysis will often be obtained. If a serious underlying condition is suspected, blood tests and abdominal X-rays will be ordered. For particularly severe vomiting some physicians may give trimetho- benzamide (Tigan) suppositories. These sup- positories are not recommended for treating uncomplicated vomiting. They should be used only for prolonged vomiting where the cause is known. The side effects of this drug include nervous system disturbances that may confuse a diagnostic evaluation. In addition, there is speculation that antivomiting drugs may con- tribute to the development of a serious illness known as Reyes syndrome. If dehydration is a problem, intravenous fluids and hospitalization may be required; this is more usual for children under the age of two. Some physicians will give intravenous fluid therapy in their offices.

Diarrhea is another common problem in children of all ages, although like constipation, it may be just a normal variation in bowel habits rather than a disease. Newborn infants who are exclusively breast-fed have more frequent and softer stools than bottle-fed infants do. Having more than a dozen of these soft stools a day is not uncommon, but despite the frequency, this is not diarrhea. Diarrhea in infants consists of a liquid, runny stool. In older children, two or three soft to runny stools a day may be considered a sign of diarrhea.

The most common cause is viral gastroenteritis. Often, there are other symptoms such as fever, runny nose, and fatigue. Like most viral infections, the problem should end in three to four days. The diarrhea is often accompanied by vomiting, which may aggravate the child's fluid losses. Because of this outpouring of fluids from both ends, it is crucial to maintain adequate hydration. Assessing dehydration is discussed on p. 141.

Diarrhea can also be caused at times by bacterial infections. The bacteria usually come from contaminated food or water, and can be particularly severe in infants. Profuse, watery diarrhea, especially accompanied with flecks of blood, should arouse a parent's suspicion of a bacterial infection.

The intestines respond to the presence of viruses and bacteria by increasing their movement. The intestines are trying to get rid of the infection and it is a natural defense mechanism of the body that produces the rapid, frequent bowel movements. There can be irritation of the lining of the intestines and some of the cells that produce enzymes necessary to digest food are temporarily damaged. Much of the ordinary digestive processes are hampered because the food does not remain long enough in the intestines to be digested.

Antibiotics, by altering the normal bacterial pattern in the intestines, often cause diarrhea. If this seems to be the case, the prescribing physician should be contacted.

Milk allergy is often blamed for diarrhea in children but is seldom the cause. If a milk allergy is suspected by you or your physician, it should be carefully documented.

Chronic diarrhea is unusual in children but when it occurs, it can be a serious problem. It requires professional medical care, especially when accompanied by weight loss.

Home Treatment

Management of diarrhea is entirely by dietary manipulation. All children have sufficient caloric reserve to withstand several days of no food intake. However, no child has sufficient *fluid* reserves to withstand several days of diarrhea without fluid intake.

Treatment of diarrhea begins with giving the child clear liquids. Products such as Gatorade or Pedialyte offer very little advantage over apple juice or flat sodas (yes, this is one time when we actually recommend the use of sodas). If the child seems to be tolerating the clear fluids, constipating foods such as bananas, rice, applesauce, and toast can be given. The first letters of the four previous words spell out "brat" and this is commonly referred to as the "brat diet." Milk should be avoided, since very often the enzyme lactase is lost during a bout of diarrhea; milk contains a great deal of lactose and cannot be digested properly. Fats should be avoided for several days, since they will not remain in the intestines long enough to be digested. Although there is

83
Diarrhea

no real evidence that the presence of undigested fat in the digestive tract is harmful, it does make the bowel movement smell badly. If the child is still having watery diarrhea after three days of clear liquid therapy, consult your physician by phone. Often, the recommendation will be to begin solid foods, since continuous liquid diets can also eventually result in diarrhea.

There are no medications that we consider safe and effective for use in children. The narcotic or narcoticlike preparations (paregoric, Parelixir, Lomotil) used by adults to control diarrhea should be avoided for children. The over-the-counter preparations such as Kao-Pectate, Kaolin, and Pectin will change the consistency of the stool from a liquid to a semisolid state but they will not reduce the amount or frequency of the bowel movements.

As soon as diarrhea begins, you may wish to protect the diaper area with petroleum jelly (Vaseline). If skin breakdown has occurred and sores are present, ointments should be avoided and efforts should be made to keep the diaper area as dry as possible.

What to Expect at the Doctor's Office
A thorough history and physical examination with special attention to assessing dehydration will be done. The abdomen will be examined. Frequently the stools will be examined under the microscope; occasionally a culture will be taken. A urine specimen may be examined to assist in assessing dehydration. In cases of bacterial infection an antibiotic may be given. Chronic diarrhea will require more extensive evaluation of the stools, blood tests, and often X-ray examinations of the intestinal tract.

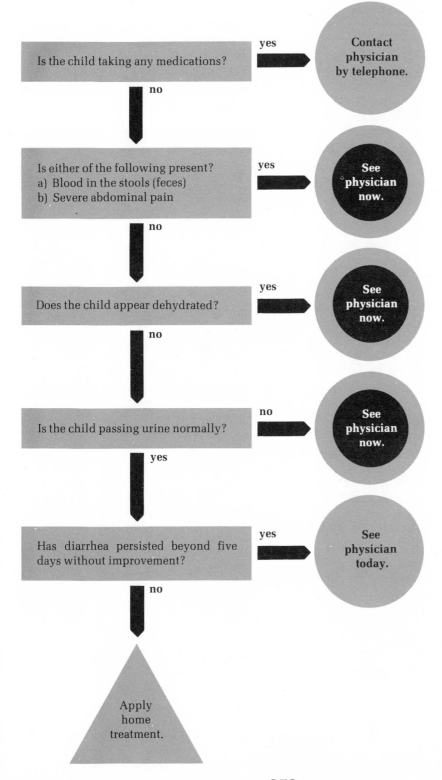

83
Diarrhea

Is the child taking any medications? — yes → Contact physician by telephone.

no ↓

Is either of the following present?
a) Blood in the stools (feces)
b) Severe abdominal pain — yes → See physician now.

no ↓

Does the child appear dehydrated? — yes → See physician now.

no ↓

Is the child passing urine normally? — no → See physician now.

yes ↓

Has diarrhea persisted beyond five days without improvement? — yes → See physician today.

no ↓

Apply home treatment.

84

Acute Abdominal Pain

Abdominal pain is one of the most common concerns of parents, and the causes for abdominal pain in children change with age of the child. During the first few months of life, colic is the most common cause and is discussed in Problem 86 (Colic).

As children become older, they often need to be reminded to have a bowel movement, and this will relieve their abdominal pain. Abdominal pain associated with vomiting and diarrhea is common with gastroenteritis or stomach flu. These problems are of greater concern in infants (see Problems 82 and 83) than in older children. Vomiting without diarrhea and especially without bowel movements is of concern because of the possibility of an obstructed or blocked intestine. Obstruction can also produce severe intermittent pain and especially violent vomiting. All these signs signal the need for a journey to the doctor. In older children, infections commonly produce abdominal pain, even though the infection itself may not be in the abdomen. Sore throats, ear infections, and excessive coughing from a cold can all cause bellyaches. Pneumonia can also cause abdominal pain, and is usually accompanied by a rapid breathing rate and fever. Hepatitis may cause abdominal pain (usually in the upper right corner of the abdomen) and is usually accompanied by nausea, vomiting, and sometimes yellow jaundice. Household members can be given potential protection from the symptoms of hepatitis by gamma globulin shots. Urinary tract infections can also be present with abdominal pain, along with discomfort or frequency in passing urine.

Appendicitis occurs less frequently than any of the problems discussed so far. While appendicitis most commonly occurs in young adults, it can occur at any age. The diagnosis of appendicitis is especially hard to make in toddlers, who cannot describe the problem but may look very sick. Older children may begin by complaining of pain in the center of the abdomen. In some, this pain will then move to the lower right part of the belly. Some children will have pain only in the lower right belly; about 20 percent will have pain elsewhere. There is usually fever, and often nausea and vomiting. Because of abdominal tenderness, children may rest with their right leg bent. Sometimes they will not bear weight on the right leg. The abdomen may be sensitive to touch. If these symptoms are present, see the doctor. If you are uncertain, waiting a few hours does not substantially increase the risk of the appendix bursting. However, waiting a long period of time (more than 12 hours) does increase the risk. Abdominal pain with unusual accompanying symptoms like joint pain and rash suggest rare illnesses like rheumatic fever and Henoch-Shonlein purpura, which require medical attention.

Ulcers are more common in adults but do occur in children. Vomiting dark material or blood should signal this as a possibility. Pain in the upper abdomen recurrent for many days needs a check.

Finally, do not overlook the possibility that your child may have swallowed some object or medicine. Always be careful with medicines and dangerous products.

Home Treatment

Watchful waiting in the first few hours is the best approach. For diarrhea, see Problem 83. For nausea and vomiting, see Problem 82. Small amounts of clear liquid can be given. Aspirin should not be given, but fever can be treated with acetaminophen if the child is uncomfortable from the fever. If pain and fever are the only problems, be sure to evaluate your child's appearance every few hours and do not hesitate to call the doctor for further advice.

What to Expect at the Doctor's Office

A thorough history and examination of ears, throat, chest, and abdomen will be made. A rectal examination will be done if appendicitis is suspected. Often a blood test and a urinalysis will also be performed. If intestinal obstruction is suspected, X-rays will be taken; they are not helpful in most cases of abdominal pain.

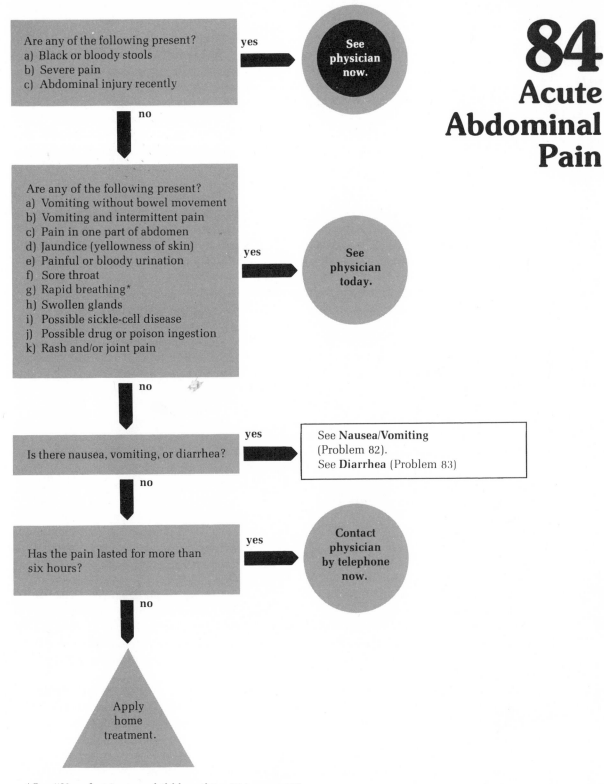

Are any of the following present?
a) Black or bloody stools
b) Severe pain
c) Abdominal injury recently

yes → See physician now.

no ↓

Are any of the following present?
a) Vomiting without bowel movement
b) Vomiting and intermittent pain
c) Pain in one part of abdomen
d) Jaundice (yellowness of skin)
e) Painful or bloody urination
f) Sore throat
g) Rapid breathing*
h) Swollen glands
i) Possible sickle-cell disease
j) Possible drug or poison ingestion
k) Rash and/or joint pain

yes → See physician today.

no ↓

Is there nausea, vomiting, or diarrhea?

yes → See **Nausea/Vomiting** (Problem 82).
See **Diarrhea** (Problem 83)

no ↓

Has the pain lasted for more than six hours?

yes → Contact physician by telephone now.

no ↓

Apply home treatment.

*See "How fast is your child breathing?" (on p. 142)

85
Recurrent Abdominal Pain

All children in the course of growing up will have a number of bouts of abdominal pain. As we have discussed in Problem 84 on acute abdominal pain, these symptoms are often related to respiratory tract infections, coughing, urinary tract infections, or stomach flu. When we refer to recurrent abdominal pain, we are talking about repeated bouts of abdominal pain for which no explanation is obvious. Somewhere between 10 and 20 percent of all children will complain of these recurrent problems.

In several studies, serious medical problems were found to be the underlying cause of pain in less than 10 percent of these children. The most common underlying medical problems were in the urinary tract. Children with medical problems often complained of pain in one particular corner of the abdomen, as opposed to diffuse or vague central abdominal pain. Some children lose the ability to digest milk as they get older. This can cause abdominal pain as well as a swelling of the belly.

The most common cause of abdominal pain in adults and children alike is stress. It is only natural for us to react to the environment in which we live. A bad day, the loss of a pet, or an argument with a friend would create stress in all of us. It is a common misconception that children's feelings are not as complex and sensitive as adults. Children become just as angry, anxious, and depressed as we do. Often, if children are permitted to talk about these feelings, the symptoms may not be as severe. Other children and adults when subjected to similar stresses may experience headaches. Stress can sometimes cause serious medical problems like ulcers; while ulcers are less common in children, they do occur.

Being subjected to numerous stresses is part of growing up. However, if abdominal pain, or any symptom for that matter, is interfering with the child's normal functioning in school, at home, or with friends, professional help should be sought.

Home Treatment

The home treatment for recurrent abdominal pain requires a common-sense approach. Care may include clear liquid feedings, some time in a hot tub, and some gentle rubbing of the belly. A child will often tell you what makes him or her feel better. In addition, an effort should be made to link the cause of the abdominal pain with the symptom. Talking with your child about what is going on in school and what may be upsetting him or her can often be profitable. Children sometimes exploit abdominal pain in order to get attention or get their own way. Your own judgment will guide you in these cases.

What to Expect at the Doctor's Office

The greatest amount of time and attention should be directed toward the medical history. A thorough physical examination should be performed, including examination of the head, chest, abdomen, and genitalia. A urinalysis and most likely an examination of the stool will be performed. Often an additional trip to the office can be avoided by arranging beforehand whether or not a stool specimen will be required. X-rays are necessary in only a few circumstances; do not expect them as part of the routine evaluation.

Is abdominal pain causing any of the
following?
a) School absenteeism
b) Disruption of family routines
c) Problems with friends

yes → Make appointment with physician.

no

Are any of the following present with
recurring episodes?
a) Fever
b) Severe pain
c) Pain localized other than around
   navel
d) Nausea, vomiting, diarrhea

yes → Make appointment with physician.

no

Have there been three or more bouts in
the past year?

yes → Contact physician by telephone.

no

Apply home treatment.

86
Colic

While colic is defined medically as "pain in the abdomen," the term colic is commonly used to mean a prolonged period of unexplained crying in infants. Abdominal pain is responsible for only some of these bouts of crying. The first episode of colic can be a disturbing experience. New babies seldom demonstrate colic symptoms while in the hospital, for several reasons. First of all, colic is very unusual within the first few days of life. Second, infants are often removed to the nursery if they are crying in the room. Once the child is home, the baby who had always seemed perfectly well behaved suddenly begins to scream. This usually occurs in the evening with both parents at home and neither is able to supply an explanation. Is the baby having terrible pain? What can you do if the baby can't tell you where it hurts? Is this an emergency? Does the baby just want to be fed? Often, neither feeding, changing, nor cuddling the infant provides comfort. Temporary relief may be found when the baby begins to suck on the fists or anything else available; often a bottle is eagerly accepted and then violently rejected. Given this insatiable crying, panic may ensue with frantic phone calls to the doctor or a frenzied trip to the emergency room. Sometimes before either of these courses of action has produced medical advice, the crying will stop, leaving the parents exhausted and baffled but thankful.

In most instances, the onset and resolution of this problem are not this dramatic. The baby simply has a crying spell that may last several hours during which nothing seems to be of comfort.

Typical colic has a number of features that usually make it easy to recognize. It begins after the second week of life and peaks at about three months of age. For this reason, it is sometimes called the "three-month" colic. Occurrences generally decrease rapidly after the age of three months. It would be unusual for colic to begin after three months of age.

Colic usually occurs in the evening. Some have postulated that the increased activity in the home during the evening hours may contribute to the colic. Parents' tolerance of such activity also is far less in the evening hours when both may be fatigued and a colicky baby can be of great concern. The attack occasionally ends with a passage of gas or stool, and "gas" is often blamed for the problem. We feel that colic is caused by gas problems in some infants, but not the majority of them.

The baby will seem perfectly well before and after these attacks and there should be no fever, vomiting, or diarrhea. Repeated episodes are the rule and may occur with great regularity at the same time each day. Some feel that colic is not related to abdominal pain at all, but is merely a characteristic that is part of the normal development of some children. While all children cry, some seem to cry longer and are more difficult to console than others. Colic can be better appreciated by a reading of the section on crying (see pp. 64–65).

Home Treatment

Colic has been treated in many ways, all of which work some of the time and none of which work all of the time. This leads us to believe that most of the time the problem cures itself and probably requires no treatment. With true colic, there is no reason for any medication to be given to the child. Parents have found that cuddling, rocking, soothing music, walking with the baby, wrapping a child snuggly, soothing talk, pacifiers, backrubs, and placing the baby on his or her stomach are sometimes effective. Many home remedies include giving a small amount of an alcoholic beverage. This makes some sense, for alcoholic beverages are sedatives and may relieve spasms of the intestines. However, we discourage relying on alcohol, or any other drug for that matter, for the relief of any but the most disturbing symptoms. Another popular home remedy is an ounce or two of warm, weak tea. Tea seems more likely to stimulate the bowel than to put it to rest, but occasionally it may provide relief.

While colic is terribly frustrating for parents to deal with, you can take heart in knowing that your child will outgrow this stage in a few

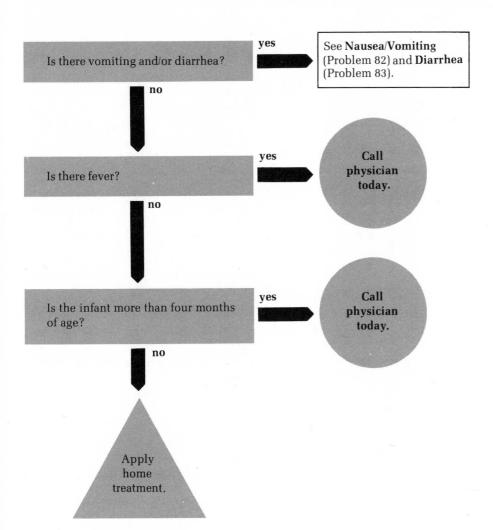

Is there vomiting and/or diarrhea? — **yes** → See **Nausea/Vomiting** (Problem 82) and **Diarrhea** (Problem 83).

no

Is there fever? — **yes** → Call physician today.

no

Is the infant more than four months of age? — **yes** → Call physician today.

no

Apply home treatment.

months. If any one attack persists beyond four hours, give the physician a call. If the attacks do not seem to be diminishing by four months of age, discuss them during a regular physician visit.

What to Expect at the Doctor's Office

If the visit is made for a single long-lasting attack, a thorough physical examination will be performed to see if there is a reason for the crying other than the colic. Particular attention will be given to ears, throat, chest, and abdomen.

If the visit is made for attacks that seem to be colic but are still occurring after four months of age, a careful history and physical examination will be performed. Most often the diagnosis will be colic that is lasting longer than usual, and a policy of watching and waiting with perhaps a dietary change may be recommended. It is very rare for serious medical problems to be present.

87
Rectal Pain, Itching, or Bleeding

Rectal bleeding is not a very common problem in children. It is most often seen during a diaper change when a few streaks of blood are noticed, usually on the surface of the stool. In newborn infants, this is most often due to a tiny tear in the rectum. This tear will usually heal by itself so long as the stools are not hard. In older infants and children, rectal bleeding is usually due to constipation, and is discussed in Problem 66.

If abdominal pain accompanies rectal bleeding, this may be a sign of a blocked intestine or a bacterial gastroenteritis; both of these require medical attention quickly.

Often a child will suddenly awaken crying in the early evening with rectal pain; there may be intense itching as well. This almost always means pinworms. Though these small worms are seldom seen, they are quite common. They live in the rectum, and the female emerges at night and secretes a sticky and irritating substance around the anus into which she lays her eggs. Occasionally the worms move into the vagina, causing pain and itching in that area. The scratching can lead to vaginal infections in girls.

You can confirm the diagnosis of pinworms by checking for them with a flashlight several hours after the child's bedtime. They are about one quarter inch long and look like white threads. While infestations with pinworms often resolve without medication, several prescription drugs that kill the pinworms will speed the process.

Home Treatment
If rectal bleeding is due to constipation, the stool should be softened. This can be accomplished by including more fruit (especially prunes or prune juice), fiber (bran, celery, whole wheat bread), and fluids in the diet. Seldom are over-the-counter laxatives (Colace, Metamucil, Maltsupex) necessary.

Temporary relief of itching may be accomplished by giving aspirin or acetaminophen. If itching is present in girls, good hygiene and tub baths will help avoid vaginal infections.

What to Expect at the Doctor's Office
Through an examination of the anus and rectum, small tears and fissures can easily be detected. Seldom are pinworms noticeable during the day. If you have seen them at night, the doctor may rely on your observation. Often, you may be asked to remove some of the pinworms with a piece of scotch tape and bring them in for evaluation. After you have collected the pinworms, fold the scotch tape over so that only the nonsticking surface is exposed. Even if you don't see the pinworms, the scotch tape applied to the area around the anus that is itching will collect the eggs, which can be identified under the microscope. Pinworms will usually be treated with one of several effective oral drugs. Treatment of the entire family is often necessary.

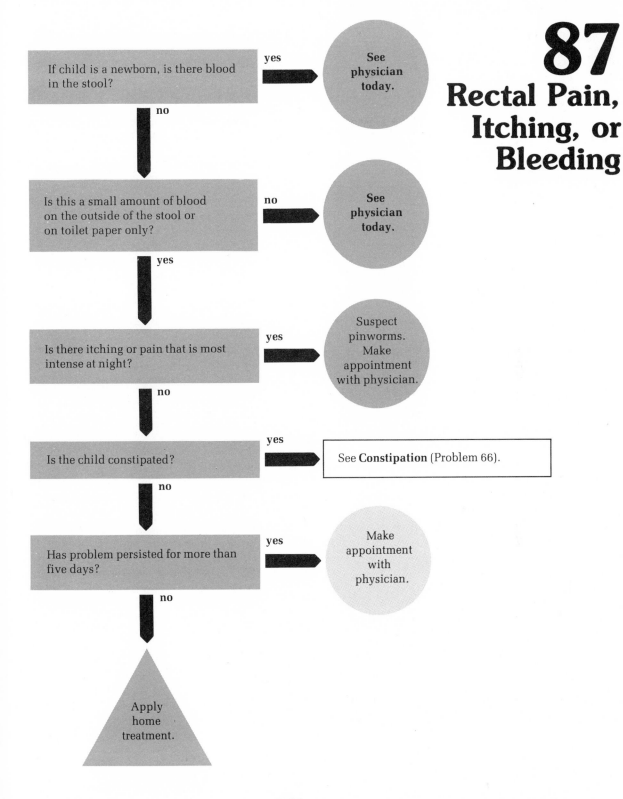

If child is a newborn, is there blood in the stool? — **yes** → See physician today.

no ↓

Is this a small amount of blood on the outside of the stool or on toilet paper only? — **no** → See physician today.

yes ↓

Is there itching or pain that is most intense at night? — **yes** → Suspect pinworms. Make appointment with physician.

no ↓

Is the child constipated? — **yes** → See **Constipation** (Problem 66).

no ↓

Has problem persisted for more than five days? — **yes** → Make appointment with physician.

no ↓

Apply home treatment.

O

The Urinary Tract

88. Painful, Frequent, or Bloody Urination　　　**364**
Usually a bladder infection.

See also

65. Bedwetting　　　**308**

88
Painful, Frequent, or Bloody Urination

These symptoms, usually indicating a bladder infection, are much more common in girls than in boys. In addition, many girls have episodes of frequency or burning on urination in which there is no infection, but only irritation of the end portion of the urethra, characterized by frequent passage of small amounts of urine. Chemical irritants such as bubble baths have been incriminated in these outside irritations of the urethra (urethritis). Both boys and girls are susceptible to urethral irritation from trauma, chronic itching from pinworms, or from masturbation.

Boys seldom have episodes of painful or frequent urination, but those that occur are more likely to be related to an infection. Sometimes infections involve not only the lower urinary tract (urethra and the bladder), but the kidneys as well. With a kidney infection, the child is likely to appear much more ill, fever is significant, and there may be nausea and vomiting, abdominal pain, back pain, or true shaking chills.

Blood in the urine can mean a problem with the bladder or the kidneys and the child should always be brought to the doctor. This can be a sign of infection or kidney stone or it can be due to injury.

The resumption of bedwetting in a previously dry child may provide a clue to a urinary tract infection (see Problem 65). If there is a fever and the bedwetting is not accompanied by any other stressful psychologic event, a urinary tract infection should be suspected.

Not uncommonly a complaint of burning on urination is accompanied by a vaginal discharge in girls. In these instances, it is likely that the vaginal irritation has involved the urethra or urinary opening. If the doctor has investigated this problem before, then following the treatment recommended by the doctor is advisable. This may include using vaginal suppositories or soaking in a bath with vinegar added.

Home Treatment
Home treatment is useful in relieving symptoms but not in eliminating infection. All new episodes of urinary burning, frequency, pain, or blood should be investigated by a physician. Drinking lots of liquids helps. Cranberry juice is better than some drinks because it contains a chemical known as quinic acid, which is transformed in the body to another chemical having antibacterial properties. However, cranberry juice does *not* provide enough of these chemicals to make it a reliable therapy. It is *not* adequate treatment for a bacterial infection. Aspirin and acetaminophen may help relieve pain. If a vaginal discharge is present, see Problem 89.

What to Expect at the Doctor's Office
The physician will perform a urinalysis and examine the back, the abdomen, the vaginal opening, and the urinary opening or urethra. The urinalysis may indicate the need for a urine culture and/or antibiotics. Sulfisoxazole (Gantrisin) and ampicillin are often prescribed. Pyridium, a medication that is helpful in relieving urethral pain, is sometimes prescribed. If there is an infection present, then X-rays of the kidney may be ordered; X-rays demonstrating damaged kidneys suggest the need for a longer course of antibiotics. Do not be surprised or discouraged if your child has a second urinary tract infection. Eighty percent of children with one infection will develop a second, but very few will have long-term problems.

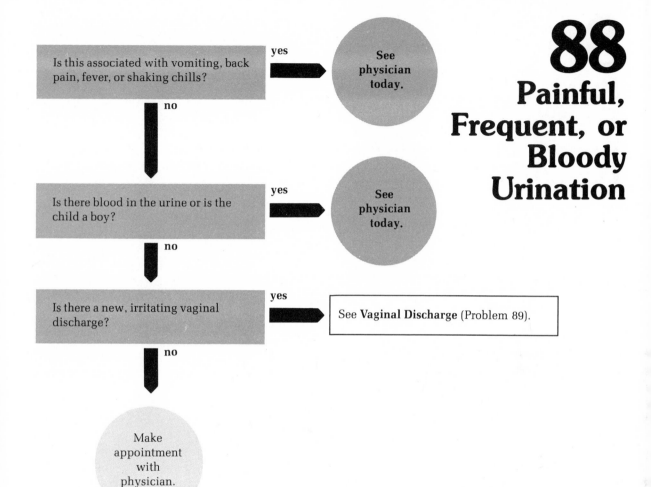

Is this associated with vomiting, back pain, fever, or shaking chills?

yes → See physician today.

no ↓

Is there blood in the urine or is the child a boy?

yes → See physician today.

no ↓

Is there a new, irritating vaginal discharge?

yes → See **Vaginal Discharge** (Problem 89).

no ↓

Make appointment with physician.

P

The Genitals

89. Vaginal Discharge   **368**
Good hygiene is important for girls.

90. Problems with the Penis   **370**
And for boys, too.

91. Vaginal Bleeding and Menstrual Problems   **372**
Understanding natural processes.

89
Vaginal Discharge

Doctors usually use the term discharge to mean something abnormal and this can be confusing. Girls have vaginal secretions (discharges) that are normal, although the amount is much less than an adult's. Adult hormones increase the amount of secreted material; children have naturally increased amounts of secretions in two situations. The first is in the newborn baby during the first week of life. Often there is some vaginal discharge or bleeding during this time due to stimulation by the mother's adult hormones. After these first two weeks, the child will have only a small amount of clear secretions until about one year before the onset of menstrual periods. At this time, the girl begins to make her own adult hormones; the amount of secretion increases and the secretions become thicker. These normal secretions are sometimes called a "normal discharge." Some secretion is normal in mid-cycle after menstruation has begun.

Poor hygiene may contribute to vaginal discharges in children. Scratching in the genital region often accompanies the rectal itching common with pinworms and can lead to a vaginal infection; pinworms occasionally reach the vagina and cause itching directly as well. Another cause of abnormal discharges in girls is a yeast infection (Candida), just as in adults. Yeast infections are likely when a child is taking an antibiotic. Other causes of discharges in children are unusual in women. Just as children stick things in their ears and noses, they may also put foreign objects in the vagina. This may lead to a bacterial infection and a discharge with a particularly bad smell. A forgotten tampon can cause the same reaction. Sand and toilet paper particles can also lead to infection and discharge. For this reason we recommend that girls be taught to wipe with toilet tissue from front to back, rather than back to front. Sometimes the chemical irritation of bubble baths will begin an itch-scratch-infection cycle.

Gonorrhea can occur at any age, although it is uncommon in younger children. In judging whether venereal disease is possible, it is important not to jump to conclusions in either direction. This is an area in which your physician can be of great help.

Home Treatment
Frequently, attention to the hygiene of the outside genital structures will be sufficient to clear the discharge. Gentle washing with soap and water, as well as warm baths, are helpful. Eliminate bubble baths if they had been used. If you suspect a foreign object in the vagina, it is possible to look for yourself. This can be accomplished by having your child lie with her chest on the ground or a table while she is on her knees. In a moment or two the vaginal opening will relax enough for you to see inside; a flashlight will help.

Yeast do not grow well in an acid environment and minor infections often respond to vinegar (3% acetic acid) sitz baths. Fill the tub with enough water to cover the child's bottom and then add one cup of white vinegar. Soak for at least 15 minutes and do this twice a day if possible. This will often clear up the problem and vaginal suppositories can be avoided. If the problem does not improve within five days, then make an appointment with the doctor.

What to Expect at the Doctor's Office
The abdomen and outside of the vagina (vulva) will be examined. The discharge will be looked at under a microscope. In adolescents, a pelvic examination may be needed. In younger children, this will be avoided if possible. If the outside of the vagina is very irritated, then an antifungal cream or ointment (Mycolog, Candeptin) may be used. If the infection inside the vagina is severe, then vaginal creams or vaginal suppositories may be prescribed. If gonorrhea is detected, then antibiotics, most often by injection, are required.

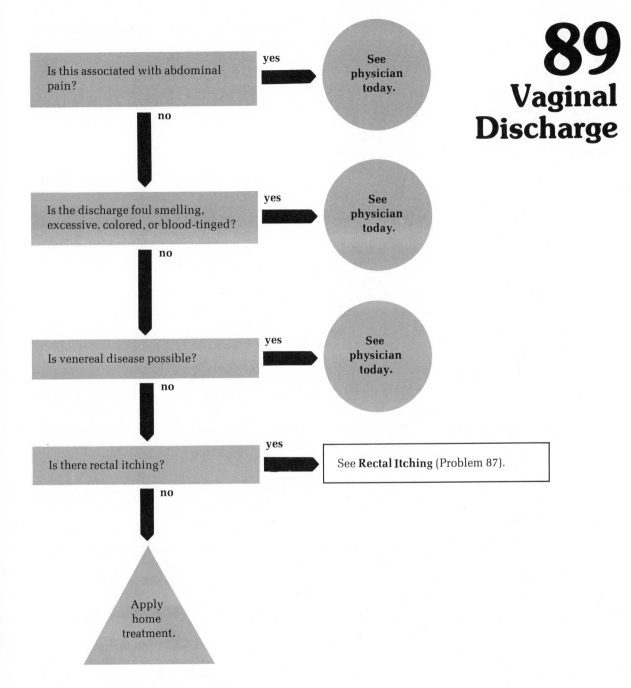

Is this associated with abdominal pain?

yes → See physician today.

no ↓

Is the discharge foul smelling, excessive, colored, or blood-tinged?

yes → See physician today.

no ↓

Is venereal disease possible?

yes → See physician today.

no ↓

Is there rectal itching?

yes → See **Rectal Itching** (Problem 87).

no ↓

Apply home treatment.

90
Problems with the Penis

Skin oils and secretions tend to accumulate underneath the foreskin of the uncircumcised penis, and this accumulation may cause irritation and may lead to infection. With a severe infection the foreskin may swell and prevent the passage of urine. To avoid these problems, parents must begin a program of foreskin hygiene. The foreskin in very young infants cannot be pulled back, but by the end of the first year it should move freely. Parents should begin to pull the foreskin back and carefully wash the area as a part of every infant's bath. Return the foreskin to its normal position after washing. As the child becomes older, this should become a part of his bath routine as well. Sometimes the foreskin is so tight that it cannot be pulled back; this problem requires the help of the doctor. If the foreskin is retracted and cannot be returned to its former position, the blood supply to the end of the penis may be impaired; this problem requires the prompt attention of the doctor.

Discharges from the urinary opening of the penis are rare before adolescence, but at any age they require the help of the physician. Sometimes an infection under the foreskin will produce enough pus so that there appears to be a discharge. If this is the case, the infection is bad enough to need the help of your physician. For minor irritation underneath the foreskin, use home treatment.

Another common problem is getting the skin of the penis caught in a zipper. This most often occurs when parents are in a hurry to zip up a younger child. Little boys seldom zip fast enough to cause this problem themselves.

Home Treatment
Careful cleaning of the area under the foreskin is essential. This is most easily accomplished with a gentle washcloth dipped in warm water. Remember to put the foreskin back in its normal position after washing. Soaking in a warm tub is also useful with foreskin problems.

What to Expect at the Doctor's Office
If the foreskin is pulled back and restricting blood flow to the end of the penis, treatment usually will consist of cold compresses and certain medications. Rarely, a minor surgical procedure will be necessary to relieve the constriction. If the foreskin is so tight that it cannot be pulled back, then it will be stretched and you will be instructed in a method of stretching the foreskin. This is a gradual process and requires some time. Circumcision is almost never necessary in dealing with foreskin problems.

If a discharge is present, it will be examined under the microscope. A culture will most likely be taken. Boys have been known to put foreign objects inside of their penis; this can be a cause of infection. Most discharges do not indicate gonorrhea, but gonorrhea can occur at any age. If gonorrhea is detected, it will require an antibiotic, which will most likely be given by injection.

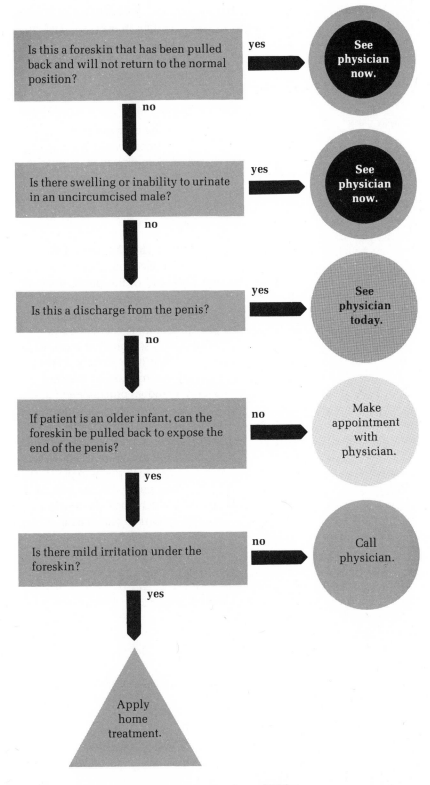

Is this a foreskin that has been pulled back and will not return to the normal position?

yes → **See physician now.**

no ↓

Is there swelling or inability to urinate in an uncircumcised male?

yes → **See physician now.**

no ↓

Is this a discharge from the penis?

yes → **See physician today.**

no ↓

If patient is an older infant, can the foreskin be pulled back to expose the end of the penis?

no → Make appointment with physician.

yes ↓

Is there mild irritation under the foreskin?

no → Call physician.

yes ↓

Apply home treatment.

91
Vaginal Bleeding and Menstrual Problems

There are a number of "problems" in this area that are really normal; however, they often concern parents and their daughters and can lead to unnecessary anxiety and avoidable trips to the doctor.

New parents are sometimes shocked to find blood coming from the vagina in the first two weeks of life. This bleeding is due to stimulation of the baby's uterus by the mother's hormones during pregnancy. When a baby is born, she is no longer exposed to these hormones and what amounts to a small menstrual period follows. This is essentially the same series of events that will cause her own periods later in life when she produces her own adult hormones. Do not be concerned about some vaginal bleeding in the first two weeks of life.

The normal time for the first menstrual period is quite variable. We have chosen the ages of 9 and 16 as the limits for this range; some feel that it should be extended to between ages 8 and 18. While a problem will probably not be found, we feel that a visit to the physician is indicated if periods begin before the age of 9 or have not begun by age 16. After periods do begin, the cycles are seldom regular for the first two years. The amount of flow also tends to vary widely, and these variations usually last for the first several years after periods begin. During this time, the help of the doctor is needed only if the periods are extremely heavy, frequent, prolonged, or have stopped altogether for more than four months.

Young women who have had several years of regular periods will often experience missed periods. Stress and pregnancy are the most common causes for missed periods. An emotionally upsetting experience is often the cause of missed periods. Missed periods can accompany rapid weight loss during crash diets. Severe illnesses can also be a cause of missed periods. Certainly, pregnancy must be considered in a sexually active adolescent who is not practicing birth control. If periods have previously been regular and one is missed, the possibility of pregnancy must be considered.

Approximately 15 percent of all women complain of some form of premenstrual tension. Included in this category are headaches, irritability, abdominal bloating, breast tenderness, and thirst. These changes are most likely due to the fluid shifts in the body brought about by changes in the hormone cycle. Approximately five percent experience *dysmenorrhea,* or severe pain during menstruation; these symptoms most often begin during the first few years of the menstrual cycles. These crampy lower abdominal and back pains usually begin shortly before the onset of the period and last for about 24 hours. Occasionally the pain may begin two days before the period and may last up to a total of about four days. Less than five percent of the women with this problem have any abnormality of their reproductive system.

Home Treatment

If the problem is irregularity alone, then no treatment is necessary other than reassuring your daughter that this is normal for the first few years and even after. An occasional heavy period may be helped by bedrest to decrease the amount of flow. Menstrual cramps may be helped by a heating pad on the abdomen and a pain reliever such as aspirin. If menstrual symptoms are accompanied by a feeling of bloating, salt restriction for several days before the expected period may be helpful.

What to Expect at the Doctor's Office

The physical examination may include a pelvic examination. A Pap smear and a pregnancy test may be needed on occasion. If the girl is 16 years or more and has never had a period, then tests of the blood and urine may be done; these tests may also be done if periods have started but have now stopped. In some situations, the doctor may elect to give hormones (by mouth or by injection) to see if a period can be begun. These hormones should never be given unless a pregnancy test is known to be negative. For

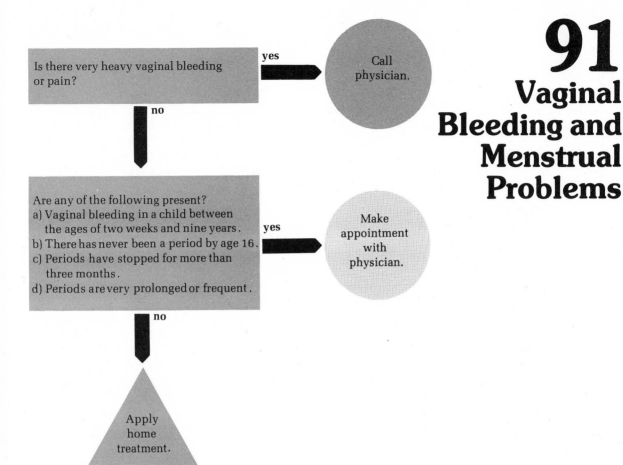

Is there very heavy vaginal bleeding or pain?

yes → Call physician.

no ↓

Are any of the following present?
a) Vaginal bleeding in a child between the ages of two weeks and nine years.
b) There has never been a period by age 16.
c) Periods have stopped for more than three months.
d) Periods are very prolonged or frequent.

yes → Make appointment with physician.

no ↓

Apply home treatment.

extremely heavy, prolonged, or frequent periods, blood tests to evaluate endocrine problems will probably be done. If the problem is one of painful and heavy periods, then hormones (most often birth control pills) may be given. Because of the risks of birth control pills, we feel adolescents should decide whether the symptoms they are experiencing are sufficiently incapacitating to warrant the use of potentially hazardous drugs.

Evaluation of periods beginning in children under the age of nine is usually quite extensive and will include evaluation of hormones (pituitary, thyroid, and ovarian) as well as X-rays. A thorough history and physical examination will be done and questions will be asked to determine if it was possible that the child may have taken some of her mother's birth control pills or other hormones.

Q
Contraception

The moral implications of sexual activity during adolescence are not traditionally the concern of the physician, although they raise many concerns with the parents and with the young adult. However, the mental and physical health of adolescents can be affected by an unwarranted pregnancy and requires discussion of contraception. An unwanted pregnancy will impose a severe psychological strain on at least one young person. More likely, it will affect another young person and his family as well. An unwanted child can be a tragedy of major proportions. Finally, the risk of pregnancy to the life and health of a young girl is greater than the risk of contraception to prevent that pregnancy.

Contraception methods vary in risk to the user, in effectiveness in preventing pregnancy, and in convenience. Methods that are most effective unfortunately tend to have the highest risks. Methods that pose little risk, such as diaphragms or condoms, are somewhat less effective. Some lack of effectiveness of these methods is largely due to inconvenience or aesthetic considerations so that they are used improperly or not at all. The amount of preparation required is especially important to teenagers. Sexual encounters at these ages often occur at erratic intervals and are unplanned. Some adolescents (and adults) do not always have strong motivation toward planning and control, especially when lovemaking has begun.

Several methods of birth control are particularly likely to fail and are not recommended. Coitus interruptus, the withdrawal of the penis just before ejaculation, is not totally effective even when practiced faithfully, and the practice can be emotionally difficult. The same thing may be said of douching immediately after intercourse. The rhythm method requires fairly regular menstrual cycles, which are often lacking in adolescence, and is often ineffective. In reality, the only advantage of these three methods is their lack of side effects and, for some, their religious acceptability.

Foams, jellies, creams, and suppositories that kill or inhibit sperm are only slightly more effective, when used without a diaphragm. There are essentially no side effects, but these methods are effective for only about 60 minutes after insertion. Many people find that these preparations are inconvenient or just plain messy. Their cost may represent a significant expense for an adolescent.

Condoms have a good deal to recommend them. If used correctly, they are 97% effective. There are no side effects, they are inexpensive and widely available, and they give some protection against venereal disease. The problem is that they don't work if they are in the wallet or on the drugstore shelf during intercourse and that's where they often are. For the male, some loss of sensation occurs. Condoms are sometimes used to help the problem of premature ejaculation because of this loss of sensation.

A diaphragm plus jelly is a compromise that is acceptable to some. It is effective in preventing pregnancy, although not as effective as birth control pills or intrauterine devices (IUD's) are. Protection lasts for twelve hours or so after insertion. It requires that intercourse be anticipated; this can be a problem. The diaphragm must be worn for several hours following intercourse as well. There are no side effects or complications of diaphragms and we highly recommend them. Diaphragms must be individually fitted.

An IUD must be inserted by a physician but requires no preparation at the time of intercourse. The IUD can be expelled from the uterus. It may also cause bleeding and cramps. It can be difficult to insert into the uterus. And there are recent reports that a particular kind of IUD (Dalkon Shield) has been the apparent cause of severe and even fatal infections. This particular type of IUD is no longer used, but these complications might be seen rarely with other types. The IUD may be expelled but the expulsion not noticed. Pregnancy can occur with the IUD in place and tubal pregnancies are more common in patients with an IUD.

Birth control pills are a frequent choice for contraception because they are the most effective means of preventing pregnancy, *if taken properly,* and because they do not require any thought at the time of intercourse. Obviously their use requires that a physician write a prescription (usually an examination is performed as well), and the patient must remember to take the pill daily. If taken regularly, protection against pregnancy is essentially complete. The risks of birth control pills are significant. They may cause blood clots and these clots have been fatal on occasion. They may cause or contribute to high blood pressure. There are many less dangerous side effects: weight gain, nausea, fluid retention, migraine headaches, vaginal bleeding, and yeast infections of the vagina. Some of the side effects can be eliminated by changing the composition of the ingredients. Most birth control pills contain combinations of two hormones: progestin and estrogen. The "mini-pill" is a progestin-only pill. It is nearly as effective as regular birth control pills but usually menstrual periods stop. The cessation of menstruation usually creates the need for periodic pregnancy testing

TABLE 1

Number of pregnancies expected for 100 women using contraceptive methods in a year. (The "average experience" group includes women who were using the method inconsistently or incorrectly.)

	Used correctly	Average experience
Birth control pills	0.340	4–10
Condoms and foam	1	5
IUD	1–3	5
Condom	3	10
Diaphragm and foam	3	17
Foam	3	22
Coitus interruptus	9	20–25
Rhythm	13	21
No protection	90	90
Douche	?	40

Source: Robert A. Hatcher, Gary K. Stewart, Felicia Guest, et al., *Contraceptive Technology, 1976–1977*. New York: Irvington, 1976. Reprinted by permission.

to see if the user is pregnant. The expense in obtaining the pills may be significant.

How safe are birth control pills and IUD's? It is impossible to predict a specific risk for a particular patient. The best information available simply boils down to this: The risk of either of these two methods is less than the risk of not using them if sexual activity is anything more than very occasional. Table 2 demonstrates the relative risks of various contraceptive methods.

Where to get reliable advice about sex and contraception is sometimes a problem. Even though the family physician or pediatrician will maintain confidentiality, embarrassment is common. Planned Parenthood clinics or public health clinics are alternatives. Planned Parenthood clinics provide competent sex advice in general and contraceptive advice in particular, as well as provide the physician services necessary for diaphragms, IUD's, and birth control pills. They do so in an atmosphere that is nonjudgmental and supportive. The teenager is often more comfortable in such an atmosphere than at the office of the family physician. Emergency rooms and walk-in clinics are not good places for this type of help.

TABLE 2

RISKS OF PREGNANCY VERSUS CONTRACEPTIVES

	Deaths per 100,000 women
Pregnancy	16
Oral contraceptive users	0.3–3
Mechanical methods (death resulting from 20 percent becoming pregnant)	3
Mechanical methods and abortion for pregnancy	0.6
Unprotected intercourse and abortion	2.6

Source: Robert A. Hatcher, Gary K. Stewart, Felicia Guest et al., *Contraceptive Technology, 1976–1977.* New York: Irvington, 1976. Reprinted by permission.

Part

III

Family Records

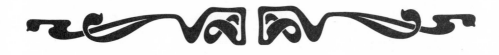

Name_____

Birth Information

Date _____ Weight _____ Mother's age _____ Length of pregnancy _____
Complications _____
_____

Medical History

	Date	Illness
Hospitalizations	_____	_____
Other medical problems (Include serious illness or injury, hearing or vision problem, positive TB test, etc.)	_____	_____
	_____	_____
	_____	_____
	_____	_____

Allergies

Medicines _____
Other _____

Family Medical History

Allergy _____   High blood pressure _____

Asthma _____   Tuberculosis _____

Diabetes _____   Other _____

Immunizations

	Date			Date
2 months			*18 months*	
DTP #1	_____		DTP booster	_____
Polio #1	_____		Polio booster	_____
4 months			*4–6 years*	
DTP #2	_____		DT booster	_____
Polio #2	_____		Polio booster	_____
6 months			*10–12 years*	
DTP #3	_____		Rubella*	_____
Polio #3	_____			
15 months				
Measles	_____			

* This vaccine should be given only to girls whose blood test shows that they do not already have immunity to rubella.

DPT = Diphtheria, pertussis (whooping cough), and tetanus (lockjaw)
DT = Diphtheria and tetanus (lockjaw)
Polio = Oral polio

Measles = Measles vaccine
Rubella = German measles (three-day measles

Note: Diphtheria and Tetanus is recommended every 10 years for life, with an additional tetanus booster for contaminated wounds more than 5 years after the last booster.

Name _____

Birth Information

Date _____ Weight _____ Mother's age _____ Length of pregnancy _____

Complications _____

_____

Medical History

	Date	Illness
Hospitalizations	_____	_____
Other medical problems (Include serious illness or injury, hearing or vision problem, positive TB test, etc.)	_____	_____
	_____	_____
	_____	_____
	_____	_____

Allergies

Medicines _____

Other _____

Family Medical History

Allergy _____	High blood pressure _____
Asthma _____	Tuberculosis _____
Diabetes _____	Other _____

Immunizations

	Date			Date
2 months DTP #1	_____		*18 months* DTP booster	_____
Polio #1	_____		Polio booster	_____
4 months DTP #2	_____		*4–6 years* DT booster	_____
Polio #2	_____		Polio booster	_____
6 months DTP #3	_____		*10–12 years* Rubella*	_____
Polio #3	_____			
15 months Measles	_____			

* This vaccine should be given only to girls whose blood test shows that they do not already have immunity to rubella.

DPT = Diphtheria, pertussis (whooping cough), and tetanus (lockjaw)

DT = Diphtheria and tetanus (lockjaw)

Polio = Oral polio

Measles = Measles vaccine

Rubella = German measles (three-day measles

Note: Diphtheria and Tetanus is recommended every 10 years for life, with an additional tetanus booster for contaminated wounds more than 5 years after the last booster.

Name_____

Birth Information

Date _____ Weight _____ Mother's age _____ Length of pregnancy _____
Complications _____
_____

Medical History

	Date	Illness
Hospitalizations	_____	_____
Other medical problems (Include serious illness or injury, hearing or vision problem, positive TB test, etc.)	_____	_____
	_____	_____
	_____	_____

Allergies

Medicines _____
Other _____

Family Medical History

Allergy _____   High blood pressure _____

Asthma _____   Tuberculosis _____

Diabetes _____   Other _____

Immunizations

2 months	Date	18 months	Date
DTP #1	_____	DTP booster	_____
Polio #1	_____	Polio booster	_____
4 months		**4–6 years**	
DTP #2	_____	DT booster	_____
Polio #2	_____	Polio booster	_____
6 months		**10–12 years**	
DTP #3	_____	Rubella*	_____
Polio #3	_____		
15 months			
Measles	_____		

* This vaccine should be given only to girls whose blood test shows that they do not already have immunity to rubella.

DPT = Diphtheria, pertussis (whooping cough), and tetanus (lockjaw)
DT = Diphtheria and tetanus (lockjaw)
Polio = Oral polio

Measles = Measles vaccine
Rubella = German measles (three-day measles

Note: Diphtheria and Tetanus is recommended every 10 years for life, with an additional tetanus booster for contaminated wounds more than 5 years after the last booster.

Name_____

Birth Information

Date _____ Weight _____ Mother's age _____ Length of pregnancy _____
Complications _____

_____

Medical History   Date   Illness

Hospitalizations   _____   _____

Other medical problems   _____   _____
(Include serious ill-
ness or injury, hear-   _____   _____
ing or vision problem,
positive TB test, etc.)   _____   _____

   _____   _____

Allergies

Medicines _____

Other _____

Family Medical History

Allergy _____   High blood pressure _____

Asthma _____   Tuberculosis _____

Diabetes _____   Other _____

Immunizations Date		Date
2 months		18 months
DTP #1 _____		DTP booster _____
Polio #1 _____		Polio booster _____
4 months		4–6 years
DTP #2 _____		DT booster _____
Polio #2 _____		Polio booster _____
6 months		10–12 years
DTP #3 _____		Rubella* _____
Polio #3 _____		
15 months		
Measles _____		

10–12 years
Rubella* _____

* This vaccine should be given only to girls whose blood test shows that they do not already have immunity to rubella.

DPT = Diphtheria, pertussis (whooping cough), and tetanus (lockjaw)

DT = Diphtheria and tetanus (lockjaw)

Polio = Oral polio

Measles = Measles vaccine

Rubella = German measles (three-day measles

Note: Diphtheria and Tetanus is recommended every 10 years for life, with an additional tetanus booster for contaminated wounds more than 5 years after the last booster.

Name_____

Birth Information

Date _____ Weight _____ Mother's age _____ Length of pregnancy _____

Complications _____

_____

Medical History	Date	Illness
Hospitalizations	_____	_____
Other medical problems (Include serious illness or injury, hearing or vision problem, positive TB test, etc.)	_____	_____
	_____	_____
	_____	_____
	_____	_____

Allergies

Medicines _____

Other _____

Family Medical History

Allergy _____   High blood pressure _____

Asthma _____   Tuberculosis _____

Diabetes _____   Other _____

Immunizations   Date

2 months
DTP #1   _____
Polio #1   _____

4 months
DTP #2   _____
Polio #2   _____

6 months
DTP #3   _____
Polio #3   _____

15 months
Measles   _____

Date

18 months
DTP booster   _____
Polio booster   _____

4–6 years
DT booster   _____
Polio booster   _____

10–12 years
Rubella*   _____

* This vaccine should be given only to girls whose blood test shows that they do not already have immunity to rubella.

DPT = Diphtheria, pertussis (whooping cough), and tetanus (lockjaw)
DT = Diphtheria and tetanus (lockjaw)
Polio = Oral polio

Measles = Measles vaccine
Rubella = German measles (three-day measles

Note: Diphtheria and Tetanus is recommended every 10 years for life, with an additional tetanus booster for contaminated wounds more than 5 years after the last booster.

Growth Charts

Here are four charts that will help you keep a permanent record of your child's growth. This information will be of interest to your child's physician on routine visits. It is also referred to several times in this book to help you decide whether a doctor's visit is necessary.

Two of the charts are for girls and two for boys. On each chart you can plot your own child's height and weight at various ages. The line for height and the one for weight will be plotted on two different scales on the same chart. As you can see, age is shown at the bottom of each chart with height on the left margin and weight on the right.

To plot your child's height, first find the vertical line for his or her age at the bottom of the chart. Next, find the horizontal line for the child's height on the left side of the page. Mark the point where the two lines cross. The next time you measure your child, mark the new age and height position on the chart. By connecting the points, you will develop a line that shows your child's growth.

To plot weight, again find the line for the child's age at the bottom of the chart. Then locate the horizontal line for the child's weight on the right side of the chart. Mark the point where the two lines cross and proceed as for the height part of the chart.

If you have more than one girl or boy, assign a different color or symbol to each one so they can be easily distinguished.

The curved lines with numbers represent "percentile" of normal children. For example, if your boy weighs 31 pounds (about 14 kilograms) at 27 months, he is in the 75th percentile. This means that about 75 percent of normal boys weigh less than he does and about 25 percent weigh more. Please remember that these are simply statistical expressions that may be helpful in certain circumstances. Being in a particular percentile does not in itself make a child "normal" or "abnormal."

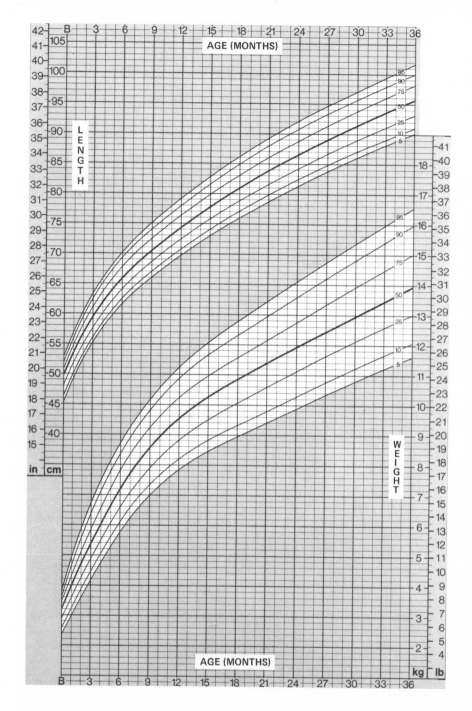

GIRLS: BIRTH TO 36 MONTHS
Physical Growth, NCHS Percentiles

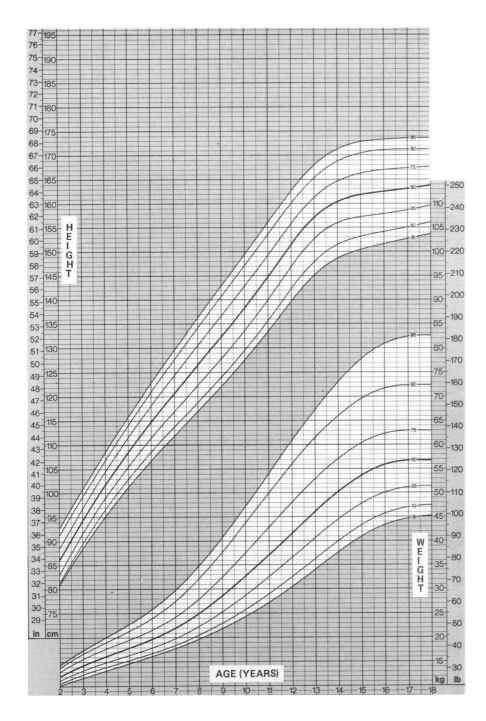

GIRLS: 2 TO 18 YEARS
Physical Growth, NCHS Percentiles

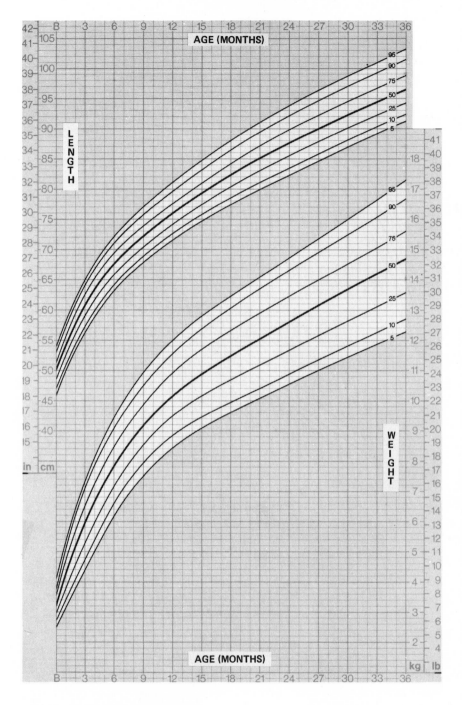

BOYS: BIRTH TO 36 MONTHS
Physical Growth, NCHS Percentiles

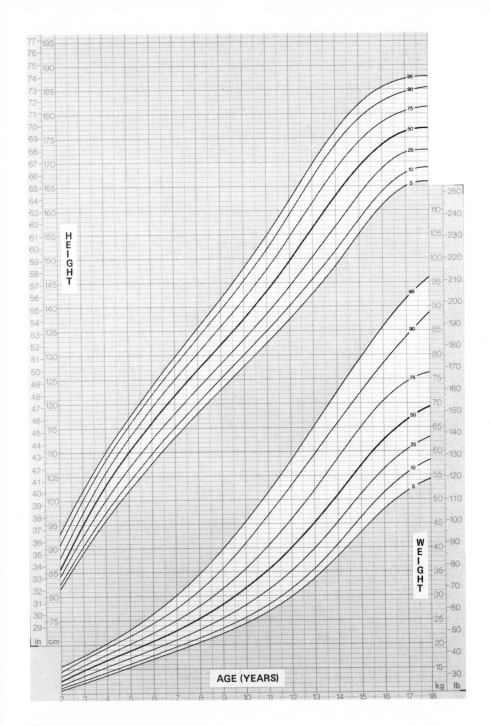

BOYS: 2 TO 18 YEARS
Physical Growth, NCHS Percentiles

Index

Where multiple page references are listed, the most detailed discussion is indicated by boldface numbers, where applicable.

A, vitamin, 7
A200, 266, 268
Abdomen, 330
    infant, 43
    injuries, 148, 150
    pain, 172, 192, 193, 200, 201,
        204, 294, 308, **354–357,**
        358, 364
    rash, 282
    swelling, 356
Abdominal pain
    acute, **354–355**
    recurrent, **356–357**
    See also Abdomen, pain.
Abortions, spontaneous and
    induced, 9
Abrasions, **154–155**
Abscess
    eyelid, 342
    lung, 226
    skin, 256
    throat, 204
    tonsils, 100
    tooth, 230
Academy of Pediatrics,
    American, 110, 113

Accidents
    automobile, 30, 105–107
    bicycle, 107
    drowning, 107–108
    head injuries, 166
    pets, 108–109
    prevention, 103–109
Ace bandage, 330. See also
    Elastic bandages.
Acetaminophen, 132, 187–188
    during pregnancy, 10
    for relief of itching, 280, 360
    See also specific complaints.
Acetone, 268
Acids, 145, 180
Acne, **258–259**
    adolescent, 54
    newborn, 43, 238
Actifed, 128, 129, 306
Action for Child Transportation
    Safety, 106
Active child, 63, 83
    hyperactivity, 83, 129, 212,
        306–307
Activity
    of infants, 39–40

of sick child, 141
Additives, food, 50, 306–307
Adenoids and adenoidectomy,
    100
Adjustment problems, 306. See
    also School.
Adolescents
    alcoholism and, 124
    athlete's foot, **260–261**
    chest pain, 330
    contraception, 375–378
    gonococcal arthritis, 294
    knee pain, 294
    low-back pain, **296–297**
    personality development,
        72–75
    puberty, 53–55
    suicide and, 124
Adrenal gland, 220, 334
Adrenalin, 172, 218, 248, 334
Advisory Committee on
    Immunization Practices,
    110
Afrin, 129, 212
Afterbirth, 22
Age, mother's, and Mongolism, 9

Airway
  obstruction, 332
  spasm, 216
  See also Breathing.
Alcohol
  alcoholism and, 123–124
  -base cleansing tissues, 250
  beverages for colic, 358
  cetyl, 196
  ingestion, excess, 348
  during pregnancy, 10
  sponging with, 186–187
  tick removal with, 268
  on umbilical cord, 43
Alco-wipe, 250
Alkalis, 145, 180
Allergens
  asthma, 193
  avoidance of, 194–195
  common, 191, 212–213
  food, 192
Allergic conjunctivitis, 338
Allergic rhinitis. *See* Hay fever.
Allergies and allergic reactions,
    144, **191–197,** 228
  additives and, 50
  asthma, 193–195, 218
  conjunctivitis, 338
  distinguishing from virus or
    bacteria, 200–201, 326
  ear infections and, 100
  eczema (atopic dermatitis),
    196–197
  to food, 192–193
  hay fever (allergic rhinitis),
    128, 195–196
  hives, **248–249**
  immunization and, 114, 156
  infant feeding and, 13, 48
  to insect bites or stings, 172
  medications for, 128–129
  to medications, 131, 133–134,
    148, 168, 187, 218, 244,
    288
  runny nose, **212–213**
  shots during pregnancy, 11
  testing and hyposensitization,
    197
Alopecia areata (hair loss),
    242–243
Aluminum chloride, 260
Ambulance, when to call,
    143–144
American Dental Association,
    120
Aminophylline, 194, 218
Amitryptyline, 10
Ammonia in urine, 240

Amniocentesis (amniotic fluid
    analysis), 9–10
Amniotic sac, rupture of, 22, 24
Ampicillin, 364
Anacin, 132
Analgesics during labor, 16, 22
Androgens, 11
Anemia
  iron deficiency, screening, 97
  sickle-cell, screening, 97–98
  weakness, tiredness, and,
    318–319
Anesthetics
  allergy to, 148, 168
  creams or sprays, 168
  during delivery, 16–17, 22–23,
    25
  oral, 228
Angel's kiss, 40
Anger, parental, 67–68
Animal bites, **152–153**
  prevention, 108–109
Animal dander, 193, 195,
    212–213
Ankle, **160–161,** 300
Anorexia nervosa, 314
Antibacterial ointment, 154, 168
Antibiotics
  and asthma, 195
  and diarrhea, 351
  overuse of, 93, 200
  during pregnancy, 11
  *See also specific complaints
    and specific drugs.*
Antibodies, breast feeding and,
    45
Antidepressants, 10
Antifungal cream or ointment,
    368
Antihistamines, 128–129, 130
  for allergy, 195, 248, 338
  and asthma, 194
  and earache, 206
  during pregnancy, 10
  for relief of itching, 172, 248,
    250, 268, 270, 280
  side effects, 70, 83, 129, 196,
    216, 250, 304, 306
Antinausea drugs, 11
Antirabies serum, 152
Antiseptics, 133, 148, 154
Antitoxin, 111
Antivomiting drugs, 350
Anus
  episiotomy and, 25
  muscular control of, 58
Anxiety, 64, 68, 73, 356
  rapid heartbeat and, 334

stress, depression, and,
    316–317
APC tablets, 132
Apgar score, 27
Apneic spell, 40
Appendicitis, 184, 200, 278, 354
Appetite
  cravings, 7–8, 52
  loss, 112
Apple juice, 351
Applesauce, 134, 350–351
Areola, 45, 55
Arms
  injuries, 148, 164–165
  rash on, 286, 288, 290
  wound healing time, 170
Arousability, 166–167
Arteriosclerosis, 121–123, 125
Arthralgia, 294
Arthritis, 115, 294
Artificial flavorings and food
    colorings, 50
Artificial respiration, 144, 186
Artificial sweeteners, 8
Aspergum, 132
Aspirin, 132, 187–188
  allergy to, 131, 187, 218
  overdosage symptoms, 132,
    332
  -phenacetin combination, 10,
    132
  during pregnancy, 10
  for relief of itching, 172, 196,
    248, 250, 268, 270, 280
  See also specific complaints.
Asthma, 193–195, 330, 332
  allergy shots, 197
  food allergy and, 192
  insect bite or sting reaction,
    172
  wheezing, **218–219**
Athlete's foot, **260–261**
Athletic supporter, 262
Athletics. *See* Sports.
Atopic dermatitis, 254–255 *See
    also* Eczema.
Attention
  getting, 57, 63
  problems, 82
Audiometry, 210
Auditory perception, 82
Automobile accidents, 30,
    105–107, 158, 160, 166
Autonomy, 65
Aveeno, 250, 264
Awakening, 69–70
  bedwetting and, 308
Axillary and facial hair, 54

Baby aspirin, 187–188
Baby food, 48
Bacitracin, 154
Back
  chicken pox on, 280
  injuries, 143, 148
  pain, 200, **296–297,** 348, 364
Bacteria
  distinguishing from virus or
    allergy, 200–201
  streptococcal, 201, 204, 244,
    256
Bacterial infections, 170, 184,
    204, 206, 208, 210, 214,
    216, 220, 222, 226, 228,
    240, 244, 250, 254, 256,
    270, 272, 280, 338,
    351–352, 368
Bad breath, **226–227**
Baking soda bath, 264, 280
Bananas, 351
Bandages, 133, 154, 170
  bandaids, 128, 133, 170
  butterfly, 148
  steristrips, 148
Barbiturates, 11, 22, 124
Barium swallow X-rays, 324
Bathing
  newborns, 26
  for rectal itching, 360
  to reduce fever, 187, 322
  for skin problems, 196, 250,
    264, 268, 280
  for urination problems, 364
Bats, 152
Beating, rhythmic, of hand or
    foot, 185
Bedbugs, **266–267**
Bedtime bottles, 70, 119
Bedwetting, 59–60, **308–309,**
    364
Beef, 192
  liver, 8
Bee stings, **172–173**
Behavior, food additives and, 50
Bellyaches. See Abdomen, pain.
Benadryl 10, 128, 172, 195,
    248, 250
Benign murmurs, 94–95
Benylin expectorant, 130
Bent-bumper syndrome, 334
Benzocaine, 264
Benzoyl peroxide, 258
Benzyl benzoate, 270
Berries, 248
Betadine, 133, 148, 154
Bicycles
  accident prevention, 107

accidents, 160, 166
  exercise and, 125
Bilingual education, 82
Bimanual examination, 96
Biopsy, 222
Birth, 19–30
  anesthesia, 22–23
  circumcision, 28–29
  delivery room procedures,
    24–25
  emotions, 19–21
  fetal heart monitoring, 24
  labor stages, 21–22
  newborn procedures, 26–28
  pitocin and induced births, 23
  premature, 25–26
  preparation procedures, 24
  rupture of membranes, 22
  taking child home, 29–30
Birth control pills, 373, 376–377
Birthmarks, 40–41
Bites
  animal, **152–153**
  dog, prevention, 108–109
  insect, 128, **172–173,** 248,
    250
  lice and bedbugs, **266–267**
  rabies, 117
  ticks and chiggers (redbugs),
    268–269
Black widow spider, 172
Blackhead, 258
Bladder
  bedwetting, 59–60, **308–309**
  infection, 364
  training, 59
Bleeding
  control of, 144
  internal, 166–167
  around joint, 162
  pumping vigorously, 148
  rectal, **360–361**
  under skin, 282
  inside skull, 166–167
  vaginal, 9, 26, 44, **372–373,**
    376
Blindness, 27, 113–114, 117,
    344
Blisters, 168, 228, 264, 266,
    270, 280
Blistex, 228
Bloating, 193, 372
Block-out, 264
Blood
  clotting problem, 282
  clotting tests, 224
  fetal, acidity of, 24
  under fingernail, 176

insects sucking, 266
  loss through intestinal tract,
    192
  removal from joint, 162
  tests, 188, 220, 222, 278, 284,
    294, 314, 320, 350, 354,
    372–373
  in urine, **364–365**
  in vomitus or stool, 141, 348,
    351, 354
Blood clots, 13, 122, 376
Blood poisoning, **170–171**
Blood pressure
  anesthesia and, 23
  high, 122–123, 129–130, 244,
    376
  measurements, 94, 167, 304,
    320
Blood vessels
  constriction of, 129–130
  injury, 149–151
Blowing nose, 224
Blows, injury from, 164, 224,
    230
Bluboro, 244, 250
Blueness
  breath-holding and, 68
  heart murmurs and, 95
  of limb, 158
Boils, 252, **256–257**
Bones
  broken, **158–159**
  See also Bones, muscles, and
    joints; injury sites by name.
Bones, muscles, and joints,
    293–301
  bowlegs and knock-knees,
    298–299
  low-back pain, **296–297**
  pain in muscles or joints,
    294–295
  pigeon toes and flat feet, 298,
    300–301
Bonine, 11
Booster shots, 111–112, 118,
    156
Bottle feeding, 47
  breast feeding or, 12–15
  formulas, 29
Bowel control, 57–59
Bowel movement, 354
  foreign object passed, 324
  frequency of, 310
  See also Constipation;
    Diarrhea; Stools.
Bowlegs, **298–299**
Boxer shorts, 262
Brace, nighttime, 298

Bradley method, 16
Brain
damage, 166
infection, 113, 278, 280, 282, 286, 323, 348
tumors, 304
Brain wave tests, 304, 307, 320, 323
Bran, 131, 310, 360
Brasivol, 258
Brat diet, 351
Braxton-Hicks contractions, 21
Brazelton, T. Berry, 64
Breast
in female adolescent, 54–55
infant's, 43
in male adolescent, 54
pumping, 45
size, breast feeding and, 14
tenderness, 6, 372
Breast feeding, 26
advantages, 12–13
baby's stools, 351
bottle feeding or, 12–15
myths, 14
polio immunization and, 113
problems and cautions, 14, 35–36, 133
techniques, 44–47
weight gain and, 314
Breastbone, 330
Breath
bad, **226–227**
holding, 68, 320, 322
shortness of, 95, 98, 143, 145, 218, 324, 330, **332–333,** 334
Breathing
breath-holding spells, 68, 320, 322
difficulty, 144, 172, 216, 218, 220, 248, 324, 330
excessive, 316
facilitating during seizure, 186
infant, 40, 42, 45
mouth, 204
normal rate, 142, 332
rapid, 132, 187, 202, 214, 332, 354
shortness of breath, 95, 98, 143, 145, 218, 324, 330, **332–333,** 334
slow, 132
tonsils, adenoids, and, 100
tube, 216, 220
Breech deliveries, 25, 27
Broken bones, **158–159.** See also injury sites by name.

Brompheniramine, 195
Bronchi, bronchioles, and bronchiolitis, 218
Bronchoscope, 324
Brown recluse spiders, 172
Bruises, 158, 160
Brushing teeth, 119–120, 226
Bubble baths, 364, 368
Buckshot wound, 150
Bumps, skin, **252–253,** 266
Burning sensation in eyes, **338–339**
Burns, **168–169**
Burping, 48
Burrow's solution, 208, 244, 250
BurVeen, 250
Butterfly bandages, 148
Buttocks
boils on, 256
discoloration around, 40

C, vitamin, 7, 11, 118
Caesarean section (C-section), 17, 23–26
Caffeine, 124, 132
Caladryl, 250
Calamine lotion, 250, 268, 270
Calcium, 7, 118
Caldesene powder, 240
Calories
overweight and, 312
required during fever, 188
required for infants, 47
Campho-Phenique, 228
Camphor, 228
Cancer
breast, 13
cervix, 28, 95
lung, 123
penis, 28
skin, 41, 252
vagina, 8, 95
Candeptin, 368
Canker sores, 228
Caput succedaneum, 41
Car sickness, 348
Carbinoxamine, 128
Carbohydrates, 7
Carbuncle, 256
Carriers
hemophilia, 9
rabies, 117
sickle-cell anemia, 98
Cartilage
rib, 330
torn, 162
Casting broken bones, 94, 158, 161, 165

Castor beans, 104
Cataracts, 42, 284
"Catch" sensation in chest, 330
Cats
bites, **152–153**
during pregnancy, 11–12
Cattle, 152
Caudal anesthesia, 23
Caustic cleansers, 181
Cauterization, 224, 252
Cavities, dental, 68, 119. See also Dental care.
Celery, 310, 360
Century Motor-toter, 106
Cephalohematoma, 41
Cereals, 48, 50, 310, 318
Cerumenex, 208, 210
Cervix
cancer, 28, 95
during childbirth, 21–22
pelvic examination, 96
Cetaphil lotion, 196, 254
Cetyl alcohol, 196
Chalazion, 342
Charring of tissue, 168
Cheeks
red, chapped, 196, 254
"slapped" appearance, 290
Cheese, 248
Chemical conjunctivitis, 338
Chest
infant, 43
injuries, 148, 150
pain, 130, 324, **330–331,** 334
rash on, 280, 282
wound healing time, 170
X-ray, 188
Chewing
painful, 278
of tongue, 322
Chicken pox, 184, **280–281**
Chiggers, **268–269**
Child abuse prevention, 67–68
Child health associates, 91–92
Childbirth, 19–30
preparation classes, 15–17
Childhood diseases, 277–291
chicken pox, 184, **280–281**
fifth disease, **290–291**
German measles, 11, 98, 114–116, 118, 222, **284–285,** 294
measles, 113–114, 118, 184, **282–283**
mumps, 116, 184, 222, 230, **278–279**
roseola, 184–185, **286–287**

scarlet fever, 201, 205, **288–289**
Childproof caps, 106, 128, 187
Chill, 186
Chip fractures, 160–161
Chlordiazepopide, 11
Chlorocyclizine, 11
Chlorpheniramine, 128, 248
  maleate, 195
Chlorpromazine, 11
Chlor-Trimeton, 128, 172, 195, 248, 270
Chocolate, 248, 258
Choking, 144
Cholesterol
  heart attack and, 122
  screening, 98
Chorionic gonadotropin, 6
Chromosomal disease, 9
Circumcision, 28–29, 370
Cirrhosis of the liver, 124
Citrus fruits, 192, 278
Clavicle fracture, 164
Cleansing
  after contact with poisonous plant, 250
  wound, 133, 148, 150, 152
  See also Washing.
Cleft palate, breast feeding and, 12
Clinics
  contraceptive advice from, 377
  free, for youths, 75
  self-help for women, 97
Clitoris, enlargement in infants, 44
Clotrimazole, 246, 262
Codeine, 130
Coitus interruptus, 375
Colace, 131, 310, 360
Cold liquids, 204, 288
Cold sores, 228
Cold water
  applications and compresses, 168, 172, 224, 228, 248, 250, 264, 370
  in ear syringe, 210
Coldness of limb, 158
Colds, common, 99, 184, **202–203,** 214, 224, 304, 318, 323, 338
  medications for, 129–130
  school avoidance and, 85, 202
  syndrome, 200, 212
Colic, 35, **358–359**
Collapse, 172
Collarbone fracture, 164
Color loss in skin, patchy, **274–275**

Colostrum, 45
Coma, 98, 144
Competitiveness, 71–72, 86
Complaints, common childhood, 137–373. See also specific complaints and specific parts of the body.
Compound W, 252
Compresses. See Cold water, applications; Heat, applications of.
Conar, 130
Conception, 6
Concepts, grasping, 70, 81
Concussion, 166
Conditioning
  cardiovascular, 86, 125
  sports readiness and, 87
Condoms, 375–376
Conduction, 187
Confidentiality, adolescent's, 74, 96
Conjunctivitis, 338
Constipation, 13, 47, 125, **310–311,** 360
  medication for, 130–131
Consumer Reports, 106
Contact dermatitis, 250
Contact lenses, 88
Contact sports, medical conditions disqualifying child from, 87–88
Contagion, period of
  chicken pox, 280
  measles, 282
  mumps, 278
  roseola, 286
Contagious diseases
  immunizations, 109–118
  impetigo, **224–245**
  See also Childhood diseases; Epidemics.
Contraception, 13, 74, 116, 375–378
Convulsions, **322–323.** See also Seizures.
Cooperation, 71–72
Coordination, 56–57
  eye, 344
  problems, 82
  sports readiness and, 87
  tests, 306
Cornea
  scraped or cut, 340
  ulcers in, 338
Coronary thrombosis, 121–122
Corticosteroid hormones, 26, 194, 208
Cortisone, 242, 272, 338

Cough, 130, 133, 144, 200–201, 212, **214–215,** 286, 324, 326, 330, 354
  barking seal, 216, 220
  dry, brassy, 282
Cough syrup and cough suppressants, 130, 330
Council on Environmental Health, 110
Cow pox, 110
Coxsackie virus, 228
Crabs (pubic lice), 266
Cradle cap, 240, **272–273**
Cramps
  IUD and, 376
  menstrual, 372–373
  See also Abdomen, pain.
Cranberry juice, 134, 364
Craniosynostosis, 93–94
Crash diets, 372
Cravings, 7–8, 52
Creams
  baby, 29–30
  contraceptive, 376
Cromolyn, 194
Crooked limb, 158–159
Crossed eyes, 42, **344–345**
Croup, 130, 133, 201, 214, **216–217,** 332
Crutches, adjustment of, 160
Crying
  colic and, **358–359**
  hoarseness, **220–221**
  infant's, 39–40, 64–65
  infections and, 206
  runny nose and, 212
  soft spot and, 41
  toddler's, 69
Cultures
  eye, 338
  mouth, 226
  penis discharge, 370
  ringworm scrapings, 246
  throat, 204, 226, 288
  urine, 364
Cuprex, 266, 268
Cuts, **148–149**
Cyanotic, 95
Cyclizine, 11
Cyst, 258

D, vitamin, 13, 30, 118, 133
  deficiency, 298
Daffodil bulbs, 104
Dalkon Shield, 377
Dander, animal, 193, 195, 212–213
Dandruff, 240, **272–273**
Datril, 132, 187

Day-care centers, 71, 79–80, 326
DDT, 14
Deafness, 114, 278, 284. *See also* Hearing loss.
Debrox, 210
Decision charts, using and interpreting, 139–141
Decongestants, 70, 128–130, 202, 206, 212, 214
side effects, 212, 304, 306
Deep knee bends, 162
Deer, ticks from, 172
Defecation
involuntary, 185
pain during, 310
See also Bowel control; Constipation; Diarrhea.
Deformities and abnormalities
birth defect, 220
bowlegs and knock-knees, **298–299**
congenital hip or spine, 296–297
German measles and, 284
injuries and, 160, 164
physical defects, 83, 114
pigeon toes and flat feet, **300–301**
Dehydration, 88–89, 141, 214, 348, 350–352
Delivery
home, hospital, and other options, 17–18
intercourse before and after, 8–9
procedures, 24–25
See also Birth.
Demerol, 22
Dennis-Browne splint, 298
Dental care, 118–121
bad breath, **226–227**
brushing teeth, 119–120
flossing, 120
fluoride, 118, 120–121
permanent teeth, 121
problems, 68, 70
tooth decay, 119
toothaches, **230–231**
toothpaste, choice of, 120
visit to dentist, first, 121
water jets, 120
Dentist, first visit to, 121. *See also* Dental care.
Depression, stress, and anxiety, **316–317,** 318, 356
Desenex, 260
Desensitization shots, 172, 197
Desitin, 240
Development

personality, 63–78
physical, 51–61
social, eating and, 49–50
Dextromethorphan, 130, 214, 330
DHS, 272
Diabetes, 122
delivery and, 25
juvenile, 98
screening, 98
Diaper rash, 30, **240–241,** 310
Diaphragm (membrane), 330
Diaphragms (contraceptive), 375–376
Diarrhea, 13, 184, 200, 314, 326, 348, **351–353,** 354
blood in, 141
delivery and, 24
lactase lack and, 192–193
medication for, 131
sick child's, 141
Diazepam, 11
Diet
brat, 351
digestive problems and, 348, 350–352, 360
heart attack and, 122
during pregnancy, 7–8
See also Nutrition.
Diet pills, 312
Diethylstilbestrol, 8, 11, 95
Digestive tract problems, 347–361
abdominal pain, acute, **354–355**
abdominal pain, recurrent, **356–357**
colic, 35, **358–359**
constipation and soiling, **310–311**
diarrhea, 13, 24, 131, 141, 184, 192–193, 200, 210, 314, 326, 348, **351–353**
nausea/vomiting, 6, 11, 98, 131, 141, 166, 172, 192–193, 200, 210, 288, 304, 314, 318, 320, 322, 324, **348–350**
rectal pain, itching or bleeding, 310, **360–361**
See also Abdomen, pain.
Dimetane, 195
Dimetapp, 306
Diphenhydramine, 10, 128, 130, 195, 248
Diphtheria, 111
Discharges
breast, 43
ear, **208–209**

eye, **338–339**
nose, 212
penis, 370
vagina, 44, 364, **368–369**
Diseases
adult, prevention of, 121–125
childhood, 277–291
Dislocations
of fingernail, 176
of shoulder and elbow, 164
Disorientation, 144–145
Disposable diapers, 240
Dizziness, 158, 210, 248, 316, **320–321,** 330
DMX, 130
Doctor consultation, urgency of, 140
See also Medical care.
Dog
bites, **152–153**
bites, prevention, 108–109
ticks from, 172
Domeboro, 244, 250
Dorcal, 130
Douche, 96, 375
Downs syndrome (Mongolism), 9
DPT shot, 110–112, 118
Drain and oven cleaners, 145, 180
Drainage
boil, 256
chalazion, 342
festering wound, 170
insect bite or sting, 172
middle-ear chamber, 101, 206
Drano, 180
Drinking from cup, 49
Drooling, 216, 220, 332
Drowning, 107–108, 144
Drowsiness, 112, 129, 131, 144, 166, 196, 212, 250, 268, 304, 322, 338
Drugs
causing hyperactivity, 306
dependence on, 124–125, 135
home pharmacy, 127–135
for mother, 10, 14, 16, 23
reactions, 248, 306
See also names of specific drugs.
Duck-walking, 300
Duo-Film, 252
Dust, 193–195, 212–213
Dyshydrosis, 260
Dyslexia, 81
Dysmenorrhea, 372–378

Ear, nose, and throat problems, 199–231

bad breath, **226–227**
colds and flu, **202–203**
cough, **214–215**
croup, **216–217**
ear discharge, **208–209**
earaches, **206–207**
hearing loss, **210–211**
hoarseness, **220–221**
mouth lesions, **228–229**
nosebleeds, **224–225**
runny nose, **212–213**
sore throat, **204–205**
swollen glands, **222–223**
toothaches, **230–231**
wheezing, **218–219**
Earaches, 70, 130, 184,
    206–207, 208, 230, 278,
    304, 318
Eardrum, 208, 210
Ears, 320
    blockage, 200, 210
    canal irritation, 208
    discharges, **208–209**
    flushing, 210
    infections, 100, 129–130, 200,
        202, 206, 210, 212, 222,
        282, 286, 320, 323, 326,
        354
    inner, dizziness and, 320
    pulling at, 206
    rash behind, 272, 282
    ringing in, 132, 187
    tubes, 101, 206
    See also Ear, nose, and throat
        problems; Earaches.
Eating
    habits and problems, 49, 52
    refusal, 316
    sick child's, 141
Ebstein's pearls, 42
Eczema, 193, 196–197,
    254–255
Effacement and dilation, 21
Eggs, 192, 248
Elastic bandages, 128, 160–162,
    330
Elavil, 10
Elbow injuries, 159, **164–165**
Electric needle, 252
Electrocardiogram (EKG), 314,
    330, 334
Electroencephalogram (EEG),
    304, 307, 320, 323
Emergencies, 143–145
    ambulance, when to call,
        143–144
    signs of, 144–145, 172
Emergency room, 143, 377

Emotions
    asthma and, 193–195
    constipation and, 310
    eczema and, 196–197
    hives and, 248
    infant's, 64–65
    nausea, vomiting and, 348
    palpitations, 334
    parental, 3–5, 16, 19–21,
        33–39
    personality development and,
        78
    preschooler's, 70–71
Emphysema, 123
Encephalitis, 278, 280, 282, 286
Endocrine problems, 373
Enema, 24, 131, 310
Enfamil, 47
Engorgement of breasts,
    preventing, 45–47
Enzymes, 192–193, 351
Eosinophils, 213
Ephedrine, 129, 194, 212
Epidemics
    conjunctivitis, 338
    fifth disease, 290
    glomerulonephritis, 244
    ringworm, 246
    rubella, 115
    scabies, 270
Epiglottitis, 216, 220
Epilepsy, 68, 322. See also
    Seizures.
Epinephrine, 194
Episiotomy, 9, 23, 25
Erections, 75
Erythema infectiosum (fifth
    disease), **290–291**
Erythema toxicum, 238
    neonatorum, 43
Erythromycin, 244, 258, 288
Esophagus, 330
Estrogens, 11, 54–55, 376
Etafron, 10
Eustachian tube, blocked, 100,
    129, 206
Evaporation, 186
Exercise
    asthma and, 195
    chest pain and, 330.
    disease prevention and,
        122–123, 125
    knock-knees, bowlegs, and,
        298
    low-back pain and, 296
    overweight, 312
    palpitations and, 334
    during pregnancy, 8, 16

runny nose and, 212
shortness of breath and, 332
sore muscles and, 294
Ex-lax, 131
Expectorants, 130
Exploration, 65
Extractions, dental, 230
Eye patch, 344
    making, 340
Eye problems
    burning, itching, and
        discharge, **338–339**
    decreased vision and crossed
        eyes, 42, **344–345**
    foreign body in eye, and pain,
        174, 338, **340–341**
    styes and blocked tear ducts,
        42, 338, **342–343**
    See also Eyes.
Eye spud, 340
Eyebrows, red and scaling, 272
Eyelids
    crusted, 338
    styes, **342–343**
Eyes
    color, 41
    crossed, 42, **344–345**
    dry, 141
    examination, 94, 320, 344
    fishhook in, 174
    infant, 41–42
    infection, 304, 338, 340
    inflamed, 282
    irritations, medications for, 131
    itching, 195, 200, 212, 282,
        326, **338–339**
    light-sensitive, 282
    muscle aches, 200
    pain, 338, **340–341**
    problems, 337–345
    pupil size, unequal, 166–167
    rolling back, 185
    sunken, 348
    yellowness of whites, 41
    See also Eye problems; Vision.
Eyestrain, 304

Face
    boils, 256
    hair, 54
    infant, 43
    injuries, 148–149, 152, 168
    rash, 274, 282, 284, 288
    wound healing time, 170
Facts of life, 77
Failing
    in school, 81–84
    in sports, 86

Fainting, 172, **320–321**
Faintness during pregnancy, 8
Falling out spells, **322–323.** *See also* Seizures.
Falls, 158, 160, 164, 166, 296, 320
Family
  planning, 6. *See also* Contraception.
  size and individual development, 60
Family practitioners, 91, 95–96
Fantasy, 70
Fat cells, 52, 312
Fathers
  childbirth preparation classes for, 15–16
  delivery and, 17
  feeding by, 14, 46
  infant care by, 38
  jealousy of baby, 34
Fatigue, 351
  in childbirth, 22
  German measles, 284
  pregnancy and, 6, 8
  toddler's, 68
  weakness and tiredness, **318–319**
Fats, dietary, 7, 98, 122, 351–352
Fear. *See* Anxiety.
Febrile seizures, 68, 185–186, 322–323
Feeding, 44–50
  bottle, 47
  breast, techniques, 44–47
  breast or bottle, 12–15
  concerns about foods, 50
  digestive problems and, 348, 350
  physical development and, 48–49
  quantity and time intervals of, 48
  social development and, 49–50
  solid foods, 48
Feet
  abnormalities, 94
  flat, and pigeon toes, **300–301**
  infant, 44
  injuries, 150
Fertility, 6
Festering, 170
Fetus
  German measles affecting, 114–115, 284

heart monitoring, 17, 24
Fever, 184–189, 332, 334, 354
  childhood diseases, 270, 280, 282, 284, 286, 288
  chill, 186
  disorientation and, 145
  doctor's treatment of, 188
  fits, 185–186, 322–323
  food and, 188
  immunizations and, 112, 114
  infection, 12, 148, 150, 154, 170, 200–201, 204, 206, 214, 218, 222, 256, 294, 308, 318, 351, 364
  medications for, 131–132
  mouth lesions and, 228
  reduction of, 186–188
  school attendance and, 99
  sick child's, 142
  temperature taking, 184–185
  tick bites, 268
  with vomiting, 304, 348
Fever blisters, 228
Fever fits, 185–186, 322–323
Fiber, 131, 310, 360
Fifth disease (erythema infectiosum), **290–291**
Fillings, dental, 230
Fine tooth comb, 266, 272
Finger foods, 48
Fingernails
  blood under, 176
  infant, 43
  skin problems and, 196, 246, 250, 254, 280
Fingers, smashed, **176–177**
First child, adjustment to, 33–36
First-degree burn, 168
Fish, 192, 248
Fishhooks, removal of, **174–175.** *See also* Puncture wounds.
Fits, **322–323**
  fever, 185–186
  See also Seizures.
Flagyl, 11
Flat-chestedness, 55
Flat feet, **300–301**
Flossing, dental, 120
Flu, 117, 200, **202–203,** 304, 318
Fluids
  bedwetting and, 308
  cold, 228
  digestive problems and, 348, 350
  intake, 188, 195, 202, 212, 218, 220, 228, 278, 288,

310, 351, 354, 356, 360
  intravenous, 218, 350
  loss, 168, 351
  retention, 376
Fluorescent stain in eye, 340
Fluoride, 118, 120–121, 133
Fluoroscope, 300
Foams, contraceptive, 376
Focusing of eyes, 41, 94
Folic acid, 7
Follicle stimulating hormone (FSH), 54
Folliculitis, 256
Fontanel, 41, 166
  bulging, 304, 348
Food allergy, 192–193, 196
Food and Drug Administration, 8, 127–128
Foods
  allergic reactions to, 192–193, 195
  concerns about, 50
  constipating, 351
  See also Diet; Feeding; Nutrition.
Forceps, 24–25
  marks from, 41
Foreign objects
  in ear canal, 210
  in eye, 174, **340–341**
  in nose, 212, 224, 226
  in penis, 370
  swallowed, 144, 214, 218, **324–325,** 354
  in vagina, 368
  in wound, 148, 150
Foreskin, 370. *See also* Circumcision.
Formula, 29, 47
  soybean, 193
  See also Bottle feeding.
Fostex, 258
Foxes, 152
Fractures, **158–159.** *See also* injury sites by name.
Fraiberg, Selma, 66
Freezing wart, 252
Frenulum, short, 42
Freon-containing nebulizers, 194
Frequent illness, 99, **326–327**
Friends and friendships, 71, 73–74
Frostbite, 168
Fruit, 192, 278, 360
Frustration
  child's, 65–66, 81
  parent's, 67–68
Functional murmurs, 94–95

Fungus infections, 246, 260, 262, 274
Furniture polish, 145, 180
Fussiness, 64, 112, 202, 206

Games, 71. *See also* Sports.
Gamma globulin
 deficiency, 326
 shots, 202, 348, 354
Gantrisin, 101, 364
Gargles, salt water, 204, 280
Gas, 48, 358
Gasoline, 145, 180
Gasping for air, 220, 332. *See also* Breathing, difficulty.
Gastro-colic reflex, 57
Gastroenteritis, 323, 354
 bacterial, 360
 viral, 200, 351
Gastrointestinal problems
 hemorrhage, 124, 131, 187
 infection, 348
 See also Digestive tract problems; Flu
Gatorade, 351
General anesthesia, 23, 25, 159
General Motors Infant and Child Love Seat, 106
General practitioners, 91
Genitals, 367–373
 curiosity about, 76
 examination of, 95
 infant, 43–44
 manipulation of, 75–76
 penis problems, 240, **370–371**
 vaginal bleeding and menstrual problems, 9, 26, 44, 368, **372–373**
 vaginal discharge, 44, 364, **368–369**
 See also Circumcision.
German measles, 11, 98, 114–116, 118, 222, **284–285,** 294
Glands
 hormonal disorders, 220
 mumps, **278–279**
 sweat, 238
 swollen, 12, 116, 200–201, **222–223,** 252, 286, 288, 294, 338
Glass in wound, 150
Glasses, eye, 88, 344
Glomerulonephritis, 244
Glycerol guaiacolate, 130
Goat's milk, 318
Gonococcal arthritis, 294

Gonococcal conjunctivitis, 27
Gonococcal infection, *eye* medication protecting against, 27, 338
Gonorrhea, 27, 368, 370
Goose bumps, 186
Goose eggs, 166
Grasp reflex, 56
Greenstick fractures, 158
Griseofulvin, 242, 246, 260
Grogginess, 186
Growing pains, 294
Growth and development, physical, 51–61
 charts, using, 381
 eating skills and, 48–49
 height, 53
 normality and, 60–61
 at puberty, 53–55
 sequence of, 56–57
 skills and, 55–57
 spurts, lags, and delays, 53
 toilet training, 57–60
 weight, 52
Growth hormone, 53
Growth plate injuries, 158, 164
Growth retardation, 194, 197
Grunting, 172
Guilt, 71, 76, 85
Gullet, 330
Gum disease, 119
Gynecologist, 96

Hair
 acne and, 258
 axillary, 54
 dandruff, **272–273**
 facial, 54
 infections around follicles, 256
 lice in, 266
 loss, **242–243**
Hairline, rash on, 282
Haloprogin, 246, 262
Halotex, 246, 262
Hand-foot-mouth syndrome, 228
Hands
 development and eating skills, 49
 infant, 43
 injuries, 149–150, 168
Hard candy, 350
Hardening of the arteries, 122–123
Hay fever, 128, 192–193, 195–196, 304, 326
 allergy shots, 197
 distinguishing from viral and

bacterial infections, 200–201
 runny nose, **212–213**
Head
 infant, 41
 injuries, 143–144, 150, 152, **166–167,** 348
 jerking, 185
 measles rash on, 282
 measurements, 93–94
 pain. *See* Headache.
 size, 52
 tilted forward, 216, 332
Headache, 16, 23, 172, 195, 200–201, 204, 244, 268, 278, 288, **304–305,** 318, 356, 372
 migraine, 304, 348, 376
Healing of normal wound, 170
Health department, reporting bites to, 152
Hearing
 assessing, 94, 210, 307
 loss, 206, 208, **210–211,** 278
 problems, 82, 306
Heart, 332, 334
 damage, 111, 204
 defects, 114
 disease, 284
 failure, 314
 inflammation, 330
 palpitations, **334–335**
 rate, sick child's, 142
 strep throat complications, 201
Heart attack, 98, 121–122, 330
Heart murmurs, 94–95
Heat, application of, 160, 162, 165, 250, 258, 268, 294, 296, 304, 330, 342, 356, 370, 372
Heat exhaustion and heat stroke, 88, 184
Heat rash, 238
Height, 52–53, 94
Hematocrit, 97
Hemoglobin, 97
Hemophilia, 9
Hemorrhaging, 25, 27
Hemorrhoids, 125
Henoch-Shonlein purpura, 354
Hepatitis, 318–319, 348, 354
Herd immunity, 115
Heredity
 allergies and, 192
 diseases and, 9, 97–98
 physical growth and, 52–53
 rickets and, 298
 tooth decay and, 119

Hernias, 43, 101

Herpes viruses, 228, 338, 340

Herpes zoster (shingles), 280

Hips
congenital abnormality, 94, 296–297
knee pain originating in, 294
pigeon toes caused by, 300

Histamines, 195, 250, 270

Hives, **248–249**
food allergies, 192
insect bite or sting, 172

Hoarseness, 200, **220–221**

Home delivery, 17–18

Homicide, 123

Homosexual encounters, 74

Hooky playing, 85

Hormones, 6, 13, 26, 101, 184
affecting newborn, 43, 238, 272, 368, 372
disorders, 220, 312
growth and, 53
menstrual problems, **372–373**
during pregnancy, 11
at puberty, 54, 258

Hospital
delivery, 17–18
discharge details, 29–30

Hotlines, parental stress, 67

Hug to remove windpipe obstruction, 324

Humidifier and humidification, 212, 218, 220. *See also* Vaporizer.

Hunger, chill and, 186

Hyaline membrane disease, 26

Hydration therapy for asthma, 195

Hydrocele, 101–102

Hydrocephalus, 94

Hydrogen peroxide, 128, 133, 148, 150, 154, 208

Hygiene
acne, 258
athlete's foot, 260
foreskin, 370
rectal itching, 360
vaginal discharge, 368

Hyperactivity, 83, 129, 212, **306–307**

Hypersensitivity response, 191

Hypertension, 125

Hyperthyroidism, 306

Hyperventilation syndrome, 145, 316, 330, 334

Hypoglycemia, 318–320

Hyposensitization, 197

Hypospadias, 28

Hypothalamus, 186

Hysteria, 70

Ice
application of, 154, 158, 160, 162, 165–166, 168, 172, 176, 224
chewing chips of, 350

Ice cream, 134

Identity
adolescent's, 73
sexual, 71

Imipramine, 308

Immobilization of suspected fractures, 158

Immune defense mechanism deficiency, 326

Immunity, breast-fed infant's, 13

Immunizations, 109–118
of breast-fed babies, 14
diphtheria, 111
DPT, 110–112, 118, 128
exposure and, 80
German measles, 114–116, 118
influenza, 117
measles, 113–114, 118
mumps, 116
pertussis (whooping cough), 111–112
polio, 112–113, 118
during pregnancy, 11
principle of, 109–110
rabies, 117
schedule for, 117–118
school entry and, 81
smallpox, 116–117
tetanus (lockjaw), 112, **156–157**

Impetigo, **244–245**

Impromine, 10

Inactivated polio virus (IPV) vaccine, 113

Inactivity, 122

Incubation period
chicken pox, 280
fifth disease, 290
German measles, 284
measles, 282
mumps, 278
roseola, 286

Independence, 73–75

Induced births, 23

Infant seats, 30, 106

Infants, 33–50
abdomen, 43
activity of, 39–40
breathing, 40

chest, 43
colic, **358–359**
eyes, 41–42
face, 43
feeding, 44–50
feet, 44
first child, adjustment to, 33–36
genitals, 43–44
growth and development, physical, 51–61
hands, 43
head, 41
maternal medications causing problems in, 10–11
mouth, 42
nose, 42
personality development, 63–65
rashes, **238–239**
second child, adjustment to, 36–39
skin and birthmarks, 40–41

Infection
asthma and, 193–195
burns and, 168
eczema and, 196
signs of, 148, 150, 154
staphylococcal, 342
streptococcal, 201, 288
viral or bacterial, differentiating between, 200–201
of wounds, **170–171**
yeast, 228, 240, 262, 272, 368, 376
See also Bacterial infections; Fungus infections; Viral infections; *infection sites by name.*

Infectious mononucleosis. *See* Mononucleosis.

Infertility, 28

Inflammation
injuries and, 158, 170
reducing, 187

Influenza, 117, 318. *See also* Flu.

Ingestion of poisons, **180–181**

Inguinal canal and inguinal hernia, 101–102

Injuries, common, 147–177
animal bites, **152–153**
ankle, **160–161**
broken bones, **158–159**
burns, **168–169**
cuts, **148–149**
fingers, smashed, **176–177**
fishhooks, **174–175**
head, **166–167**

infected wounds and blood poisoning, **170–171**
insect bites and stings, **172–173**
knee, **162–163**
puncture wounds, **150–151**
scrapes and abrasions, **154–155**
tetanus shots, **156–157**
wrist, elbow, and shoulder, **164–165**
Innocent murmurs, 94–95
Insect bites and stings, 128, **172–173,** 218, 248, 252
lice and bedbugs, **266–267**
relief of itching, 172, 248, 250
ticks and chiggers (redbugs), **268–269**
Insect repellents, 268
Insecticides, 180, 266
Intelligence
development rate and, 61
testing, 84–85
Intercourse, sexual
conception and, 6
during pregnancy, 8–9
pubic lice and, 266
trends in, 77
Internists, 91
Intestine
blockage, 348, 354, 360
irritation, 351
perforated, 324
Intrauterine devices (IUDs), 376–377
Iodine, 148, 154
allergy, 133
Ionil, 272
Ipecac, syrup of, 128, 132, 180
Iritis, 338, 340
Iron, 7, 46–47
sources, 318
Iron deficiency anemia, 97, 318–319
Irritability, 112, 114, 206, 304, 318, 348, 372
Isoproterenol, 194
Itching, 172, 244, 248, 250, 254, 266, 268, 270
chicken pox, 280
ears, 208
eyes, 195, 200, 212, 282, 326, **338–339**
measles, 282
rectal, **360–361**
relief of, 172, 195–196, 250
vaginal, 368
See also Skin and skin problems.

Jaundice, 14, 41–42, 348, 354
Jaw
injury, 230
jutting, 216, 220
swollen, 230
Jealousy, father's, of baby, 34
Jellies, contraceptive, 376
Jello, 350
Jenner, 110
Jerking of head, 185
Jock itch, **262–263**
Jockey shorts, 262
Jogging, 125
Joints
ankle injuries, **160–161**
bones, muscles, and, 293–301
finger, 176
jaw, 230
knee injuries, **162–163**
pain in, 115, 204, 284, **294–295,** 354
painful, swollen, 204
wrist, elbow, and shoulder injuries, **164–165**
Juice
apple, 351
cranberry, 134, 364
fruit, for infants, 48
iced frozen, 228
orange, 278
prune, 130–131, 310, 360
Junior foods, 48
Junk food, 50, 122
Justice, child's code of, 71
Juvenile diabetes mellitus, 98

K, vitamin, 27
Kanamycin, 11
Kaolin, 131, 352
Kaopectate, 131, 352
Karo syrup, 47, 310
Keratin plugs, 258
Kerosene, 180
Ketones, 7
Kidney
disease, 278
impetigo complication, 244
infection, 364
strep throat complications, 201, 204
Kidney stone, 364
Knee
injuries, **162–163**
knock-knees, **298–299**
pain, 294
Knock-knees, **298–299**
Koplik's spots, 282
Kwell, 266, 268, 270

Labor
induced, 23, 26
premature, 9
prolonged, 25
stages, 21–22
Laboratory tests, 92
routine for children, 97–98
See also tests by name.
Labyrinthitis, 320
Lacerations, **148–149**
Lactase, 192–193, 351
Lactic acid, 252
La Leche League, 15, 44, 46
Lamaze method, 16
Lamb, 248
Lancing
boil, 256
stye, 342
Language, 49, 61, 66, 70, 81–82, 84–85
Lanolin, 45
Larvae, red, 268
Laryngitis (hoarseness), **220–221**
Larynx, 216
Lateral stability of knee, 162
Laughing, infant's, 40
Laxatives, 131, 310, 360
Lazy eye, 82, 94, 344
Learning problems
factors contributing to, 81–83
hyperactivity, **306–307**
investigating, 83–84
Legs
bowlegs and knock-knees, **298–299**
injuries, 148, 158, 160–163
pain traveling down, 296
rash on, 290, 294
wound healing time, 110
See also Ankle injuries; Knee injuries.
Lemons, 278
Lentils, 318
Lesions
mouth, **228–229**
skin, 117, 254, 272
Letdown reflex in nursing, 35–36, 45
Lethargy, 132, 166, 282, 286, 348. *See also* Drowsiness; Weakness.
Librium, 11
Lice, **266–267**
Lidocaine, 149
Ligaments
injuries, 160–165
pain, 330
Lightheadedness. *See* Dizziness;

Fainting.
Lima beans, 318
Limping, 296
Lipomas, 252
"Liquid aspirin," 187
Liquiprin, 132, 187
Lip lesions, 228
Liver
  beef, 192
  cirrhosis of, 124
  damage, 188
  newborn, 41
  tenderness over, 348
Local anesthetics, 23, 149, 154,
    168, 174
Lockjaw. See Tetanus.
Lomotil, 131, 352
Lotions, creams, and oils, 29–30
Lotrimin, 246, 262
Low-back pain, **296–297**
Low blood sugar, 318–320
LSD, 11
Luminal, 22
Lumps, skin, **252–253**
Lungs, 330, 332, 334
  abscess, 226
  disease, 30
  fluid in newborn's, 27
  infection, 214
  wheezing and, 193, 195
Lymph glands, nodes, and
    channels, 170, 222, 284,
    294, 338

Magic Years, The, 66
Malabsorption, 314
Malaria, 98
Malathion, 266
Maltsupex, 131, 310, 360
Marezine, 11
Marijuana, 124
Massage, 304, 342, 356
Mastoid, 206
Masturbation, 76–77, 364
Maturational lag, 82, 84
Measles, 113–114, 118, 184,
    282–283, 338
Measles immune globulin, 114
Meclizine, 11
MEDEX, 92
Medical care, 91–102
  choosing medical professional,
    91–93
  frequent illness, screening for
    cause of, 99
  laboratory tests, 97–98
  pelvic examination, first,
    95–97
  surgery, 99–102

well-baby examinations,
    93–95
Medications
  fever reduction and, 187–188
  giving, 133–134
  home pharmacy, 127–135
  for mother, 10–11, 22
  oral poisoning and, 144–145,
    180–181
  See also Drugs.
Melanoma, 252
Memory loss, 166, 186
Meningitis, 113, 184–185, 304,
    322, 348
Meningo-encephalitis, 116
Menstruation
  child's impressions about, 77
  conception and, 6
  headache and, 304
  low-back pain and, 296
  onset, 54–55, 372
  problems, **372–373**
  temperature and, 184
Mental health centers, 316
Mental retardation, 27, 284, 306
Mercurochrome, 133, 148, 154
Merthiolate, 148, 208
Metabolic disease, 9
Metamucil, 131, 310, 360
Metatarsus adductus, 94, 300
Mica Tin, 246
Miconazole, 246
Migraine headaches, 304, 348,
    376
Miliaria, 238
Milk
  cow's, allergy and digestion
    problems, 192, 196, 248,
    351, 356
  goat's, 318
  to neutralize poisons, 180
  soybean substitute for, 193
  See also Bottle feeding; Breast
    feeding.
Milk of magnesia, 131, 180
Mineral oil, 131, 208, 310
Minerals, 7, 133
Minimal brain dysfunction
    (MBD), 306
Mini-pill, 376
Ministers, 316
Missed periods, 372
Mites, 270
Mold, 193, 212–213
Moles, 41, 252
Mongolism, 9
Mononucleosis (mono), 200,
    204, 222, 318–319
Montessori, Maria, 79

Moral Judgment of the Child,
    The, 71
Motion
  ankle, abnormal, 160
  eye, 344
  knee, range of, 162
  limitation caused by injuries,
    164
Motion sickness, 195, 348
Motor skills, 70
Mouth
  bad breath, **226–227**
  breathing, 204
  chicken pox in, 280
  difficulty opening, 204
  dry, 141, 348
  eating skills, 48–49
  infant, 42
  lesions, **228–229**
  spots in, 42, 228, 282, 288
Mouthwash, 226
Mucus
  asthma and, 193, 195
  bloody, before labor, 21
  excess in nostrils, 42, 212, 214
Multiple births, 25
Mumps, 116, 184, 222, 230,
    278–279
Murine, 131, 338
Muscle relaxants, 297
Muscles
  bones, joints, and, 293–301
  chest, 330
  eye, 344
  pain, 117, 200–201, **294–295**
  spasms, 296, 304
Mustard to induce vomiting, 180
Mycolog, 368
Mycostatin, 240
Myocardial infarction, 122

Naps, 69, 80
Narcotics, 352
Nausea, 6, 98, 200, 304, 320,
    348–350, 354, 364, 376
  drugs against, 11
  drugs producing, 131
  injury and, 172
  See also Vomiting.
Nebulizers, 194
Neck
  rash on, 282, 286
  stiff, 282, 304, 348
Negativism, 58, 65
Nembutal, 22
Neosporin, 27, 154
Neo-Synephrine, 129, 212
Nerve
  injury, 150

testing function of, 296, 304
Nervousness, 318
Neurasthenia, 318
Neutralizing poisons, 180
Newborn procedures, 26–28.
    See also Infants.
Nicotine, 123–124
Night lights, 69–70
Night terrors, 70, 316
Nightmares, 316
Nipples
    inverted, 14, 55
    tenderness or lump, in male
        adolescent, 54
Nits, 266
"No," child's negativism and,
    58–59, 65
Normal discharge, 368
Normality of development,
    60–61
Noscapine, 130
Nose
    bleeding, **224–225**
    ears, throat, and, 199–231
    infant, 42
    picking, 224
    runny, 129, 195–196,
        200–201, **212–213,** 286,
        326, 351
    stuffy, 212
    white dots on infant's, 238
Nose drops, 129, 202, 206, 214
    side effects, 212
Nosebleeds, **224–225**
Novahistine, 130
Numbness, 148, 150, 158, 316
Nurse practitioners, 92
Nursery schools, 71, 326
Nursing Mothers Association, 44
Nursing Your Baby, 46
Nutrition
    child's selection and, 49
    infant, 48
    junk food and, 50
    maternal, 7–8, 12, 118
    physical growth and, 52
    weakness, tiredness, and, 318
Nuts, 192, 248, 318
Nystatin, 228

Oatmeal bath, 250, 268
Obesity, **312–313**
    breast feeding and, 13
    fat cells and, 52, 312
    low-back pain and, 296
    male adolescent, 54
    risk factor for heart attack, 122
Odor, body, 54

Oil
    baby, 29–30, 272
    skin, 238, 258, 272
    for tick removal, 268
Oleander, 105
Olive oil, 208
Ophthalmologist, 174, 338, 340,
    344
Ophthalmoscope, 344
Optometrist, 344
Orabase, 228
Oral polio virus (OPV) vaccine,
    113, 118
Oral thermometers and oral
    temperature, 184
Oranges, 310
Orgasm, fertility and, 6
Orthopedic surgeon, 298
Osgood-Schlatter's disease, 294
Otitis externa, 208
Otitis media, 206. *See also*
    Earache.
Ovaries, 54
    hormones, 373
    infection, mumps and, 278
    inflammation, 116
    pelvic examination, 96
Overdosage and drug reactions.
    See Poisoning, oral; *drugs
    by name.*
Overweight, 13, 52, 54, 122,
    296, **312–313**
Ovulation, 6, 184
Oxygen, 143
Oxymetazoline, 129
Oxytocin, 23

Pabafilm, 264
Pabonal, 264
Pacifiers, 68–69, 118, 358
Packing nose with gauze, 224
Pain
    abdominal, 172, 192–193,
        200–201, 204, 294, 308,
        324, 348, **354–357,** 358,
        364
    breast feeding and, 35–36
    breath-holding spells and, 68
    chest, 130, 324, **330–331,**
        334
    childbirth and, 16, 22
    crying, 65
    behind ear, 278
    eye, 338, **340–341**
    flu and, 200
    foot, 300
    injuries and, 154, 158, 160,
        162, 164–165, 168, 170,

174, 176
    joints, 115, 204, 284,
        294–295, 354
    low-back, **296–297**
    medications for, 131–132
    menstrual, 372–373
    muscle, 117, 200–201,
        294–295
    rectal, 310, **360–361**
    severe, 145
    toothache confused with other
        pains, 230
    urination and, **364–365**
    See also pain sites by name.
Painless Childbirth, 16
Palate, soft, spots on, 288
Paleness, 158, 166
Palm, cuts in, 148
Palpitations, **334–335**
Pancreas
    infection, 278
    inflammation, 124
Pancreatitis, 278
Pap smears, 95–97, 372
Paracervical anesthesia, 23
Paralysis, 111, 113, 186, 268
Parapectolin, 131
Paregoric, 131, 352
Parelixir, 131, 352
Parent skills and concerns, 3–135
    childbirth, 19–30
    growth and development,
        51–61
    medical care, 91–102
    medications, 127–135
    newborn care, 33–50
    personality development,
        63–78
    pregnancy, 3–18
    prevention of illness, 103–125
    school, 79–80
Parotid glands, 278
Peas, 318
Pectin, 131, 352
Pedialyte, 351
Pediatricians, 27, 91, 95
Peeling, skin, 258, 264, 288
Pelvic examination
    first, 95–97
    vaginal problems and, 368,
        372
Pelvic injuries, 158
Penicillin, 111, 134, 200–201,
    244, 288
    allergy, 134, 244, 288
Penis, 54
    circumcision, 28–29
    hygiene, 28

problems, **370-371**
rash, 240
Perforation
of eardrum, 208
of intestine, 324
Pericardium, 330
Peripheral neuropathy, 115
Permanent teeth, 121
Pernox, 258
Personality changes, 166, 304
Personality development, 63-78
adolescent's, 72-75
infant's, 63-65
preschooler's, 70-71
school years, early, 71-72
sexuality, 75-78
toddler's, 65-70
Pertussis, 111-112
Petechiae, 43
Petersen Safety Shell, 106
Petit mal, 83
Petroleum jelly, 240, 352
Petroleum products, 180
Pets
asthma and, 194
bite prevention, 108-109
during pregnancy, 11-12
ticks and, 268
Phenacetin, 132
Phenergan, 11, 130
Phenobarbital, 194
Phenol, 228
Phenylephrine, 129
Phenylketonuria, 27-28
Phimosis, 28
Phororus, 118
Physician
consultation, urgency of, 140
See also Medical care.
Physician's assistants, 92
Physicians for Automotive
Safety, 106
Piaget, 71
Pickles, 278
Pigeon toes, 94, 298, **300-301**
Pimples, 258, 280
Pink eye, 338
Pinning fractures, 159
Pinworms, 360, 364, 368
Pitocin, 23
Pituitary gland, 53-54
hormones, 373
Pityriasis alba, 274
Placenta, 22, 25
Plaque, 122, 272
Planned Parenthood clinics, 377
Plastic pants, 240, 254
Play, 70, 80

Playing doctor or house, 76
Pneumonia, 113, 184, 202, 214,
218, 282, 330, 332, 354
Pneumothorax, 330
Poinsettia leaves, 104
Pointing of abscess, 342
Poison control center, 128, 132,
143, 180
Poison ivy and poison oak,
250-251
Poisoning
blood, **170-171**
contact, 250
oral, 132, 144-145,
180-181, 348
prevention, 104-105
Poisonous plants, 104-105, 180,
250
Poisonous spiders, 172
Polio, 109, 112-113, 118
Pollen, 193, 195, 201, 212-213,
248, 338
Pollutants, 191, 338
Polybrominated biphenyls
(PBB), 14
Polychlorinated biphenyls (PCB),
14
Popsicles, 228, 348
Pork, 248
Portwine stains, 41
Position, sudden changes in, 321
Possums, 152
Post-ictal state, 322
Postnasal drip, 212, 214
Postural hypotension, 320
Potassium hydroxide solution,
246
Potassium iodide, 11
Powders, 30, 240, 260, 262
Prednisone, 194, 250
Pregnancy, 3-18
breast feeding or bottle
feeding, 12-15
care during, 6-12
childbirth preparation classes,
15-17
conception, 6
contraception, 375-378
delivery options, 17-18
drugs to avoid during, 10-11
emotions during, 3-5
German measles, 114-116,
284
missed periods and, 372
test, 372
Premarital sexual experience,
77-78
Premature births, 25-26

Premature ejaculation, 376
Premature infant, breast feeding,
45
Premature labor, 21, 26
Prenatal care, 6-12
amniocentesis, 9-10
diet, 7-8
drugs to avoid, 10-11
exercise, 8
foods to avoid, 8
immunization and allergy
shots, 11
pets, 11-12
sexual activity, 8-9
travel, 8
Prepping, 24
Preschool years
day-care centers, 79-80
personality development, 70-71
Presun, 264
Prevention, 103-125
accidents, 103-109
adult diseases, 121-125
asthma attack, 194
dental care, 118-121
immunizations, 109-118
poisoning, 180
sunburn, 264
Prickly heat, 238
Progestins, 11, 376
Promethazine, 11
Prophylactic sulfisoxazole, 101
Proteins, 7
Prune juice and prunes,
130-131, 310, 360
Pryor, Karen, 46
Pseudoephedrine, 128-129, 212
Psoriasis, 272
Psychiatric disorders, 306
Psychiatrists and psychologists,
316
Puberty
acne, **258-259**
growth at, 53-55
Pubic hair, 54, 266
Pubic lice, 266
Pubic region, 262
Pudendal block anesthesia, 23
Pulled elbow, 164
Pulse
fast or irregular, 334
sick child's, 142
slow or irregular, 166-167
Puncture wounds, 112,
150-151. *See also*
Fishhooks.
Pupil of eye, 166-167, 338, 340
Pus, 148, 150, 154, 170, 256,

338, 342, 370
Pustular stage of chicken pox, 280
Pyribenzamine, 195
Pyridium, 364
Pyridoxine, 11

Q-tips, 30
Quiet child, 63
Quinic acid, 364

Rabies and rabies vaccine, 117, 152
Raccoons, 152
Radiation, 300. *See also* X-rays.
Ragweed, 195
Raking, 56
Rashes, 204, 205, 268, 354
    allergic, 192
    aspirin, 187
    baby, 43, **238–239**
    chicken pox, 280
    dark, blotchy, on legs, 294
    diaper, **240–241**
    fifth disease, 290
    German measles, 284
    immunizations and, 114
    insect bite or sting, 172
    measles, 282
    roseola, 286
    scarlet fever, 288
    skin symptom table, 236–237
    See also Skin and skin problems.
Readiness
    for school, 80–81
    for sports, 87–88
Rectal fissure, 310
Rectal thermometers and rectal temperatures, 184
Rectum
    examination, 96, 354
    irritations, 13
    pain, itching or bleeding, **360–361**
    tear in, 310
Red measles, **282–283**. *See also* Measles.
Redbugs, **268–269**
Redness, 148, 150, 154, 168, 230, 270
"Reds," 124
Regression toward the mean, 53
Removing stitches, 148
Rescue squad, 143
Respiratory distress syndrome, 26
Respiratory infections, 113, 356

ear, nose, and throat problems, 199–225
influenza, 117
upper, 99
Respiratory rate, normal, 142, 332
Rest, 202, 204, 296
Resuscitation, 108, 143
Retardation
    growth, 194–197
    mental, 27, 284, 306
Retin-A, 258
Retina, 42
Retinoblastoma, 42
Retinoic acid, 258
Rewards and punishments
    food as, 49–50
    toilet training and, 57–59
Reyes syndrome, 350
Rh sensitization, 9
Rheumatic fever, 204–205, 288, 294, 354
Rheumatoid arthritis, 294
Rhinitis medicamentosum, 212
Rhus plant family, 250
Rhythm method, 375
Ribs, 330
Rice, 248, 310, 351
Rickets, 298
RID, 266
Ringworm, 242, **246–247,** 272, 274
Ritalin, 307
Robitussin and Robitussin-DM, 130, 214, 330
Rocky Mountain spotted fever, 172, 268
Romilar, 130, 214, 330
Rondec and Rondec-DM, 128–130
Rooming in, 28
Root canals, 230
Rooting reflex, 45, 64
Roseola, 184–185, **286–287,** 323
Roughage, 119
Rubber gloves, 254
Rubella, **284–285**. *See also* German measles.
Runny nose, **212–213**. *See also* Nose, runny.
Rupture of amniotic fluid sac, 9, 22, 24

Sabin vaccine, 113
Safety
    automobile, 30, 105–107
    bicycle, 107

home, 104–105
    pet, 108
    sports, 88–89
    water, 108
Safety lenses, 88
Salicylates, 307
Salicyclic acid plasters, 252
Salivary glands
    infection, 278
    swelling, 116, 222
Salivation
    drooling, 216, 220
    excess, 204
Salk, Jonas, 113
Salmon patch, 40
Salt
    gargle, 204, 280
    restriction, 372
Sassafras, 8
Scabies, **270–271**
Scabs, 170
Scalds, 168
Scalp
    abnormalities, 242
    chicken pox, 280
    dandruff, 240, **272–273**
    infection, 222, 246
    lice, 266
    oiliness and flaking, 272
    ticks, 268
Scarlet fever, 201, 205, **288–289**
Scarring, 168, 280
School, 79–89
    adjustment problems, 306
    athletics, in childhood, 86–89
    attendance, fever, colds, and, 99, 202
    avoidance, 85, 316
    changing frequently, 83
    day-care centers, 79–80
    early years, personality development during, 71–72
    failing in, 81–84
    hyperactivity, **306–307**
    intelligence testing (IQ), 84–85
    readiness for, 80–81
Schwarz strain vaccine, 114
Sciatica, 296
Scotch broom, 105
Scrapes, **154–155**
Scrotum
    swelling, 43–44, 101–102
    undescended testicles, 101
Seat belts and safety restraints, 106
Sebaceous gland hyperplasia, 238

Seborrhea, 240, 270
Sebucare, 272
Sebulex, 272
Seconal, 22
Second child, adjusting to, 36–39
Second-degree burn, 168, 264
Second opinion, 93
Sedatives, 22
Seizures, 41, 68, 83, 111–113, 144–145, 185–186, 282, 286, 304, 320, **322–323**
   hyperactivity, **306–307**
Selenium sulfide, 272
Selsun and Selsun Blue shampoos, 246, 272, 274
Separation, easing shock of, 80
Separation, shoulder, 164
Septicemia (blood poisoning), **170–171**
Serous otitis media, 206
Serum, body, 170, 280
Serum immunity, 116
Serum injections, 111
Setting bone, 159, 161
Seven-day measles, **282–283.** *See also* Measles.
Sex, determining fetus's, 9
Sex roles and sexual identity, 71, 75, 77
Sexuality and sexual activity
   adolescent's, 74
   before and after childbirth, 8–9
   contraception, 375–378
   development, 75–79
Shaking, 172
Shellfish, 248
Shingles, 280
Shivering, 186
Shock
   as allergic reaction, 192
   signs of, 158
Shoes, 260, 300
Shortness of breath, 95, 98, 143, 145, 218, 324, 330, **332–333,** 334
Shots. *See* Immunizations; Pregnancy.
Shoulder, **164–165,** 280
Sick child, recognizing, 141–142
Sickle-cell anemia, 294
   screening, 97–98
Silk, 254
Silver fork deformity, 164
Silver nitrate, 27, 42
Similac, 47
Sinuses and sinusitis, 129–130, 212–213, 230, 304
Sitting, 61, 296

Sitz bath, 368
Size, physical, 53
   school problems and, 83
   sports readiness and, 87
Skills
   development, 55–57
   verbal and performance, IQ and, 84
Skin and skin problems, 233–275, 330
   acne, **258–259**
   athlete's foot, **260–261**
   baby rashes, **238–239**
   birthmarks and, 40–41
   boils, 252, **256–257**
   dandruff and cradle cap, 240, **272–273**
   diaper rash, **240–241**
   discoloration, 197, 244
   dryness, itching, weeping, crusting, 196–197
   eczema, 193, 196–197, **254–255**
   hair loss, **242–243**
   hives, 172, 192, **248–249**
   impetigo, **244–245**
   jock itch, **262–263**
   lesions, 117
   lice and bedbugs, **266–267**
   lumps, bumps, and warts, **252–253**
   patchy loss of skin color, **274–275**
   poison ivy and poison oak, **250–251**
   ringworm, 242, **246–247,** 272, 274
   scabies, 270–271
   sunburn, **264–265**
   sunlight and, 42
   symptom table, 236–237
   ticks and chiggers, **268–269**
   turgor of sick and of normal child, 141
   See also Childhood diseases.
Skin grafts, 168
Skunks, 152
"Slapped cheek" appearance, 290
Sleeping, 334
   antihistamines and, 129, 196, 212, 250
   cough suppressants and, 130
   difficulty falling asleep, 316
   excessive, 316
   infant's, 39
   low-back pain and, 296
   through night, 46–48

position, 64
post-ictal state, 322
school problems and, 83
tiredness, **318–319**
toddler's, 69–70
See also Drowsiness.
Sling, 165
Slit lamp, 344
SMA, 47
Smallpox, 109–110, 116–117
Smiling, 60–61, 64
Smoking, cigarette, 122–123
Sneezing
   hay fever, 195, 200, 326
   infant, 42, 212
Soaking
   boils, 256
   penis, 370
   scabies, 270
   tick bite, 268
   urination problems, 364
   wound, 150, 170
Soap, abrasive, 258
Social workers, 316
Socialization and social skills
   eating, 49–50
   school readiness and, 81
   school-ager's, 72
   toddler's, 71
Soda, flat, 351
Soft spot (fontanel), 41, 166
   bulging, 304, 348
Soiling, constipation and, **310–311**
Solid foods, 48
Sore throat, **204–205.** *See also* Throat, sore.
Sour foods, pain and, 278
Soybeans, 193, 318
Sparine, 22
Speculum, 96–97
Speech
   defect, 81
   difficulties, 304
   hearing loss and, 210
   interference by adenoids, 100
"Speed," 124
Sperm, 54
Spider bicycles, 107
Spiders, poisonous, identifying, 172
Spinach, 318
Spinal anesthesia, 23
Spinal cord infection, 323, 348
Spinal tap, 188, 282, 323
Spine, 296–297, 330
Spitting up, 348
Spleen enlargement, 204

Splinting, 158, 165, 176
Sponging to reduce fever, 186–187, 322
Sports
  childhood, 86–89
  foot placement and, 300
  injuries, 162, 164, 166
  readiness, 87–88
  safety, 88–89
Spots
  in mouth, 42, 228, 282, 288
  See also Childhood diseases; Skin and skin problems.
Sprains, 160, 162, 164–165
Standing with low-back pain, 296
Starch, 119
Stealing, 71–72
Steam, 133, 216, 258. *See also* Vaporizer.
Sterility, 116, 278
Sterilization
  of formula, 15
  of wound, 133
Steristrips, 148
Sternum, 330
Steroids, 40, 194, 196, 240, 250, 254, 258, 264, 312, 340
Stiffening of body, 185
Stiffness
  back, 296
  neck, 282, 304, 348
Stings, insect, **172–173,** 218
Stitches, 148
Stomach flu, 200, 318, 354, 356
Stomach pump, 180
Stomachache, 288. *See also* Abdomen, pain.
Stools
  analysis, 192, 314, 352, 356
  blood in, 141, 348, 351, 360
  of breast-fed baby, 13
  greasy, smelly, 314
  hardening, 131
  pain in passing, 310
  softening, 131, 360
  See also Bowel control; Constipation; Diarrhea.
Stork bite, 40
Strabismus, 82, 94, 344
Strains, 160, 162, 164–165, 296–297
Strawberry marks, 40
Strep throat, 200–201, 204, 304, 326
Streptomycin, 11
Stress
  anxiety, depression and, **316–317**

bedwetting and, 308, 364
child's, 68
digestive problems and, 348, 356
headaches and, 304
heart attack and, 122
menstrual problems and, 372
overweight and, 312
palpitations and, 334
parental, 67
school avoidance and, 85
suicide and, 124
weakness, tiredness, and, 318
Stroke, 122–123
Strolee Wee Care Car Seat, 106
Stupor, 144
Styes, blocked tear ducts and, **342–343**
Subdural hematoma, 166
Subungual hematoma, 176
Sucking, 48, 64, 68
  affecting mother, 23
  bottle feeding and, 15
  breast feeding and, 45
  thumb, pacifiers and, 68–69
Sudafed, 129, 212, 306
Suffocation, 68–69
Sugar, 47, 50, 119
Suicide, 123–124, 180
Sulfa drugs, 11, 14
Sulfisoxazole, 101, 364
Sunburn, 168, 258, **264–265**
Sunlamps, 258
Sunlight
  acne and, 258
  jaundice reduction and, 41
  vitamin D and, 13
Sunscreens, 264
Sunstroke, 264
Supplements
  to bottle feeding, 47
  to breast feeding, 13, 30, 46
  during pregnancy, 7
  fluoride, 120–121
Suppositories
  aspirin, 187, 322
  contraceptive, 376
  drugs to open breathing tube, 218
  glycerine, 310
  trimethobenzamine, 350
  vaginal, 364, 368
Suppressants, cough, 130, 330
Surgery
  acne, 258
  birthmarks, 40
  breast reduction, 54–55
  chalazion, 342

circumcision, 28–29
crossed eye correction, 344
finger injuries and, 176
frequently performed procedures, 99–102
knock-knee correction, 298
penis, relieving constriction of, 370
perforated intestine, 324
pinning fractures, 159
torn ligaments, repairing, 161–163
Suturing, 148
Swallowed foreign objects, 144, 214, 218, **324–325,** 354
Swallowing
  difficulty, 204, 220
  painful, 278
  to relieve ear pressure, 206
  of tongue, 322
Sweating, 158, 166, 172, 196, 254, 318
Swelling
  belly, 356
  epiglottis, 216
  genitals, 43–44, 101–102
  glands, 12, 116, 200–201, **222–223,** 278, 286, 288, 294, 338
  in infants, 41–44
  at infection site, 148, 150, 154
  at injection site, 111–112
  injuries and, 158, 160, 162, 166, 170, 176
  jaw, 230
  joints, 204
  mouth and lips, 192
  skin, 248, 270
  See also swollen sites by name.
Swimmer's ear, 208
Swimming
  asthma and, 195
  classes, 107–108
  eczema and, 254
  as exercise, 125
Swollen glands, **222–223.** *See also* Glands, swollen.
Swyngomatic American Safety Seat, 106
Symptoms, skin, table of, 236–237
Syringe, ear, 208, 210
Systemic reactions
  hives, 248
  insect bites or stings, 172

Tailbone, 296
Talc, 30, 240

Talking, 82. *See also* Language.
Tampon, forgotten, 368
Taping ankle injury, 161
Tay-Sachs disease, 9
Tea, 204, 358
Tear duct, blocked, 42, 338, **342–343**
Tearing, excess, 42
Teddy Tot Astroseat, 106
Teeth
  brushing, 119–120
  permanent, 121
  See also Dental care.
Teething, 118–119
Television, educational, 81
Temper tantrums, 65–66
Temperature
  of formula, 47
  of water in ear syringe, 210
Temperature, body
  dangerous, 185
  factors affecting, 184
  newborn's, 27
  ovulation and, 6
  taking, 184–185
  See also Fever.
Tempra, 10, 132, 187
Ten-day measles, **282–283.** *See also* Measles.
Tendon injuries, 149
Tension
  headaches, 304
  premenstrual, 372
Terminal phalanx, 176
Terrible twos, 66
Testes, inflammation of, 116
Testicles, 54
  mumps and, 278
  undescended, 95, 101
Testosterone, 54
Tetanus (lockjaw) and tetanus shots, 112, 149–150, 152, 154, **156–157,** 174
Tetanus immune globulin, 112, 156
Tetracycline, 11, 14, 118, 258
Thalidomide, 10
Therapy
  for anxiety and depression, 316
  for asthma patient and family, 195
Thermometers, oral and rectal, 184
Thigh injuries, 158
Third-degree burns, 168
Thirst, 158, 372
  excessive, 98

See also Dehydration.
Thorazine, 11
Three-day measles, **284–285.** *See also* German measles.
Three-in-one shot, 110–112
Three-month colic, 358
Throat
  culture, 204
  ears, nose, and, 199–231
  infection, 100
  red, 286, 288
  sore, 100, 184, 200–201, **204–205,** 222, 226, 230, 282, 304, 318, 354
  strep, 200–201
Throwing ability, 56
Throwing up, **348–350.** *See also* Vomiting.
Thrush, 228
Thumb sucking, 68–69
Thyroid
  disorder, 220, 312–313
  hormone, 53, 373
  hyperthyroidism, 306
Tick paralysis, 268
Ticks, 172, **268–269**
Tigan, 350
Tine test, 97
Tinea cruris (jock itch), **262–263**
Tinea versicolor, 274
Tingling, 148, 150, 172, 316, 330
Toast, 351
Tiredness, **318–319.** *See also* Fatigue; Weakness.
Toddler's personality development, 65–70
Toeing in, 94, 300
Toenails, 260
Tofranil, 10, 308
Toilet training, 57–60
  bedwetting, 59–60, **308–309**
  bladder, 59
  bowels, 57–59
  constipation and, 310
Tolnaftate, 246, 260, 262
Tongue
  chewing or swallowing of, 322
  fuzzy, white, 288
Tongue thrust, 118
Tongue-tied, 42
Tonsils and tonsillectomy, 99–100, 204
Tooth decay, 119, 226, 230. *See also* Dental care.
Tooth eruption
  baby teeth, 118

permanent teeth, 120
Toothaches, **230–231,** 304
Toothpaste, choice of, 120
Torn ligaments, 160–162, 164
Toxoid, 111
Toxoplasmosis, 11–12
Trachea (windpipe), 144, 214, 216
Trait, genetic, 98
Tranquilizers, 11, 22, 124
Transition stage of labor, 21
Travel during pregnancy, 8
Trench mouth, 228
Triaminic, 306
Trimethobenzamide suppositories, 350
Tripelennamine, 195
Triprolidine, 128
Trunk, rash on, 286, 288
Tubal pregnancy, 376
Tuberculosis, 110
  screening, 97, 114
Tumor of eye in newborns, 42
Turpentine, 145
Twitching, 172
2-G, 130
Tylenol, 10, 132, 187

Ulcer
  cornea, 338
  mouth, 228
  stomach, 124–125, 354, 356
Ultraviolet light, 242, 246, 340
Umbilical cord, 43
Umbilical hernia, 43, 101
Unconsciousness, 144, 166, 172
  dizziness and fainting, **320–321**
  See also Seizures.
Underweight, 52, **314–315,** 326
Undescended testicles, 54, 101
United States Department of Health, Education, and Welfare (HEW), 110
United States Public Health Service, 117
Unresponsiveness, 132, 166
Upper respiratory infections, 99, 199–225. *See also* Colds, common.
Urethra and urethritis, 364
Urinalysis. *See* Urine, urinalysis.
Urinary tract infections, 184, 296–297, 308, 314, 348, 354, 356, 363–365
Urination
  bedwetting, 59–60, **308–309**
  bladder training, 59

burning, 308
discomfort during, 354
frequent, 6, 98, 308, 354
infrequent, 141
involuntary, 185
painful, frequent, or bloody,
364–365
Urine
dark, 348
dark brown, 244
dark yellow, 141
diaper rash, **240–241**
scant, deep yellow, 348
urinalysis, 6, 98, 188, 308,
314, 320, 350, 352, 354,
356, 364
See also Urination.
Uterus, 13
contractions, 16, 21, 23–24,
26
pelvic examination, 96
Uveitis, 338

Vaccines. *See* Immunizations;
vaccines by name.
Vacuum around nipple,
breaking, 45
Vagina
bleeding and menstrual
problems, 9, 26, 44, 368,
372–373
discharge from, 364, **368–369**
episiotomy, 25
infections, 360, 368
lubricants, fertility and, 6
pelvic examination, 96
Validol, 10, 132, 187
Valium, 11, 14, 124
Values, development of, 71, 73
Vaporizer, 128, 130, 133, 195,
204, 212, 214, 216, 218,
220, 224, 282
Variability limits for development,
60–61
Vaseline, 240, 264, 352
Veal, 192
Venereal disease, 27, 95, 368,
376
Verbal ability. *See* Language.
Vergo, 252
Vernix caseosa, 40
Vertigo, 320. *See also* Dizziness.
Vesicles, chicken pox, 280
Vinegar, 240, 364, 368
Viral gastroenteritis, 200, 351
Viral infections, 80, 99, 184, 204,
210, 214, 216, 218, 220,
222, 224, 228, 252, 278,

280, 282, 284, 286, 320,
326, 338, 348, 351
arthralgia accompanying, 294
Viral URI (Upper Respiratory
Infection), 200, 202. *See
also* Colds, common.
Virus
distinguishing from bacteria or
allergy, 200–201
immunizations and, 109–110
problems caused by, 202
See also specific complaints.
Visine, 131, 338
Vision
decreased, **344–345**
disturbances, headaches and,
304
infant, 42
interference with, 338
loss, 344
problems, 82, 94, 306
test, 307, 340
Vistaril, 250
Visual acuity. *See* Vision.
Visual motor ability problems, 82
Vitamins, 7
excess during pregnancy, 11
for infants, 30
supplements, 133
See also vitamins by name.
Vlem-Dome, 258
Vocal cords, 220
Voice box, 216
Voice changes
adolescent, 54
hoarseness, **220–221**
Vomiting, 98, 172, 200, 210,
288, 314, 320, 322, 324,
348–350, 351, 354, 364
blood in, 141, 354
decreasing, 195
with fever, 304
inducing, methods for, 132,
180
lactase lack, food allergies,
and, 192–193
not inducing, in poisoning,
128, 145, 180
persistent, 166, 318
sick child's, 141
See also Nausea.
Vulva, 368

Walking, 61
bowlegs and knock-knees,
298–299
difficulties, 304

pigeon toes and flat feet, 298,
300–301
Wandering eye, 82, 94
Warts, **252–253**
Washing
acne, 258
athlete's foot, 260
diapers, 240
eyes, 338, 340
penis, 370
vaginal discharge and, 368
See also Cleansing, wound.
Water, fluoridated, 120
Water jets
dental care, 120
ear care, 208, 210
Water safety, 108
Wax, ear, 30, 208, 210
Weak eye, 82, 94
Weakness, 166, 204, 278, 282,
288, **318–319**
in limb, 148, 186, 296, 304
Weight, 52
bearing, on limb, 160, 162,
354
control, 122–123
gain, 7, 49, 316, 376
loss, 89, 222, 296, 312, 314,
316, 351, 372
measurement, 94
See also Overweight;
Underweight.
Well-baby examinations, 93–95
Wheat, 192, 248
Wheel covers for bicycles, 107
Wheezing, **218–219,** 324, 332
aspirin-induced, 131
asthmatic, 193
insect bite or sting reaction,
172
White cell immunity, 116
Whole wheat bread, 360
Whooping cough, 111–112
Windpipe
infection, 216
object in, 144, 214, 218, 324
Wisdom teeth, 121
Withdrawal, weakness, tiredness,
and, 318
Wobbling of knee, 162
*Womanly Art of Breastfeeding,
The,* 46
Wood in wound, 150
Wood's lamp, 242, 246
Wool, 196, 254
Working mothers, 79
World Health Organization, 109,
117

Worm infestation, 226, 360, 364, 368
Wounds
  infected, **170–171**
  normal healing, 170
  See also Bites; Cuts; Fishhooks; Puncture wounds; Scrapes.

Wrist injuries, **164–165**

X-rays, 92. *See also specific complaints and specific parts of the body.*
Xylocaine, 23, 149, 228

Yeast infections, 262, 272, 376

candida, 240, 368
monilial, 228, 240
Yellow jaundice. *See* Jaundice.
Yellowness of whites of eyes, 41

Zen macrobiotic diet, 318
Zinc oxide ointment, 240
Zyradryl, 250